PREFACE

Feeling deprived is the dieter's downfall, whether health or appearance is the underlying motivation. It is clear to me, after working with thousands of patients as a consulting nutritionist for the past 25 years, that people like to eat in their own way. Dietary success is associated with freedom to choose rather than restricted choice. Since most "diets" foster deprivation and lead to unbalanced eating, it is no wonder that so many fail.

This is not the case with *Controlling Your Fat Tooth*. There is no such thing as "good," "bad" or "disallowed" food. You can easily see how to nurture your food cravings and still maintain a sense of dietary balance.

This book offers a sensible, do-it-yourself approach so that you can make more informed choices within your food preferences. The fat budgeting system helps you to select foods at home, in a supermarket or at a restaurant. Even if you don't need to lose weight or reduce cholesterol, you'll find that this book is packed full of useful information and tasty recipes.

I have known the Piscatellas since Joe went through coronary bypass surgery, and have followed their progress in making dietary changes in the real world. What they have learned about changing food habits to reduce saturated fat and cholesterol is shared in their two excellent books, *Don't Eat Your Heart Out Cookbook* and *Choices for a Healthy Heart*. *Controlling Your Fat Tooth* takes the logical next step: changing habits to reduce total fat.

After reviewing the information, suggestions, and every single recipe for nutritional content, I can tell you that these authors know what they're doing. Furthermore, as one who is concerned with taste (I grew up in the catering business) as well as health, I can say that you're in for some wonderful, delicious food.

I can heartily recommend *Controlling Your Fat Tooth* for anyone who wants to eat delicious food in a healthful way. This is a take-charge book!

Evette M. Hackman, Ph.D., R.D.
Nutrition and Food Editor, *Shape* magazine

FOREWORD

The evidence is clear. Americans eat too much fat. Excess fat consumption has been linked to chronic ill health, including coronary heart disease, obesity, and breast and colon cancers. Fat-rich diets are known to promote weight gain and interfere with successful weight reduction. Expert nutrition advice has been unanimous: "Eat less fat."

All dietary guidelines issued in recent years recommend a reduction in fat intake, yet many people seem unwilling to exchange their hamburgers, pizza and French fries for fresh vegetables, fruit and cereal grains. This is not merely a question of education, habit or willpower. Preferences and cravings for high-fat foods are so deeply ingrained that mere exhortations to eat less fat may not be enough. We need a better understanding of what makes high-fat foods so irresistible and a clear and coherent strategy for controlling the fat content of our diet.

Controlling Your Fat Tooth provides such a strategy by focusing on the concept of fat preferences. Past studies of food preferences have been limited to a single ingredient, sugar, and the notion of a "sweet tooth." We have been conditioned to think of carbohydrates and "sweets" as the most fattening foods imaginable, without stopping to realize that ice cream and cookies are rich not in sugar but in fat. It is fat that provides the bulk of calories. So, for many people, the attraction to certain foods is not because of a "sweet tooth." Rather, a "fat tooth" dictates food preferences. And, since oral perception of fats can be unreliable, many consumers do not realize that their favorite foods are rich in fat.

Preferences for high-fat foods may involve both body and mind as well as cultural factors. There is evidence that some of our food preferences are under metabolic as well as psychological control. Cultural factors also play a major role. Some food habits are acquired in early childhood and others are dictated by social norms. Recent societal changes, including an increased pace of life, have made high-fat foods a staple of the American diet. The net result is that the combination of "fat tooth" preferences and a fat-rich environment has produced deeply rooted eating habits that are remarkably resistant to change.

Controlling Your Fat Tooth examines the American diet, provides current information on fat preferences and eating habits, and offers a promising new approach to making better food choices. Operating in the real world, Mr. Piscatella gives us a step-by-step plan for offsetting fat cravings. This includes the establishment of a personal fat budget and the use of that budget as a management technique for making smarter food choices. In doing so, the book does away with the concept of "good" and "bad" foods. Instead, it offers suggestions for small dietary changes, cooking tips and tasty recipes that can result in a lot less fat without deprivation or prohibition.

Cutting dietary fat is a public health priority well understood today by physicians, nutritionists and the general public. No one argues the positive effect of low-fat dietary habits on weight control, cancer and cardiac health. The only question is how to make it happen. *Controlling Your Fat Tooth* is a scientifically sound, effective tool for translating into everyday actions what we know we should do: eat less fat.

Adam Drewnowski, Ph.D.
Director, Program in Human Nutrition
The University of Michigan

CONTENTS

PART II: HOW TO BEAT THE ODDS
IN A PRO-FAT ENVIRONMENT

COOKBOOK

The information in this book is provided for information only and should not be construed as medical advice or instruction. Always consult your physician or other appropriate health professionals before making any dietary changes.

INTRODUCTION

I've been a keen observer of American eating habits since 1977, when open-heart coronary bypass surgery at age 32 made me understand the link between diet and health. The way I'd chosen to eat had played a significant role in the development of high cholesterol, coronary artery blockages and the need for surgery. As my dietary habits began to change dramatically, I again became aware of their effect on my health—this time in positive terms. My blood cholesterol dropped from 300 mg/dl to 180 mg/dl, and I lost 22 pounds. What I learned about the relationship between dietary choices and health, and how to put that information to work in the real world, are the main themes of my books *Don't Eat Your Heart Out Cookbook* and *Choices for a Healthy Heart*.

I mention this so the reader will know I have more than an academic curiosity about diet. I have a deep personal interest, and am therefore troubled by the strange incongruity in American dietary habits that has recently become evident. On the one hand, we have become more nutrition-conscious, especially about the need to restrict dietary fat, and there is even a public perception that we are "eating light." On the other hand, data on eating habits do not reflect this change. To be sure, the intake of some fatty foods—beef and whole milk, for example—has dropped during the last decade. But this change has been offset by an increase in other fatty foods such as cheese, frozen meals and fast foods. The net result has been a less than monumental reduction in the overall fat content of the U.S. diet—from 40% to 37% of total calories. Contrary to public belief, fat continues to be at the center of our dietary pattern. Says Dr. Mark Hegsted of Harvard University, long a leader in the movement to institute a more healthful diet, "Despite heightened nutritional awareness, Americans seem to have an insatiable appetite for fat. It is clear that we haven't made much progress in getting people to eat less total fat."

There is a gap between what is known about a healthful, low-fat diet pattern and what is practiced in real life. This book is about that gap, why it exists, and what can be done to bridge it. We live today in a fast-paced society that has traded nutrition for convenience, encouraging fast foods, take-out, microwave meals, snack foods and other components of a high-fat diet. In addition, people concerned about cholesterol have reduced their intake of saturated fats (such as butter) yet have increased their consumption of unsaturated fats (such as margarine). But environment isn't the only factor. New research suggests that brain chemistry can dictate a strong craving for fatty foods—a physiological "fat tooth." In its mildest form, the "fat tooth" may simply make an ice-cream cone more attractive than a carrot; taken to the extreme, however, it can produce an addiction to fat.

Controlling Your Fat Tooth deals with both the environmental and physiological factors by offering a simple, effective, do-it-yourself approach to managing dietary fat without deprivation or prohibition. Its methodology acknowledges different lifestyles and emphasizes freedom of choice. With this approach, no food is "good" or "bad." "This makes good sense," says James Heimbach, administrator of the USDA's Human Nutrition Information Service. "It puts the stress on a total diet rather than on specific nutrients or individual foods." Most important, the book provides a specific program for mitigating "fat tooth" cravings with exercise, and for better-managing food choices with a personal fat budget. It also includes over 200 delicious low-fat recipes to help you start and maintain a healthy diet.

Eating too much dietary fat is the most significant reason for the dramatic increase in diet-induced diseases in North America, particularly heart disease, cancer and obesity. I learned that the hard way in 1977. It is my intent to provide information and tools to help you control your own "fat tooth" and manage your own dietary habits in the hope that you'll never have to face a similar learning experience.

Joseph C. Piscatella

PART I

THE AMERICAN DIET AND ITS CONSEQUENCES

CHAPTER 1

THE GREAT AMERICAN DELUSION

I f Rip Van Winkle had fallen into his deep slumber 20 years ago and awakened today, he would be amazed at the many changes in the way we live. From computers to cable television, day-care to drugs, numerous factors have fundamentally altered the American culture. And at the forefront of social change is a burgeoning concern about food and health. Judging from media headlines, advertising, medical pronouncements, and cocktail conversation, it's obvious that people have come to recognize the relationship between what we eat and how we look and feel.

Twenty years ago, we lived in a culture that subscribed to "three squares" and equated a "balanced diet" with red meat and whole milk at virtually every meal. Bacon and eggs constituted a healthy breakfast. A favorite family dinner included slabs of rare prime rib, baked potato drowned in butter and sour cream, salad thick with Thousand Island dressing, and gooey chocolate cake washed down with creamy whole milk. Indeed, the prevailing nutritional theory of the day was a legacy from the Great Depression: all food is good food.

Today, we live in an era of nutritional awareness. Bookstores offer a multitude of titles on healthy eating. Monthly magazines devote pages to food and health. Television news now includes regular segments on health complete with resident physician/broadcaster. According to Gallup research, approximately 25% of the U.S. population today claims to know more about nutrition than the average person—and roughly 70% wants even more information.

In particular, there is more awareness of the detrimental health impact of excessive dietary fat. Sources ranging from the National Research Council's Committee on Diet and Health to medical experts writing in popular magazines have driven home the point: *Eat less fat!* And, for the most part, that message has been clearly understood. Because of our cholesterol mania, or the national fantasy to be thin, people today know that too much dietary fat is harmful. According to Dr. Alan Levy of the U.S. Department of Agriculture, 55% of the American public cites fats and fatty foods as a prime risk for coronary disease. In 1983, only 29% could do so. Indeed, the fat content of food, according to the Food Marketing Institute, is now the greatest nutritional concern for Americans, topping salt and cholesterol.

Public attention has focused on the contribution of our fat-rich diet to a variety of diseases and conditions prevalent in Americans, including stroke, diabetes, some forms of cancer (breast, prostate, colon), and specifically to the twin national epidemics of heart disease and obesity. These problems are not insignificant:

- In America, breast cancer is the most common cause of cancer death in women.
- In America, someone dies of cardiovascular disease every 32 seconds.
- In America, there are an estimated 40 million overweight people.

In modern life, it seems, "high-fat" is out, "low-fat" is in. But a closer look at our dietary habits reveals a curious dichotomy: despite the prevailing information that reducing fat intake is critical to losing weight, lowering cholesterol and maintaining good health, we continue to consume high-fat foods. For each of us, the average daily intake is six to eight tablespoons of fat—800 to 1,000 calories, or the equivalent of one full stick of butter. We may be more aware of the need to eat a low-fat diet, and in an abstract sense "buy in" to low-fat eating, but in reality our actions demonstrate a deep preference for fatty foods.

THE FAT EXCHANGE

The combined finger-wagging of doctors, nutritionists, health writers and fitness magazines has led to some dietary changes. After all, nobody wants to have the bulging thighs or cholesterol-clogged arteries produced by a high-fat diet. In 1980, about 40% of calories on the U.S. diet came from fat. Today the figure stands at about 37%. That's better, but it's still a long way from the level recommended by most health professionals: 30% or fewer calories from fat.

The chief reduction has been in foods rich in saturated fat and cholesterol, a response to an increase in heart disease education. According to the *New England Journal of Medicine*, in the past 20 years red meat consumption has fallen by 38.8%, butter by 33.3%, and whole milk and cream by 24.1%. In practical terms, this means that Americans who used to drink 110 quarts of whole milk each year—the national average—are now consuming just 50 quarts. And it's paying off. Although heart disease is still epidemic, since 1978 the number of people dying from heart disease in the United States has dropped by 29%.

At first glance, this seems like a tremendous step forward. An examination of the entire diet pattern, however, provides a truer picture. According to an analysis of eating habits by the USDA, the intake of certain fatty foods has decreased while the intake of other fatty foods is on the rise. In other words, one set of high-fat foods has been exchanged for another set. "We Americans want to have our own cake and eat it, too," says Dr. Herman Hellerstein, a noted cardiologist. People are eat ng more unsaturated fat and far less of the saturated type. But the overall fat content of our diet has not been significantly reduced.

ARE AMERICANS EATING LESS FAT?
YES... ...AND NO

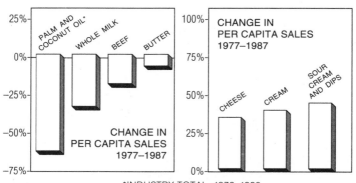

*INDUSTRY TOTAL, 1976–1988

Source: Milk Industry Foundation, National Livestock and Meat Board, Dept. of Agriculture, Frito-Lay.

Red Meat, Poultry and Fish

No two ways about it, Americans have cut back on red meat over the last two decades, reducing individual consumption by about 10 pounds per year. That's the good news. The bad news is that each of us still eats over 60 pounds of beef annually. No better illustration of our love for beef exists than a statistic offered by the Beef Industry Council: Americans eat 33 billion hamburgers a year, about three per week for every person in the country.

The consumption of pork has remained steady over the past 10 years at about 45 pounds per person. Apparently, a number of people have been taken in by the industry's misleading ads, which refer to pork as "the other white meat" and intimate that it's as low in fat as poultry. Consumption of beef and pork combined stands at just over

100 pounds per person per year, slightly less than a decade ago. Overall, the reduction in red meat can only be called moderate.

Many nutritionists also believe the data to be skewed by gender. According to the USDA's report "Nationwide Food Consumption for Individuals," most of the reduction in red meat is the result of dietary changes made by females. In general, males have continued to eat red meat, listing steaks, hot dogs and hamburgers as their most frequently consumed foods. This preference was confirmed by a study of U.S. Army personnel, in which males over age 20 selected steak as their favorite food and those under 20 selected pizza with meat topping. Females, on the other hand, get their fat from margarine, dairy foods, mayonnaise and salad dressings. This sex difference may be less a matter of taste buds than of gender roles. "Women are more

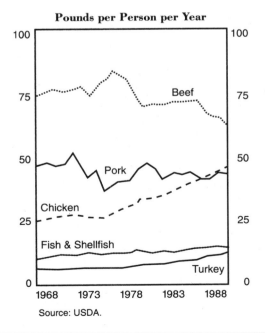

Pounds per Person per Year

Source: USDA.

weight conscious, and are socialized not to eat heavy, fattening foods," says Dr. Adam Drewnowski, director of the Human Nutrition Program at the University of Michigan School of Public Health, which conducted a fat-preference study. "Instead of ordering a steak or burger, women opt for a 'lighter' choice, such as tuna salad—which is loaded with mayo." So, while it can be said that the popularity of red meat has fallen off somewhat, the drop may not represent a change for all of society.

Poultry has been gaining steadily in consumption, but again the figures are misleading. Although Americans eat chicken twice as often today as in 1970, cooking methods transform it from a low-fat to a high-fat food: fried chicken, greasy fast-food nuggets, chicken hot dogs, frozen entrées in fat-rich sauces. The same basic problem exists with turkey. A skinless white turkey breast is a low-fat food; ground turkey, however, packaged with skin, dark meat and fat, has a higher fat content than does ground round. Turkey sausage, turkey bologna and turkey pastrami only give the illusion of being low in fat.

The consumption of fish and shellfish has remained steady over the last decade, which is good because fish is a heart-healthy food. On the other hand, most fish is eaten in restaurants, where it's fried and/or served with butter, mayonnaise or tartar sauce—a far cry from low-fat fare.

Milk and Dairy Products

The greatest change in the consumption of dairy products is a sharp decrease in whole milk and an equally sharp increase in "low-fat 2%" milk. Unfortunately, this is a shift that produces only a marginal decrease in fat. Whole milk provides 51% of calories from fat, or about 8.5 grams of fat per cup; so-called "low-fat 2%" milk (which means that fat constitutes 2% of *total weight*) provides 38% of calories from fat, or about 5.2 grams of fat per cup. A change has been made, but not one that has led to a substantial fat reduction.

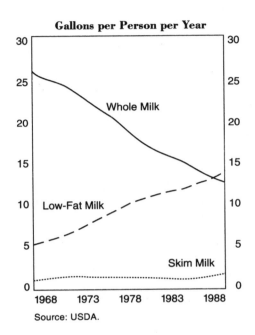

Gallons per Person per Year

Source: USDA.

Ice cream consumption has remained steady at about 18 pounds per person per year, but the type has changed. High-fat super-premium brands such as Häagen-Dazs, Ben & Jerry's, and Frusen Glädjé have increased sales from 20% to 50% of the market at the expense of brands lower in fat. We may be eating the same amount of ice cream, but the fat content of what we're eating has soared.

Since 1968, the consumption of high-fat hard cheese has more than doubled to about 22 pounds per person per year. One reason is the growth in popularity of fast-food cheese-burgers and pizza. Because many types of cheese are actually higher than red meat in fat content, this shift is significant.

Experts see a gender-related situation with whole-milk products similar to that with red meat, but this time it's

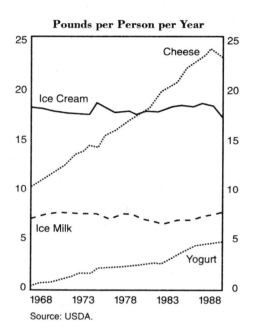

Pounds per Person per Year

Source: USDA.

reversed. In general, males have moderated their intake of dairy foods. This has not been too difficult to achieve, since males have not shown a propensity for these foods. American females, according to the USDA, continue to list cheese and ice cream among their most frequently eaten foods.

Fats and Oils

Consumption of butter and lard is lower, and that's good for our cholesterol levels, but we're eating more salad oils and cooking oils—about 27 pounds per person per year. Margarine has stayed at about 10 pounds per year. The net result is that we're eating healthier fats but in unhealthy quantities.

Most of the problem with fats and oils comes from a

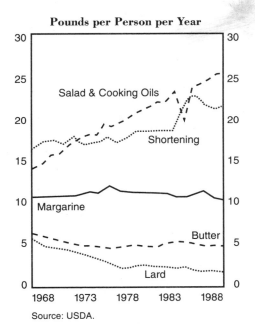

Pounds per Person per Year

Source: USDA.

dramatic increase in our consumption of commercially baked goods, snack foods and junk foods. Croissants, a particularly fatty bakery item, for example, have become a supermarket staple, accounting for $700 million in yearly sales. According to the American Dietetic Association, a four-inch croissant can contain as much as four teaspoons of butter! One plain 3.5-ounce doughnut is about 50% fat and contains as many calories as four slices of bread with jam. Candy consumption has risen to 20 pounds per person per year, while sales of commercial cheesecakes are at record levels. Walk through any mall in the country, and you'll find further evidence of our love for snacks: shoppers waiting in long lines for marshmallow-studded brownies, frisbee-size cookies, and waffle-cornucopias of ice cream.

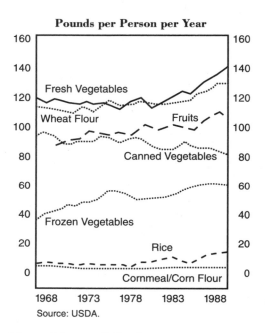

Pounds per Person per Year

Fresh Vegetables
Wheat Flour
Fruits
Canned Vegetables
Frozen Vegetables
Rice
Cornmeal/Corn Flour

1968   1973   1978   1983   1988

Source: USDA.

Fruits, Vegetables and Grains

Americans are now eating about 17% more high fiber, high-carbohydrate foods than we did a decade ago, chiefly because of an increase in consumption of fresh fruits, vegetables, wheat flour and rice. Again, on the surface, this is very good news. But potatoes account for almost 40% of the vegetables we consume, and we eat our potatoes with a lot of fat. Sixty-five percent of the potato crop each year is processed into chips, instant mixes or frozen items such as French fries. We still eat less than half as much bread, cereal, pasta and rice as our grandparents did in 1910.

KNOWLEDGE VS. ACTION

It is evident from an analysis of food habits that a certain ambivalence exists toward dietary reform. Says Bonnie

Liebman, a nutritionist at the Center for Science in the Public Interest, "If the United States got a Food Report Card, it would barely be pulling a C+. The Surgeon General and other 'teachers' say to eat less fat. So we're eating more chicken instead of beef, but it's fried chicken; more grains, but they're in fatty baked goods; more salads, but they're smothered in oily dressings."

While the consumption of certain fatty foods has been reduced, low-fat foods have not filled the void. Instead, other foods rich in fat have been substituted. "What's happened in terms of diet trends these last 10 years," says Dr. Drewnowski, "is that we've gone away from a hamburger and a glass of milk as the staple American food, to pizza and a Diet Coke. Perhaps this is somewhat better than the diet we used to have, but it's still not good. The average woman eats about 65 grams of fat a day, and the average man about 100 grams. That's too much."

SCIENTIFIC EVIDENCE

The gap between knowledge and action is well illustrated by a University of North Carolina study that compared the eating patterns of 5,400 women in 1977–78 with those of over 1,000 different women eight years later. The study showed that some positive dietary changes had been made. Fewer women in the second group consumed fatty cuts of beef and pork or drank whole milk. Furthermore, they were far less likely to eat chicken that had been fried or still had the skin on.

On the negative side, however, some less than favorable shifts were discovered. More women in the second group ate potato, corn and tortilla chips as well as buttered popcorn. And more indulged heavily in ice cream, cakes, cookies, pies, doughnuts and granola bars. These shifts were surprising to many of the researchers because the second group of women were better educated about diet and health. Adept at absorbing nutrition information and "translating" it appropriately, they were still unsuccessful in developing low-fat eating habits. Fatty foods were merely exchanged—cheese for red meat, margarine for butter—so that the fat content of their diet remained too high.

"I've found the same results in our studies," says Dr. Barbara Levine, assistant professor of nutrition at Cornell University Medical College. "If you look at groups of affluent, more educated women, they do eat more salads. But they also use more salad dressing and eat higher-fat cheeses."

POOR COMPLIANCE

What has become clear is that changing food behavior requires more than nutritional information or diet-disease links. As Winston Churchill once stated, "The lightning of cause has not been followed by the thunderclap of effect." This point is illustrated by a Los Angeles *Times* survey in which 96% of the respondents identified excessive dietary fat, particularly saturated fat, as a risk for heart disease. Yet fewer than 40% were willing to make *any* low-fat changes in diet. And of those who were willing to make changes, less than 20% thought they could stick with them.

Even more amazing is that many people with life-threatening conditions show poor compliance with low-fat eating. For example, if anyone should be motivated to eat healthier foods, it's someone who has a heart problem. There is nothing like a heart attack or bypass surgery to get your attention. But it doesn't always work that way. My friend John had a heart attack at age 45 and received dietary instruction in a cardiac rehabilitation program. He ate a low-fat diet for about three months, and his cholesterol dropped. Then he started to cheat. "One Big Mac won't kill me," he rationalized. The cheating became more regular, until finally he was back on a high-fat diet. John knew better. After all, for him the link between diet and disease was no longer a theoretical concept. It was a reality. And yet he couldn't stay away from high-fat foods.

And John is not alone. According to a survey conducted by the National Institutes of Health, over 50% of heart patients are no longer on a low-fat diet within six months of their coronary event. Cardiac rehabilitation programs cite "dietary noncompliance" as the single greatest problem in instituting heart-healthy lifestyle habits among patients. Doctors report the same results in trying to get patients to comply with dietary restrictions. The NIH survey showed that more than 85% of doctors feel they are unsuccessful in helping patients achieve lasting dietary changes.

The same situation exists among people who cut down on dietary fat for weight loss. Over 10 million people in the United States are enrolled in weight-loss programs involving diets, and millions·of others reduce calories on their own. However, fewer than 30% who go on low-fat diets are on them for more than one year. Many fall off the diet, get back on for a time, then fall off again, as illustrated by the fact that the average American dieter goes on and off 2.3 diets a year. "Yo-yo" dieting is a primary reason that weight loss can be an up-and-down, roller-coaster affair. Perhaps the inability to stick to a low-fat diet pattern is why weight-loss programs have so many repeat customers.

THE CRITICAL QUESTION

Many people today know that excessive dietary fat constitutes a major health risk, yet the United States continues to have a national appetite satisfied mainly by French fries, doughnuts, cheeseburgers, ice cream, frozen meals and other fatty fare. Our dietary habits reflect a schizophrenic mixture of increased health-consciousness and high-fat indulgence. Despite knowing better, Americans continue to eat too much fat.

The critical question is: Why?

CHAPTER 2

THE "FAT TOOTH" ENIGMA

The U.S. Department of Agriculture boasts that "America has the most abundant food supply in the world." While this is true, availability of food appears to have little bearing on well-balanced nutrition. The fact is, Americans eat too much fat in general, too much artery-clogging saturated fat in particular, and too much refined sugar. Too much sodium and alcohol, along with too many calories, round out the excesses. At the same time, we are seriously short in the consumption of high-carbohydrate, high-fiber foods, particularly vegetables, fruits, grains and legumes.

The single greatest problem in this litany of dietary disasters is excessive fat, which provides almost 4 out of every 10 calories eaten by Americans. The favored position of high-fat foods has been graphically illustrated by the National Cancer Institute, whose data show that children and adolescents are two to five times more likely to eat fatty baked goods than fruits or vegetables, while adults are five to six times likelier to make the same choice. A slice of apple pie, it seems, is far more popular than an apple.

Type of Food	% of People Who Eat These Foods Every Day		
		Children	
	Adults	12–17	6–11
Doughnuts, cakes, cookies	40–45%	21–24%	32–37%
Apples, bananas, oranges	7–12	5–8	8–18
Carrots, peas	7–8	4–6	3–9

Why are fatty foods so attractive? If we know that a high-fat diet will raise our risk of heart disease and cancer, and make us overweight, why do we wolf down chocolate bars and overdose on pastries?

The problem is, of course, that food selection is seldom based on rational concerns. Rather, emotional, environmental and physiological forces work together in a complex mixture to shape our dietary habits. Emotional stress, for example, may be an underlying reason for bingeing on high-calorie foods. It is axiomatic that when a compulsive eater is under stress, "all roads lead to the refrigerator." Depression, anger, loneliness and even joy can affect what and how much a person eats. Says Dr. Katherine Halmi of New York Hospital, "In our society, food serves as a psychological panacea for much of the population. Stress is somewhat assuaged by eating." Indeed, studies show that people under emotional stress often find relief in foods rich in fat and sugar, such as ice cream and chocolate.

Environment and lifestyle also play an important role, often determining the range of foods from which selections will be made. A post–World War II push for protein and calcium, for example, helped to establish red meat and whole milk, each high in fat, as the twin nutritional foundations of the modern American diet. Today, an increased pace of life has altered dietary styles. Free time has been diminished an estimated 37% since 1970, allowing less time for shopping, cooking and even eating. Many people have reacted to time constraints by designing a diet based on convenience foods (frozen meals, take-out, snack and fast foods), most of which are extremely rich in fat.

While the impact of emotional and environmental factors on dietary habits is well demonstrated, scientists have recently begun to understand a third factor: the existence of a physiological basis for food preferences. Simply put, research shows that cravings for certain food tastes may be governed by brain chemicals; i.e., some people may be predisposed naturally to prefer certain foods.

According to Dr. Judith Wurtman of the Massachusetts Institute of Technology, the hunger for pastry, chocolate, ice cream and other sweet-tasting treats may be regulated in part by serotonin, one of several brain chemicals that appear to control many physiological functions. When such foods are eaten, the brain responds by releasing increased amounts of serotonin. This causes a feeling of satisfaction, sometimes to the point of sleepiness. Dr. Wurtman speculates that some people, particularly the obese, may crave sweet-tasting foods because they "need" extra serotonin, even though these foods may produce an overindulgence of calories that contributes to their obesity. According to such research, their craving for cake or cookies is chemically based in the brain, rather than a matter of "weak will."

The scientific study of the link between brain chemistry and nutrition has led to a better understanding of what is actually being craved. For many years, it was thought that the attractiveness of ice cream, candy and desserts was the result of a craving for sugar, the so-called "sweet tooth." New data, however, show the underlying desire for sweet-tasting foods to be more complicated. Researchers at the University of Michigan suggest that the basic craving may really be for fat—or, more accurately, for sweetened fat. Characterized as a "fat tooth," this craving predisposes some people to select foods rich in fat. In doing so, it exercises a great impact on the establishment of long-term dietary habits. Says Dr. Drewnowski, an expert on food preferences, "In most people, the 'fat tooth' creates an inclination for fatty foods, such as the desire for a chocolate dessert after dinner. Sometimes the craving is satisfied, sometimes it is not. But with other people, the 'fat tooth' produces a craving so strong that it must be satisfied. These people literally become fat junkies and will sometimes go on thousand-calorie binges. Indeed, studies show that these strong fat cravings may be triggered by the physiological mechanism that is responsible for drug addiction."

FAT, NOT SUGAR

According to scientists, the "fat tooth" is not a new concept. In the past, however, it has often been confused with the more familiar "sweet tooth," a heightened responsiveness to sweet-tasting foods easily recognized by most people. It is theorized that many "sweet tooth" food choices are actually governed by "fat tooth" cravings.

To be sure, the "sweet tooth" does exist. No other animal, with the possible exception of cats, has such an inclination. But in humans the preference for sweet-tasting foods is sufficiently strong to influence dietary decisions. Even though many people try to avoid candy bars, cookies, milk shakes and other treats for weight or health reasons, sweets rank high on the list of our most commonly consumed foods. Refined sugar consumption is more than twice the amount eaten 75 years ago. Indeed, on average adults in the United States consume about 130 pounds of refined sugars (cane and beet sugar, high-fructose corn syrup, glucose and dextrose) and artificial sweeteners (saccharin and aspartame) per person per year. The figures are even greater for children. According to Dr. Alexander G. Schauss of Washington State University, children consume on average about 274 pounds of sweeteners per year.

The influence of physiological cravings on the food selection process is seen even in early childhood. Dr. Mary Story of the University of Minnesota School of Public

Health points out that when children are given a choice between nutritious food and sweet-tasting but nutrient-lacking items such as ice cream and pastry, chances are they will opt for the "goodies." Children are born with a "sweet tooth," an innate preference for sugary foods. This should not be news to many mothers and fathers who have found that, when left to their own devices, their toddlers snatch cookies, munch on sugar cubes or indulge in chocolate Kisses. In fact, researchers have found that even infants who are only two hours old prefer a sugary taste to any other taste.

The influence of the "sweet tooth" seems to peak during childhood. Studies show that as we mature, we have less tolerance for higher concentrations of sugar and a diminishing desire for foods with an overriding sweet taste. Children, however, have a higher level of tolerance and are not put off by intensely sweet solutions. This is why children like the extremely sweet frosting on commercial birthday cakes, while adults generally do not. Some children even fail to arrive at the standard saturation breakpoint, where something tastes "too sweet." The more sugar, it would seem, the better. It should be no surprise that sugar contributes over 25% of all calories to the preadolescent diet.

Though moderated in adulthood, the "sweet tooth" is certainly not totally lost. Adults of all ages report cravings for sweet foods. But is it sugar that is being craved? Studies conducted at UCLA, the University of Washington, the University of Michigan and MIT suggest that the real attraction for adults may be fat, not sugar, and that sugar may be used simply to make it taste better. This may be because pure fats, such as salad oils, are not particularly palatable.

If this is the case, it may not be an independent craving for sugar that causes a person to drive 10 blocks out of the way for a hot-fudge sundae. It may be predilection for fat. In a taste preference study conducted at the University of Washington, researchers created different mixtures of chilled milk, cream and sugar to be sampled and rated by obese and normal-weight women. The range of choice included skim milk, whole milk, half-and-half, heavy cream, and heavy cream with an admixture of safflower oil. Sugar (sucrose) was added in varying degrees, and the women were asked to choose the most palatable "milk shake" drink. Obese subjects selected a mixture of 4% sugar and 34% fat as optimal, whereas the normal-weight subjects selected a mixture of 9% sugar and 20% fat.

The study made three important points. First, a preference for straight sugar or straight fat did not exist; indeed, much higher ratings were obtained for mixtures of sugar and fat than for either ingredient separately. Second, while it took a minimal amount of sugar to make the mixture palatable, a high concentration of fat was necessary. Obese subjects, for example, disliked a mixture of 10% sucrose in skim milk but liked the same concentration in heavy cream. And third, the obese women in the study did not prefer sweeter mixtures than their normal-weight counterparts but did prefer fattier mixtures.

These results contrast with the popular belief that obese and overweight individuals have a sensory "sweet tooth" responsible for their overeating of sweet, high-calorie foods. The research shows that these foods are selected in response to their elevated fat content, with sugar playing only a supporting role as a condiment to make the fat taste better. Ultimately, then, it may actually be a "fat tooth" that dictates a preference for calorically dense foods.

WHAT WE KNOW ABOUT THE "FAT TOOTH"

Many nutrition experts support the position that the "sweet tooth" may exist only to make fat more palatable and may thereby help to introduce fat into the diet of children and adolescents. By the time adulthood is reached, the "sweet tooth'' has done its job and has evolved into a "fat tooth.'' The underlying mechanism that promotes this metamorphosis is not well understood. Much more needs to be known about the role of brain chemistry and the influence of cravings on the food selection process. Still, at this juncture, scientists believe that certain aspects of the "fat tooth" are well demonstrated.

The Craving for Fat Is Natural

The "fat tooth," it seems, is a natural physiological occurrence in certain people. Some scientists hypothesize that fat is craved as an opiate. Studies by Dr. Elliot Blass at Johns Hopkins University and Dr. Roy Martin at the University of Georgia found that dietary fat has a painkilling effect in test animals. Other studies have shown that when calories in massive amounts are delivered quickly via sweetened fat, test animals respond with a higher degree of pleasure.

It may be, however, that by fighting a natural inclination for fatty foods (particularly those foods identified with overweight and other health problems) many people set themselves up for pendulum-like swings between abstention and bingeing, which result in frustration and noncompliance. Indeed, it may go a long way toward answering the question as to why we know more about the risk of a high-fat diet, yet continue to eat it.

This is particularly true in the case of sweets and other high-calorie treats, often eaten in reaction to cravings. Most people are familiar with cravings that are fairly benign, such as the simple desire for an ice-cream cone while strolling through a park on a sunny day. Other cravings, however, are much stronger, capable of producing extremely powerful urges for certain tastes and foods. Any chocoholic can describe in detail the feeling of intense need that leads to the abandonment of all good sense and the consumption of an entire one-pound package of chocolate chips. When such a craving hits, health risks and weight loss be damned! Nothing will stand in the way of satisfaction. Food selection then becomes far less a product of nutritional concern than a response to an overwhelming, immediate need.

For many years the inability to control cravings and avoid fatty, high-calorie foods was seen as a character flaw. Food choices were a matter of willpower. While thin people were praised for having the moral fiber to pass up a Twinkie, overweight people were condemned for giving in all too easily to the desire for a hot-fudge fix. Today we know this Calvinistic view oversimplifies the process. People do not choose to eat certain foods simply because of flabby willpower. In many instances, they may be responding to a natural craving.

I can identify with this situation from my own experience. As a 32-year-old survivor of bypass surgery, I had everything going for me—motivation, knowledge and support—and yet there were times when the craving for chocolate was so strong that I could have killed for an M&M. I'd often give in, eat the whole package, and be plunged into a state of guilt. Was it weak will? I don't think so. After all, I had the willpower to exercise daily at six o'clock in the morning. In retrospect, what was lacking was an understanding that by establishing "good" and "bad" foods I was working against a natural craving and that the solution was to work with nature, not against it.

Sugar Masks Fat Content

A second impact of the "fat tooth" is that sugar often masks the fat content of foods, so that people are not able to identify them as high-fat. Thus, they have a problem in meeting their own dietary standards because of a lack of knowledge. In a survey conducted by Procter & Gamble, respondents had no trouble identifying butter and French fries as high-fat foods. A significant number, however, incorrectly labeled pastries, candy and many other sugary foods as being low in fat. The general perception was that sugar was the main element in these foods. Such a survey, while not conclusive, suggests that when sugar is an over-riding taste, there is confusion in the perceived fat content of individual foods. As a result, a person could eat a great amount of dietary fat without even knowing it.

This concept becomes clearer with an examination of the caloric mix of many "sweet tooth" foods. A good example is a peanut butter and jelly sandwich. Of the 225 calories supplied by two tablespoons of Skippy peanut butter and two teaspoons of Smucker's jelly, an average sandwich mixture, sugar accounts for just 25%. Fat produces a whopping 75% of calories. How, then, can it be said that the attraction to this sandwich is due to a craving for sugar? According to many scientists, a craving for fat is the compelling factor in this case. Jelly simply sugar-coats the fat in the peanut butter, making it taste better.

The same relationship is true for other foods commonly identified as being sugar-rich. Compare the sugar and fat calories in a variety of popular chocolate candies:

Food Item	Total Calories per Package/Bar	% of Calories from:	
		Sugar	Fat
M&M's Plain Chocolate Candies	237	45%	52%
M&M's Peanut Chocolate Candies	241	36	45
Hershey Milk Chocolate Bar with Almonds	226	35	56
Hershey Special Dark Chocolate Bar	222	36	49
Nestle Crunch Bar	156	38	46

In reality, these candies contain more fat than sugar. "They are sweetened fat," says Dr. Paula Geiselman of the UCLA medical school, "not fatty sweets. This distinction is important."

The masking of fat by sugar is a greater problem with solid foods than with liquids. In taste preference tests at the

University of Pennsylvania, subjects selected a liquid mixture of 13% sugar and 20% fat as optimal; however, when presented with sugar/fat mixtures in solid foods, they chose a mixture of 16% sugar and 35% fat. In other words, their tolerance for fat was increased by the solid state of the food. This may explain why there has been such little change in the fat content of the American diet, even in the face of greater awareness of dietary fat as the number one nutritional issue. It may be that consumers are merely replacing obvious fat sources (whole milk, cream) with foods in which fat is difficult to detect by sensory means (cheese, frozen desserts).

The "Fat Tooth" Can Be Regulated

There is evidence that exercise and dieting may have opposite effects on the craving for fat. Studies have shown that regular exercise may offset such cravings at the brain chemistry level. This is more fully discussed in Chapter 8. There is also evidence that chronic dieting may actually enhance the craving for fat.

According to Dr. Kelly Brownell at the University of Pennsylvania, a pattern of "yo-yo" dieting (cyclically losing and regaining weight two or three times a year) increases the craving for fat, particularly in obese people. Says Dr. Judith Stern of the University of California at Davis, "Quick weight loss in obese people does not produce normal eating habits. If anything, their 'fat tooth' is enhanced, and they end up with worse food selections— higher in fat and calories." Clinical studies involving laboratory rats illustrate this phenomenon. Ordinarily, rats will select a diet in which 35% to 40% of calories come from fat; however, after being subjected to forced weight loss and gain, their food selection changes to a diet of 50% to 60% fat. The dieting process, it seems, exercises a degree of independent influence that may result in an increased preference for fat.

This means that many of the people who most need to

avoid fatty foods to lose weight may, as the result of chronic dieting, have the greatest inclination to eat fatty foods. It's a Catch-22 situation.

PREDISPOSITION IS NOT DESTINY

The "fat tooth" may very well exist as a physiological trigger that predisposes people to crave fat and, in doing so, shapes attitudes about food and food choices. Like a genetic tendency toward obesity, it sets up many people to choose high-fat foods and may explain the prevalence of fat in the U.S. diet.

However, with few exceptions, no one selects a high-fat diet pattern exclusively because of "fat tooth" cravings. These cravings may predispose a person to choose fatty foods, but it takes an environment where high-fat choices can easily be made to produce a fat-rich diet. Just as the person with genetic tendencies toward obesity can control environment to offset these tendencies, so can the person with "fat tooth" cravings. By understanding that fat cravings may exist as the result of brain chemistry, we are in a much better position to control environment and to design and implement a healthy, balanced diet pattern that takes such cravings into consideration.

Ultimately, "fat tooth" cravings are controlled by working with and not against nature. Later chapters provide information on how to control the "fat tooth" with a combination of exercise (to offset fat cravings) and a personal fat budget (to manage the environment).

CHAPTER 3

FEEDING THE "FAT TOOTH"

The contemporary American diet is seriously out of balance, but it wasn't always that way. A comparison of foods consumed in 1910, when the U.S. Department of Agriculture first started to keep figures on the food supply, with those consumed today shows a dramatic shift in calorie sources. In 1910, dietary fat made up just 27% of calories; today it accounts for 37%. The consumption of refined sugar has doubled in that period, while that of high-carbohydrate, high-fiber foods has fallen by about 25%. The result is a modern diet in which fat contributes far too many calories. On any given day, according to data compiled by the USDA, almost 30% of the adult population will eat a hot dog, ham or luncheon meat; 26% will devour a hamburger, cheeseburger or meat loaf; 41% will eat a doughnut, cookies or a piece of cake; 23% will put away at least one serving of steak or roast beef; and 41% will down two glasses of whole milk.

The "fat tooth" may predispose us to choose these foods, but inherent physiological cravings alone are not responsible for fat-rich dietary habits. Since the end of World War II, a pro-fat environment has made fatty foods available and acceptable.

A HISTORY OF GOOD INTENTIONS

The roots of fat's primacy in the American diet can be traced to three distinct time periods, each characterized by a prevailing nutritional philosophy and a high degree of nutritional naïveté, particularly with regard to food labeling and health claims. Says Dr. Mark Hegsted, "We ought to recognize that the high-fat menu we happen to eat today was never planned. It just grew as the result of our affluence, the efficiency of the American farmer, the growth of the processed food industry, the emergence of sophisticated advertising techniques, and the increased pace of life. The fact that we consume it today is obviously no indication that it is desirable."

1948-1963:
IKE, SPOCK, JFK, AND THE PUSH
FOR ANIMAL PROTEIN

Prior to World War II, many people could not afford to eat red meat regularly. A Sunday roast was still a special meal. After the war, however, an expanded middle class had more money to spend on food, and they spent it on meat. Freezers became common. Red meat became the entrée of choice, often served at two or more meals a day. According to the World Health Organization, in virtually every nation that experiences increased income, an increase in red meat consumption follows.

The affordability of meat coincided with one of the main nutritional philosophies of the day: Eat a lot of red meat for protein. Savvy food advertisers were quick to emphasize protein content to promote their products as being essential for strong muscles, a legacy that continues today. The Beef Industry Council, for example, advertises beef as "a super source of complete, high-quality protein," and Oscar Mayer & Company has bragged that one of their hot dogs contains "as much protein as an egg."

The fact that dietary fat came along as part of the deal was ignored. So, with the increase in red meat consumption for protein came a rise in the intake of dietary fat as well.

Protein: Too Much of a Good Thing

Asked to identify the most important component of a healthy diet, most people would answer: "Protein." There is a foundation for this belief, since protein is required throughout life to maintain and build body tissues, form antibodies, make hemoglobin in the blood, and produce important enzymes and hormones. In addition, because it cannot be stored in the body for later use, protein must be consumed on a regular basis.

Unfortunately, the amount needed to be eaten each day has been overestimated. Important as it is as a nutritional "building block," protein is not required in abundance. The Recommended Daily Allowances for protein are:

Population	Age	Grams of Protein
Children	1–3	23
	4–6	30
	7–10	34
Males	11–14	45
	15 +	56
Females*	11–18	45
	19 +	44

*Pregnant females should add 30 grams to the figure given for their age group; breastfeeding women should add 20 grams.

For an adult, the RDA is no more than 0.8 grams of protein per kilogram (2.2 pounds) of body weight, or about 56 grams for an average-size man and 45 grams for an average-size woman. (Athletes need about 1.2 grams per kilogram of weight.) To put this in perspective, 56 grams of protein are provided by a meal containing 4 ounces of white-meat turkey, two slices of whole-wheat bread, an 8-ounce glass of skim milk, and a banana.

Far more protein is consumed in the United States than is needed for good nutrition. According to government statistics, infants and children consume about twice the RDA for protein. The average middle-aged man consumes 60% more than the recommended level; the average middle-aged woman, about 25% more. This is too much of a good thing. Because the body uses only what it needs, excessive protein can strain the kidneys and liver (which have to process it for excretion) and can cause calcium loss in bones. And, if red meat is the source, too much protein means a diet too rich in fat.

The amount of protein found in the U.S. diet today is about the same as that consumed in the early 1900s: approximately 12% of calories. So, while Americans have overconsumed protein for about 100 years, it was not a significant problem until food sources changed. During the first half of this century, most protein was supplied by low-fat foods such as flour, cereal products and legumes. Since that time, there has been a steady trend away from low-fat vegetable protein and toward high-fat animal protein. Today, about 70% of protein consumed comes from animal meat and dairy products. Nutritionists believe the proper ratio to be just the opposite: about one-third from animals and two-thirds from plants.

Red Meat: More Fat than Protein

While red meat is rich in protein, it's an even richer source of undesirable fat—the most critical dietary problem for Americans. As Dr. William E. Connor of the Oregon Health Sciences University says, "It's the company that protein keeps that is the health issue." According to the USDA, about 20% of the calories in prime rib come from protein and 80% from fat. Yet prime rib is often promoted as a "high-protein" food. With over three-quarters of the calories derived from fat, it is neither accurate nor fair to label this cut of meat "high-protein" without acknowledging that it is "high-fat" as well.

Red meat supplies three of the top five sources of fat on the U.S. diet, or about 23% of total fat and 27% of saturated fat consumed. Good efforts have been made by meat producers to provide leaner animals, and this is reflected in the lower fat content of some cuts. Three ounces of roasted eye of round, for example, can be as low as 155 calories and 32% fat. Despite these efforts, most red meat still contains far more fat than protein. The following analysis shows the dominant position of fat:

Food (3 oz.)	Total Calories	% of Calories as Protein	% of Calories as Fat
Bacon	159	17%	81%
Beef, ground, regular	263	21	77
Beef steak, T-bone	275	30	68
Beef, ground, lean	223	28	70
Ham, cured	244	23	74
Lamb, chop	305	24	74
Lamb, leg	237	36	62
Pork, chop	255	33	65
Rib roast, beef	329	23	76
Sausage, pork	396	6	93
Spareribs, pork	338	29	69

Source: USDA.

Luncheon Meats and Sausages: The Same Story

These are among America's most favorite foods—from pastrami sandwiches at the Stage Deli in New York, to bratwurst at the Summer Festival in Milwaukee, to hot dogs at Dodger Stadium in Los Angeles. And every day millions of schoolchildren eat bologna sandwiches as standard fare. Luncheon meats and sausages are fun foods, tasty and easy to eat, and they do contain protein. Unfortunately, they're loaded with fat (as well as sodium and, in many instances, dangerous additives). In addition, people forget that these foods belong in the red meat category. Says Dr. Evette

Hackman, a registered dietitian in private practice and a nutrition editor for *Shape* magazine, "Many of my patients will eat a hot dog or a bologna sandwich and tell me that they don't eat red meat."

How much fat do these foods contain? A look at the percentage of calories from fat in the following items shows their grease content to be sky-high, with protein running a distant second.

Over 60% Fat: Beer salami, pork; bologna, turkey; corned beef; hot dog, chicken; picnic loaf.

Over 70% Fat: Bratwurst; bologna, pork; hot dog, turkey; ham, chopped; Italian sausage; Kielbasa sausage; pastrami, beef; salami; sausage, smoked link; summer sausage.

Over 80% fat: Beer salami, beef; bockwurst; bologna, beef; liverwurst; hot dog, beef and pork; knockwurst; pepperoni; Polish sausage; beef sausage stick.

Source: USDA.

Fortunately, a number of low-fat sources of protein do exist. Small pieces of fish, skinless poultry or extra-lean beef added as a condiment to pasta, rice or vegetables can contribute valuable protein. So can beans (kidney, black, lima, navy, garbanzo), legumes (peas, lentils, soybeans) and tofu (bean curd) added to soups, rice, and salads. Skim and low-fat dairy foods are also excellent sources. The salient point is that prodigious amounts of high-fat red meat are not needed to ensure sufficient protein intake for good health.

Increased animal protein was once a legitimate dietary goal. Indeed, it still is for many places in the world that suffer from malnutrition. In Ethiopia, all food *is* good food. But this concept no longer applies in the United States. By meeting protein needs primarily with red meat, we consume too much fat and perpetuate the fatty American diet.

1964-1979:
THE BEATLES, HO CHI MINH, AND
THE PUSH FOR CALCIUM

This 15-year period saw a tremendous boost in the consumption of whole-milk dairy products sparked by the theory that people need a lot of milk to ensure adequate calcium for strong bones and healthy teeth. Food manufacturers responded with slick advertising campaigns for a wide range of "high-calcium" dairy foods—whole milk, cheese, ice cream and yogurt. Dairy foods were established as a daily nutritional necessity, and an elevated fat intake level was guaranteed.

Calcium: A Legitimate Need

No question about it, calcium is essential in building strong bones and teeth. The body gets this mineral from the diet and stores about 98% of it in the bones. This supply is not static, however, and each year about 20% of calcium is removed from the bones. This means we have to replenish the supply on an ongoing basis. A diet consistently short of calcium can result in bone deterioration, a condition known in adults as osteoporosis and afflicting about 50% of post-menopausal women. Research shows that osteoporosis results from many factors (such as lack of estrogen and lack of exercise), but none plays a more important role than a long-standing calcium deficiency.

The recommended daily calcium intake for adults, according to the National Institutes of Health, is 800 milligrams. For pregnant and nursing women, the requirement increases to 1,200 milligrams. Caucasian women are estimated to take in only about 650 milligrams of calcium a day. The picture is even worse for black women, whose daily intake averages just 450 milligrams. Therefore, although it must be recognized that many high-calcium foods are also rich in fat, the effort to boost calcium intake is a valid one.

Whole-Milk Products: More Fat than Calcium

The best sources of calcium are milk and other dairy products. Recently, researchers at the University of Pittsburgh found that calcium had the most protective effect on the bones of older women who reported high milk consumption throughout life but particularly when they were young. While it's possible to get calcium from canned sardines and salmon, which contain edible bones, and from dark green vegetables such as spinach, these foods are too impractical to be a main calcium source for most people.

Unfortunately, whole-milk products are high in fat, a fact often overlooked in advertising. A cup of whole milk provides a quarter to a third of the recommended daily calcium level for adults, but half the calories in the milk come from fat. Even 2% milk derives about 38% of calories from fat. Better choices are skim (or non-fat) milk, 1% milk and non-fat buttermilk. Happily, skim milk fortified with dry milk solids is higher than whole milk in calcium and lacks excessive fat. A cup of skim milk has essentially the same nutritional value as a cup of whole milk, but the whole milk contains the equivalent of two pats of butter! If you drink three glasses of milk daily, the difference in fat calories between whole and skim milk is 210—enough to produce 22 pounds of excess body fat in one year. Cream for coffee, whipped cream for desserts, evaporated milk and condensed milk are also very rich in fat calories.

The following comparison of the fat and calcium content of various types of milk illustrates the wide range available:

Type (1 cup)	Total Calories	% of Calories from Fat	Milligrams of Calcium
Whole milk	150	51%	288
2% milk	125	38	287
1% milk	104	22	300
Skim milk	81	2	302
Skim buttermilk	88	2	285

Three cups of fortified skim milk provides about 906 milligrams of calcium, or more than 100% of the RDA. The point here is that you don't have to consume huge amounts of full-fat milk to ensure sufficient calcium intake.

Cheese. On the average, we eat about 22 pounds of cheese a year in sandwiches, casseroles, snacks and pizzas. Many women in particular look to cheese as a primary source of calcium. Indeed, one ounce of Swiss cheese provides 262 milligrams of calcium, while the same amount of American cheese provides 198 milligrams.

The problem, of course, is that most varieties of whole-milk cheese are as fat as or even fatter than red meat. Whole-milk cheese is a concentrated form of milk (about eight pounds of milk will make one pound of cheese), so most of the calories come from fat. This means that two slices of American cheese, about one and a half ounces total, contains as much fat as three and a half pats of butter! The following is a short list of many of the most commonly consumed types of cheese that are more than 60% fat:

American	Mozzarella
Brie	Provolone
Camembert	Ricotta
Cheddar	Romano
Cream cheese	Swiss
Feta	
Havarti	
Monterey Jack	

Cheese spreads, dips, sauces and imitation cheese offer no break. Most of these foods are also over 60% fat. The key point is that if full-fat cheese is used as a primary calcium source, other fat sources in the diet should be moderated. (This point will be discussed more fully in Chapter 9.) Fortunately, choices do exist, such as low-fat and non-fat cottage cheese, hoop, farmer's, quark and part-skim ricotta.

Yogurt. A cup of plain, low-fat yogurt contains 415 milligrams of calcium, while the same amount of non-fat yogurt contains 452 milligrams. But not all yogurt is low in fat. Custard-style yogurts made with milk, cream, and milk solids can be over 30% fat. Most "low-fat" yogurts are about 18% fat, while non-fat yogurts—the best choice— range from 0% to 3% fat. Frozen yogurt also comes in a wide range of fat content.

Ice cream. A cup of ice cream, or two average scoops, contains 194 milligrams of calcium but also about 270 calories, 130 of them from fat. The same amount of premium ice cream (Häagen-Dazs, Ben & Jerry's, Frusen Glädjé) has twice the calories, more than half from fat. Clearly, America's best-loved dessert is simply too rich in fat to be a primary calcium source. Some non-dairy frozen desserts are low in saturated fat, but not in total fat and calories. One cup of Tofutti contains 460 calories and is 58% fat.

Type (1 cup)	Total Calories	% of Calories from Fat
Frusen Glädjé, vanilla	550	61%
Häagen-Dazs, vanilla	500	61
Lady Borden, butter pecan	360	60
Ben & Jerry's, vanilla	587	55
Breyers, chocolate	320	45

Source: Individual food companies.

1980-PRESENT: REAGAN, GORBACHEV, YUPPIES, AND CONVENIENCE FOODS

The modern era of high-speed living and traumatic societal shifts has brought about dramatic changes in eating habits. On one hand, we know more about good nutrition. "Like all the kids of my time," says Mary Prather, a registered dietitian, "I was guided by the Nutrition Food Health Chart. At every school, there was a chart on the wall with a picture of four foods that would give you strong young bodies and glowing health for life: white bread, whole milk, eggs and red meat. Today we know better."

On the other hand, thanks to the hurried pace of life in contemporary America, convenience has taken precedence over nutrition.

The major contributor to fat intake today is a pro-fat environment shaped by a drastically increased pace of life. Extended work hours, longer commuting times, two-income families, single-parent households—these are some of the factors that have produced a serious shortage of time. People are eating on the run, no longer inclined to shop, cook, or make food choices based on good nutrition. They are settling for "what is available" from restaurants, take-outs and food stores. And what is available is typically high in fat.

"We're become a nation that has denigrated the role of preparing, serving, and sharing food in society. We've moved from eating to grazing to refueling," observes Joel Weiner of Kraft General Foods. Consequently, nutrition has taken a back seat. Says Dr. Lilian Cheung of the Harvard School of Public Health, "I think the rat race in America has a lot to do with the disengagement from the emotionally satisfying aspects of food that existed in the past. For example, many people fall into the trap of recognizing that they are hungry, they didn't have a decent breakfast, and so they just grab anything to eat and eat it at their desks. Then they go home and find that, although physically they ate, psychologically they really didn't. So it's easy to snack or to eat again."

The marketplace has responded to this situation with a proliferation of new convenience foods, snack foods and fast foods designed for life in the fast lane. These foods are easy, quick, tasty, "fun"—and rich in fat.

Prepared Foods

The last decade has seen a dramatic increase in the availability and variety of processed, ready-made foods. Bottled sauces and dressings, boxed meals, frozen desserts, microwavable snacks—a few years ago half the manufactured food items didn't exist. But today, in response to our hurried and harried lifestyle, they have become dietary staples. Yearly sales for frozen meals alone are over $1 billion.

While convenience foods are quickly prepared and may taste acceptable, too many of them are high in fat. Stouffer's Frozen Beef Pie, for example, contains 560 calories, 60% of which come from fat. Two tablespoons of Marie's Ranch Salad Dressing provide 200 calories and are 95% fat. A half-cup serving of Noodle Roni Fettuccini Sauce contains 300 calories and is 54% fat. While you might expect the fat content of beef pie, salad dressing and fettuccine sauce to be somewhat high, fat calories in a number of other prepared foods are not so readily identifiable. Drink two cups of General Foods premixed International Coffees, and you'll deposit six grams of artery-clogging hydrogenated coconut oil into your system. Oscar Mayer's line of Zappetites Microwave Snacks, from mini-cheeseburgers to chili cheese dogs, average about 56% fat. A typical serving of Bachman Air Popped Pop Corn, inexplicably soaked in oil after it's air-popped, is 62% fat.

Even "low-fat" processed foods can be affected by hidden fat in the form of vegetable oils, cheese and butterfat. Good examples include granola cereal, non-dairy creamers, packaged potato mixes, prebasted turkeys, stuffing/bread mixes, gravies, refried beans, crackers and instant breakfast drinks.

The advent of microwave ovens has made both cooking and reheating easy. Speed is no longer the privilege of the wealthy. Microwaves are now owned by two-thirds of American households, including nearly half the households with incomes under $10,000. Even many college dormitory rooms today boast both a refrigerator and a microwave. Unfortunately, microwaves are used mostly for reheating rather than for cooking. Far fewer people cook a turkey breast in a microwave than heat up a frozen turkey meal. The problem is that the majority of foods designed for microwaves are rich in fat. Pillsbury's Heat n' Eat Microwave pizza gets 48% of its calories from fat. Swanson's Great Starts Eggs, Sausage and Potatoes breakfast is 72% fat. Betty Crocker's Microwave Yellow Cake is 48% fat.

Perhaps the greatest tragedy here is the missed opportunity with frozen meals, many of which have converted healthful, low-fat poultry and fish into high-fat meals:

Food Item	Total Calories	% of Calories from Fat
Chicken breast, skinless (4 oz.)	122	10%
Stouffer's Creamed Chicken (6½ oz.)	320	68
Beatrice's Chicken Kiev (6 oz.)	400	54
Turkey breast, skinless (4 oz.)	124	8
Banquet Family Entree Turkey with Gravy (8 oz.)	296	67
Tyson's Frozen Turkey Patties (3 oz.)	220	57
Cod (3 oz.)	69	9
Halibut (3 oz.)	129	17
Gorton's Crispy Fillet (1 fillet)	250	58
Van de Kamp's Light & Crispy Fish Sticks (4 sticks)	270	67
Mrs. Paul's au Gratin Fillets (5 oz.)	250	42

Source: USDA and individual food companies.

Snack and Junk Foods

The average American, according to the National Eating Trends Report, consumes about 200 snack foods per year. To appreciate the impact of these foods on eating habits, consider the following:

- $3.9 billion is spent annually on packaged, store-bought cookies.

- Over 100 million M&M's are produced each day.
- More than $8 billion worth of potato chips, pretzels, corn chips and tortilla chips are bought annually.

It isn't that people have just discovered candy, potato chips and cookies. Admittedly, we have a long history of snacking. But the role of snacking has changed. In the past, it was something done between meals; today, it may *be* the meal. The pace of everyday life at home and in the workplace often disrupts the schedule of regular, balanced meals, so we eat snack and junk foods on the run. In such a situation, "fat tooth" cravings often dictate food selection. Indeed, many people don't realize how high in fat snacks can be. A couple of Hershey chocolate bars with almonds in place of lunch means an intake of 460 calories and 28 grams of fat.

Snacking also contributes to a modern phenomenon called the "work out, pig out" mentality, often described as "the yuppie diet." These folks run five miles a day or do aerobic dance for an hour, then reward themselves with fatty snack foods. Says Richard T. O'Connell, president of the National Confectioners Association, "This is a prime reason why annual candy consumption has recently jumped from 19 to 25 pounds per person. . . . there is more nutritional averaging by those who consume candy as a reward."

Chips are among the worst offenders. Some 50% to 60% of the calories in potato chips come from fat. Eating 8 ounces of chips is like adding 12 to 20 teaspoons of vegetable oil to a baked potato. A single, one-ounce serving of Pringle's Regular chips or Cheezums, for example, gets 69% of calories from fat. Just 15 chips provide 15% of the fat an average person should consume in an entire day. It's the same for corn and tortilla chips. Fritos Dip Size or Bar-B-Q Corn Chips, for example, get 62% of their calories from fat. Commercially baked goods fare no better. Sara Lee Carrot Cake is 45% fat; Hostess Ding Dong's and Pepperidge Farm chocolate-chip cookies are 48% fat.

Restaurants

More people are eating in restaurants today. The American Restaurant Association reports that some 38% of all food dollars currently are being spent at restaurants and estimates that three-quarters of all meals eaten in the 1990s will be consumed away from home.

Much restaurant food is very high in fat. Consider the typical restaurant breakfast of bacon (81% fat), ham (70% fat) or sausage (93% fat), eggs (63% fat) fried in butter (100% fat), potatoes fried in lard (100% fat), toast with butter (100% fat), and coffee with cream (96% fat)—a fat disaster! A Big Country Breakfast with sausage at Hardee's contains 1,005 calories and is 66% fat.

Restaurant sandwich lunches can also be high in fat. Most luncheon meats are more than 60% fat, and that's before mayonnaise (100% fat) goes on the bread. Even salad bars can be a problem since many offerings are made with fat-rich dressings and condiments (cheese, bacon bits, avocados, seeds and nuts, olives and croutons). A typical small ladle at a salad bar holds about two tablespoons of dressing, or about 400 or so calories, almost all derived from fat; in comparison, the same amount of hot fudge has slightly fewer calories and far less fat. The following table shows how many calories can be packed into a small amount of certain salads:

Salad	Calories per ½ Cup
Macaroni	217
Coleslaw	212
Chicken	200
Tuna	190
Potato	124

Source: USDA.

Too many restaurant dinners are rich in red meat, deep-fried fish, creamy sauces, butter, oil and fatty desserts.

Even healthy ethnic foods have been changed into high-fat foods. Pasta, served in Italy with a simple marinara sauce, comes in the United States with sausage, meatballs and cream sauce. A dinner of chicken, rice and beans found in Mexico is transformed into deep-fried burritos and tacos. And the fish-and-rice dinners of Japan are traded for a steak in the U.S. version of a "Japanese" restaurant.

Of particular concern is the number of meals supplied by the 75,000 fast-food restaurants in the United States. Every day, an estimated one-fifth of the population eats at a fast-food restaurant. The quintessential example of success is McDonald's, which spends more than $1.7 million a day in advertising to attract customers, particularly young children. And it works. McDonald's serves over 18 million people daily—more than the entire combined populations of Michigan, Wisconsin and Minnesota.

Fifty-five percent of the calories in a McDonald's Big Mac come from fat. A Wendy's cheese-stuffed potato contains an amount of fat equal to nine pats of butter. A Burger King Chicken sandwich has as much fat as one and a half pints of ice cream. And the Jack in the Box Ultimate Cheeseburger contains over 15 teaspoons of fat.

Chain/Food Item	Total Calories	% of Calories from Fat
Arby's		
Chicken Salad Croissant	460	70%
Potato Cakes	201	63
Sausage & Egg Croissant	499	59
Super Roast Beef	501	40
Arthur Treacher's		
Cole Slaw	123	60%
Fish, fried (2 pcs.)	355	50
Shrimp, fried	381	57
Burger King		
Bacon Double Cheeseburger	510	55%
Double Beef Whopper with Cheese	970	59
Hash Browns	162	61
Specialty Chicken Sandwich	688	52

Chain/Food Item	Total Calories	% of Calories from Fat
Carl's Jr.		
Bacon 'n Cheese Omelette	290	87%
French Fries, regular	250	54
Scrambled Eggs	150	72
Zucchini, fried	311	55
Dairy Queen		
Dilly Bar	210	56%
Hot Dog with Chili	320	56
Onion Rings (3 oz.)	280	51
Hardee's		
Apple Turnover	282	44%
Canadian Sunrise Biscuit	482	55
Shrimp n' Pasta Salad	362	72
Jack in the Box		
Cheese Nachos	571	55%
Jumbo Jack with Cheese	630	50
Sausage Crescent	584	66
Taco Salad	377	56
Kentucky Fried Chicken		
Cole Slaw	176	50%
Extra Crispy or Spicy Thigh	371	64
Kentucky Nuggets (6 pcs.)	276	57
Original Recipe Drumstick	147	54
Long John Silver		
Breaded Clams (1 order)	526	53%
Fish Dinner, fried (3 pcs.)	1180	53
Seafood Salad	426	63
Tartar Sauce	119	83
McDonald's		
Big Mac	570	55%
Biscuit with Sausage and Egg	585	61
Egg McMuffin	340	42
McD.L.T.	680	58
Wendy's		
Ham & Cheese Omelet	250	61%
Home Fries	360	55
Ranch Salad Dressing (1 Tbs.)	80	100
Triple Cheeseburger	1040	59

Says Dr. Cheung, "We can talk our heads off as to what we should be eating, but without the help of the fast-food industry, we're not going to get very far." Fortunately, there are a few good choices that can fit into your fat budget. These will be discussed in Chapter 13.

What Happened to Three Squares?

Nothing has suffered more in the exchange of nutrition for convenience than the practice of eating three balanced meals every day. A good example is breakfast. While health professionals tell us that this is the most important meal of the day, the message falls on deaf ears. In about 50% of American families, one or more persons skip breakfast regularly. Says Nancy Clark, a sports nutritionist, "People tell me they don't have time for breakfast. What they don't realize is that by skipping this meal, they can become ravenous later in the day and make all the wrong food choices." Even when breakfast is eaten, it often consists of foods that are low on the nutritional ladder. The Coca-Cola Company estimates that 965,000 Americans drink $237 million worth of Coke at breakfast each year.

Even school lunches suffer. Although the USDA's National School Lunch Program describes meals as "tasty, attractive and nutritious," a close look reveals that a typical school lunch is no better (and may be worse) than a typical fast-food lunch. Indeed, many of today's school menus are built around fast-food-style items. At the elementary school in my neighborhood, the menu for one week was:

Monday—Chicken Nuggets
Tuesday—Macaroni and Cheese
Wednesday—Corndogs
Thursday—Cheeseburgers
Friday—Pizza

Chances are, these school lunches are as high in fat as comparable foods served in fast-food restaurants.

NUTRITIONAL INFORMATION OR MISINFORMATION?

In the last few years, no topic has received more media coverage than diet and health. It seems as though a "new" scientific study is reported every week. With free time reduced to a hurry-up lifestyle, Americans appreciate such information. For the most part, it has worked to our benefit by raising levels of nutritional awareness and knowledge. The National Institutes of Health's landmark cholesterol study in 1984, for example, led to a sharp increase in public awareness about the need to reduce cholesterol levels. But sometimes, as in the oat bran controversy, such studies can add to our confusion.

Research conducted at the University of Kentucky and at Northwestern University found that the soluble fiber in oat bran caused the body to excrete cholesterol and therefore would have an independent cholesterol-lowering effect when added to the diet. The public responded with oat bran mania, mixing up oat bran muffins, downing batches of oat bran cereal, and sprinkling oat bran on frozen yogurt. Sales of the stuff went from one million pounds to 24 million pounds in less than two years. But then a study at Brigham & Women's Hospital in Boston yielded a different finding. Oat bran did not reduce cholesterol independently, said the researchers. Rather its true value was in displacing high-fat breakfast foods such as bacon and eggs. The same result could be accomplished with wheat or rice cereals.

Each study was conducted by respected, credible scientific professionals. Each showed a different and opposite result. Whom should we believe?

All too often, the public is caught in the middle. According to Gallup research, 53% of the population feels there are too many reports on various health risks, yet still are not sure what to eat and what to avoid. Many people simply remain on—or revert to—the comfortable, contemporary high-fat diet. "I think the confusion starts from a good place," says Dr. James Rippe of the University of Massachusetts. "The idea is that knowledge is power. But we've probably gone too far. We have too much knowledge, too much media exposure of 'breakthroughs' and controversies. What we need is more common sense." Says Dr. Katherine Halmi of New York Hospital, "One of the problems is that as soon as scientists have done a study, the commercial element takes hold of that information and promotes it. A lot of this is done for economic benefit rather than a concern about what's most healthful."

Modern confusion over "good nutrition" cannot be attributed solely to overzealous and premature reporting on the part of the media. Advertisers and food manufacturers who have traded nutritional information for hype on food labels bear some responsibility. And, in all fairness, so does a public that wants easy answers to complex problems. The result has been a huge increase in pop nutritionists with revolutionary cures, "food-as-medicine" products, and materials ranging from books to dietary supplements. "We are too willing to put our faith in quick fixes," says Dr. Sarah Short of Syracuse University. "Many of the most popular books offering crash diets or magical ways to cure cholesterol should be on the fiction list." This is echoed by Dr. Paul Saltman of the University of California at San Diego: "Our lifestyle has produced a bumper-sticker mentality when it comes to food. 'Eat my oat bran muffin and it will cure your heart disease,' or 'Buy my lite dinner and pounds will melt away.' It doesn't work that way. Americans are all to ready to accept quick solutions that may in reality aggravate the problem. We need to return to basics. There is no shortcut to a low-fat lifestyle."

THE TRUTH ABOUT DIETARY FAT

One misconception concerning nutrition is that dietary fat is inherently harmful. Nothing could be farther from the truth. In itself, fat is not bad.

Like proteins and carbohydrates, dietary fat plays a legitimate and important role in maintaining good health. It is essential because it is not manufactured by the body and must therefore be provided by foods. Polyunsaturated fats (mostly from vegetable oils) supply the body with linoleic acid, an essential fatty acid. Dietary fat is also used in the transportation of important fat-soluble vitamins into the body. Without fat in the diet, we would not be able to absorb vitamins A, D, E and K.

And finally, dietary fat provides the body with a concentrated source of energy (calories). At 9 calories per gram, fat supplies more than twice the calories as the same amount of protein or carbohydrate. This is especially important for children—particularly those under two, who can use the higher energy from fat to meet increased growth needs.

Dietary fat also makes food more palatable. Graham Kerr, the former "Galloping Gourmet," told me that when he learned to cook, commercial kitchens kept butter in nut-size chunks. The rule was, he said, "when in doubt about the recipe, throw in a nut of butter. The extra fat made everything taste better." Besides enhancing flavor, dietary fat helps to distribute flavors throughout the mouth, keeps them there longer, and provides texture. It also makes food moister, causing it to literally "melt in the mouth." And, because fat is digested slowly, it provides an enjoyable feeling of satisfaction after a meal. This is why a high-fat American meal (beefsteak, French fries and a salad with dressing) will often satisfy the appetite longer than a low-fat Oriental meal (dishes that emphasize more rapidly digested carbohydrates such as vegetables and rice).

Consumed in the proper amount, there is nothing wrong with dietary fat. It is an overabundance of fat that constitutes a health issue. From a nutritional standpoint, the daily requirement for fat can fully be satisfied by consuming the equivalent of one tablespoon of vegetable oil. The average person, however, eats eight times that amount. According to the USDA, the top five sources of dietary fat are:

1. Hamburgers, cheeseburgers, meat loaf
2. Hot dogs, ham, processed meats
3. Whole-milk dairy products
4. Commercially baked goods, such as muffins, doughnuts and cookies
5. Beef steaks and roast beef, French fries, fried chicken

Other sources include cooking oils, margarine, snack foods such as chocolate, potato chips and candy, and convenience foods such as cream soups, chili con carne and frozen dinners.

What's Wrong with Fat?

More than two centuries ago, the German poet Goethe observed: "You are what you eat." Today, scientists are validating this observation. As data from numerous studies accumulate, it becomes clear that what and how much you eat can have a direct impact on your health, appearance and longevity.

Nowhere is this more true than in the United States, where a high-fat diet contributes to the development of an imposing list of typically American diseases. These include heart disease, cancer, stroke, diabetes and high blood pressure, not to mention the less threatening but still serious problems of gout, osteoarthritis, gallbladder disease and the nation's leading ailment—obesity.

Public interest in diet and disease has existed throughout the 20th century. In the early 1900s there was widespread concern about contamination of foods and alteration of food products. "Germs" were in their heyday. In books and newspapers, reformers brought attention to unsanitary conditions and methods of handling food. The government responded by creating the Food and Drug Administration, which was responsible for the institution of great improvements in food inspection, sanitation and uniform standards of identity.

In the late 1930s and early 1940s, interest in food was

again peaked by the discovery of vitamins and essential elements. At this time, deficiency diseases such as rickets, scurvy and beriberi, arising from inadequate diets, were a significant public health problem. This led to the establishment of "Recommended Dietary Allowances," the creation of the Food and Nutrition Board, and widespread programs of food fortification and enrichment.

Today the emphasis has changed from nutritional deficiency to fat excess. Says former surgeon general C. Everett Koop, "As the diseases of nutritional deficiency have diminished, they have been replaced by diseases of dietary excess and imbalance—problems that now rank among the leading causes of illness and death in the United States."

HALF THE LEADING CAUSES OF DEATH ARE AFFECTED BY DIET*

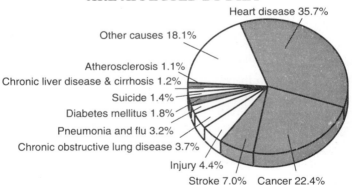

Heart disease 35.7%

Other causes 18.1%

Atherosclerosis 1.1%
Chronic liver disease & cirrhosis 1.2%
Suicide 1.4%
Diabetes mellitus 1.8%
Pneumonia and flu 3.2%
Chronic obstructive lung disease 3.7%

Injury 4.4%

Stroke 7.0%   Cancer 22.4%

* Shaded segments show direct related causes.

The impact of the modern diet on health is the subject of the 1988 Surgeon General's Report on Nutrition and Health. The report, which paints a picture of the United States gobbling its way to the grave, found a causal link between a high-fat diet and 5 of the 10 leading causes of death: "After smoking, the choice of diet can influence long-term health prospects more than any other factor.'' While Koop condemned the modern diet for its role in fostering chronic disease, he also held out hope. Just as risk goes up with a poor diet, so can it be reduced with a healthy diet. This means that to a great extent the avoidance of life-threatening disease is within our control, as can be seen in the clear relationship between certain dietary changes and the risk of chronic disease.

	Reduce Risk of:				
Dietary Change	Heart Disease	Cancer	Stroke	Diabetes	Gastro-intestinal Diseases
Reduce fats	X	X	X	X	X
Reduce calories	X	X	X	X	X
Increase fiber, complex carbohydrates		X		X	X
Reduce sodium	X		X		
Control alcohol		X	X		X

In addition, the report stated that a decrease in dietary fat was crucial to maintaining proper body weight.

The Surgeon General is not alone in being concerned about the national diet. Since 1958, some 17 major health organizations have called for changes in the way America eats. Dietary guidelines have been issued by the American Heart Association, the U.S. Senate Select Committee on Nutrition and Human Needs, the National Cancer Institute and the National Cholesterol Education Program. In 1990, 10 major voluntary and governmental agencies agreed on dietary concepts for the American public, issued in a special report entitled ''The Healthy American Diet.'' The report called on people to improve their health by eating a balanced diet with less total fat and saturated fat, by increasing the consumption of complex carbohydrates and fiber, and by maintaining a reasonable body weight.

Although the sheer number of reports and standards on

the makeup of a healthy diet can be overwhelming, there is a consensus when it comes to the nation's highest dietary priority: *Reduce the intake of dietary fat to no more than 30% of calories, saturated fat to no more than 10% of calories.* The 1989 National Research Council's Committee on Diet and Health Report sums up the rationale succinctly: "There is clear evidence that the total amounts and types of fats in the diet influence the risk of cardiovascular diseases, certain forms of cancer, and obesity. While it is evident that dietary patterns are important factors to the cause of several major diseases, dietary modification can reduce such risks."

It is important, therefore, to clearly understand the connection between excessive dietary fat and chronic disease. This understanding provides both a rationale for change and a motivation for success.

CHAPTER 4

DIETARY FAT, CHOLESTEROL, AND HEART DISEASE

If six fully loaded 747s were to crash tomorrow, by nightfall newspapers throughout the country would carry four-inch headlines shouting about the 2,000 people killed. Every television network would preempt regular programming to bring on-the-spot special reports. And for weeks after, talk-show hosts would interview anyone remotely connected to the tragedies. No two ways about it, when 2,000 people die from a single cause in one day, it's big news. Or is it?

The fact is, 2,000 Americans die every day, 365 days a year, from a single cause—coronary heart disease. By far the number one killer of Americans, outnumbering cancer and auto accidents combined, this disease is rampant throughout the country. Consider the following:

- One person suffers a heart attack every minute.
- Each year there are 1.5 million heart attacks producing some 600,000 to 800,000 deaths.

- The chance of an American dying of heart and blood vessel disease is about 1 out of 2.
- By age 60, every fifth male in the United States has suffered a heart attack.
- Twice as many women die each year from cardiovascular disease as from all types of cancer.

In America, virtually no family escapes coronary heart disease. Says Dr. Edward Schneider of the University of Southern California, "A hundred years from now, people will look back on this century and realize there was an epidemic of coronary heart disease in the Western world that was unique in history. The tragedy is that much of it was—and is—preventable."

WHAT IS CORONARY HEART DISEASE?

Coronary heart disease is a condition in which blood flow to the heart is restricted due to the buildup of cholesterol blockages, or plaque, on the inner walls of the coronary arteries. It is the product of a disease called atherosclerosis, which is translated from the Greek as "hard mush"—an apt description of artery blockages that start out as soft, mushy accumulations of cholesterol and end up as deposits of hard, encrusted material. The process, which takes place over time, is akin to the buildup of rust inside an old water pipe; ultimately, corrosion will narrow the diameter, resulting in a reduced flow of water through the pipe. As cholesterol deposits form on the artery walls, the interior becomes narrower and the flow of blood to the heart is impeded.

The seriousness of this situation stems from the fact that the only supply route to the heart is through the coronary arteries. Like the rest of the body, the heart needs a continuous supply of oxygen- and nutrient-rich blood in order to function. It pumps a tremendous amount of blood to the body (beating about 100,000 times a day to send out the equivalent of some 1,800 gallons of blood), but it can't use any of the blood moving through it. So, nature has devised an ingenious system. Every time the heart pumps, 95% of the blood goes to the body and 5%—a commission of sorts—comes back to the heart through the coronary arteries. When cholesterol builds up in these arteries, and blood supply is inadequate for the needs of the heart, chest pain called angina, or angina pectoris, often results. This is usually felt as a discomforting sensation of tightening in the chest, heavy pressure behind the breastbone, or a burning sensation in the lungs. It can also be felt as a sharp pain in the jaw, neck, arm or shoulder. Angina is a warning sign that the coronary arteries are clogged.

Should blood be cut off to the heart completely, a heart attack results. This is called a myocardial infarction. When a heart attack takes place, the area of heart muscle denied blood dies of suffocation and is replaced by scar tissue. Since scar tissue cannot contract, the heart loses some of its ability to pump.

THE ROLE OF CHOLESTEROL

For most Americans, coronary heart disease is not preordained. To be sure, some people do have a genetic predisposition to heart attack, but research shows that they make up less than 15% of the population. The majority of us have the power to control the three greatest risk factors for coronary heart disease and heart attack—smoking, high blood pressure and elevated blood cholesterol.

Unfortunately, these risks do not add up arithmetically. Instead, there is a geometric progression that significantly increases the chances of coronary heart disease with each additional risk factor. If you have any one of the risk factors—you smoke, have high blood pressure, or have elevated blood cholesterol—you have two times the risk of someone with no risk factors. If you have two risk factors, your risk goes up four times. And if you have all three factors, your risk goes up eight times.

While all three major risk factors are significant, none is more important than elevated blood cholesterol. Indeed, without the buildup of cholesterol blockages, coronary heart disease would not take place. Smoking and high blood pressure are associated with high rates of heart attack primarily in populations where elevated cholesterol levels are very common. Italians, for example, smoke more than people in the United States, and Japanese have a greater incidence of high blood pressure. But elevated levels of cholesterol are not usually found in Italians or Japanese— and neither are high rates of heart attack. Says Dr. Robert Wissler of the University of Chicago, "Cigarette smoking and hypertension have little influence on heart disease except as added factors. In other words, the primary problem is what is happening in terms of cholesterol."

The amount of cholesterol contained in the blood, then, is the cardiovascular bottom line. As Dr. Robert Levy, director of the National Heart, Lung and Blood Institute, observed, "There is no controversy that cholesterol is the chief risk factor for heart attack." Dr. Richard Carleton of the National Cholesterol Education Program, describes the evidence of a link between cholesterol and heart disease as "enormous and compelling."

One of the most important cholesterol studies is in Framingham, Massachusetts, where investigators have continuously monitored the cardiac health of the population since 1948. Their findings are conclusive: as blood cholesterol rises, so does the incidence of heart attack. According to Dr. William Castelli, director of the Framingham Study, for every 1% rise in cholesterol above 150 mg/dl, the risk of heart attack goes up by 2%. This makes blood cholesterol level a key predictor of future incidence of heart attack. Researchers at the National Cholesterol Education Program estimate that about 60 million people in the United States over age 20 are at risk for coronary heart disease because of elevated blood cholesterol.

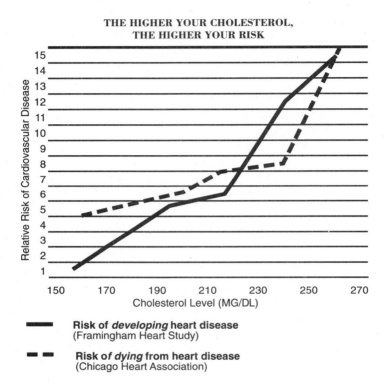

THE HIGHER YOUR CHOLESTEROL, THE HIGHER YOUR RISK

━━━ **Risk of *developing* heart disease**
(Framingham Heart Study)

■ ■ **Risk of *dying* from heart disease**
(Chicago Heart Association)

CHOLESTEROL LEVEL

In the appropriate amount, cholesterol is not harmful. It is necessary for cell wall construction, for the transmission of nerve impulses, and for the synthesis of important steroid and sex hormones. Indeed, no cell could exist without it. The critical concern is not cholesterol per se, but how much and what type is in the bloodstream. The higher a person's cholesterol "count," the greater the risk for heart disease. But the opposite is just as true. Lowering blood cholesterol level reduces the risk for heart disease.

Cholesterol level is determined by analyzing a blood

sample and expressing the results as the number of milligrams (mg) of cholesterol in one deciliter (dl) of blood. For example, a person with 220 milligrams of cholesterol in a deciliter of blood has a cholesterol level of 220 mg/dl, popularly referred to as a cholesterol "count" of 220.

The table below shows the risk at different levels according to the National Institutes of Health.

| | Cholesterol Level | | |
Age	Moderate Risk	High Risk	Goal Level
< 20	> 180	> 200	< 180
20–29	> 200	> 220	< 180
30–39	> 220	> 240	< 200
> 40	> 240	> 260	< 200

The public health goal for the nation is a "desirable" cholesterol level below 200 mg/dl. And the lower, the better. Indeed, studies by Dr. Jeremiah Stamler of Northwestern University have shown that cardiac risk drops dramatically with levels below 180 mg/dl. Part of the problem in complying with these guidelines stems from confusion over what is a "normal" cholesterol level. In the past, people with levels well over 200 mg/dl were told they were normal. This happened to me, just a few months before my bypass surgery, with a cholesterol level of 250 mg/dl. It wasn't that my doctor was trying to mislead me. It was that I was confusing statistical norms with norms for good health. Statistically speaking, my cholesterol was "normal," which really meant that it was "average" for an American. If your cholesterol is around 220 mg/dl, you are normal (average) by today's standards. But remember, it's also normal for Americans to die of heart disease. In this respect, "normal" is not necessarily "healthy."

The optimal, or ideal, cholesterol level for good health is actually around 150 mg/dl. It is in this context that the NIH goal of "under 200 mg/dl" makes sense.

GOOD AND BAD CHOLESTEROL

Type of cholesterol also has an impact on cardiac risk. Low-density lipoprotein, or LDL cholesterol, endangers cardiac health; high-density lipoprotein, or HDL cholesterol, promotes cardiac health. One of the chief distinctions between these two main types of cholesterol involves chemical packaging. Cholesterol in a pure state is a waxy substance that does not mix with water and therefore must combine with fat and protein molecules in order to be transported in the bloodstream. The chemical packages formed in this manner are called lipoproteins.

Low-density lipoproteins are considered "bad" cholesterol because they unravel quite easily. Should an LDL penetrate an artery wall, its cholesterol could be released and deposited, thus beginning the clogging process. High-density lipoproteins are considered "good" for two reasons. First, should an HDL penetrate an artery wall, the package remains intact and no cholesterol is released. Second, HDLs act as arterial Drano, removing harmful LDLs from the lining of blood vessels and helping the body to excrete them.

While elevated LDL cholesterol is an unequivocal risk for coronary heart disease, low levels of the protective HDL cholesterol can be equally dangerous. Of 1,000 patients at Johns Hopkins University, 185 men and 47 women had coronary heart disease even though their total cholesterol levels were under 200 mg/dl. Of those individuals, 68% of the men and 32% of the women had HDL levels less than 35 mg/dl. These figures show that total cholesterol doesn't tell the entire story. If two people have cholesterol counts of 220 mg/dl, but one has an HDL level of 60 and the other an HDL level of only 25, the difference in coronary risk is substantial. The person with higher HDLs has significantly less risk. The table that follows expresses the link between HDL levels and cardiac risks according to NIH data.

| Degree | HDL Cholesterol | |
of Risk	Men	Women
Very low	>65	>75
Low	55	65
Average	45	55
Moderate	25	40
High	<25	<40

Medical experts now believe that the ratio of HDL to total cholesterol is more significant than the total cholesterol number by itself. (This ratio is obtained by dividing total cholesterol by HDLs. For example, a person with a total cholesterol of 200 and an HDL of 40 has a 5:1 ratio.) According to Dr. Ken Cooper, HDL should constitute no less than 20% of total cholesterol in males (a ratio of 5:1) and no less than 22.5% in females (a ratio of 4.5:1). The lower the ratio, or the greater the percentage of HDL, the more protection against coronary disease.

There are two ways to improve the HDL ratio:

1. Increase HDLs. This can be done by losing excess weight and by giving up cigarette smoking. Exercise is one of the best ways to increase HDLs. As few as three workouts a week for 20 minutes can improve HDL ratio. Studies find that joggers and brisk walkers who cover just 11 miles per week have significantly higher HDLs than their sedentary counterparts.

2. Decrease LDLs. The most effective way to lower LDLs, apart from medication, is to reduce saturated fats in the diet.

THE IMPACT OF DIETARY FAT

Three factors contribute to the level of blood cholesterol. First, all the cholesterol the body needs for good health is produced by the liver. Second, an excessive intake of foods rich in dietary cholesterol, such as eggs and organ meats, can cause blood cholesterol level to rise. And third, the intake of foods rich in dietary fat, particularly saturated fat, can cause the body to increase cholesterol production. The third factor—dietary fat intake—is the most important.

SATURATED FAT

Saturated fat is found in animal foods such as meat, poultry, fish, and dairy products, and in three vegetable oils: palm oil, palm kernel oil and coconut oil. This is the most harmful type of fat, since it works in the body to increase blood cholesterol level. The more saturated a fat, the greater its impact on cholesterol. Coconut oil is 92% saturated fat, for example, while palm kernel oil is 86%, butterfat is 59%, beef fat is 54%, and palm oil is 51%.

The emphasis on saturated fat is a change from the past, when the elimination of dietary cholesterol such as eggs and organ meats was the main concern. This is not to say that dietary cholesterol is unimportant, for it is. The American Heart Association recommends no more than 300 milligrams per day. But today we know that cholesterol-rich foods are responsible for only about one-third of excessive cholesterol in the arteries. The rest comes from saturated fat. Says Dr. Ernst J. Schaefer, chief of the lipid metabolism laboratory at Tufts University's Human Nutrition Research Center on Aging, "Reducing saturated fat consumption by 50% may lower blood cholesterol twice as much as a similar drop in dietary cholesterol." According to Dr. Mark A. Kantor, a nutrition specialist at the University of Maryland, "The amount of cholesterol produced by the body and the rate it is removed from the bloodstream is controlled to a great extent by saturated fat in the diet."

An additional problem occurs when unsaturated vegetable oils are hydrogenated, or hardened, as in stick margarine and shortening. A study by Dr. Ronald Mensink at the Agricultural University in Wageningen (the Netherlands), reported in the *New England Journal of Medicine*, states that hydrogenated unsaturated fats, called trans fatty acids, increase LDL cholesterol and are as likely as saturated fats to increase the risk of heart disease. This means that stick margarine made from corn oil, for example, may not be that much better than butter in terms of cardiac health.

POLY- AND MONOUNSATURATED FATS

Polyunsaturated and monounsaturated fats, found in vegetables in the form of oil, are seen to be more healthful because they lower cholesterol in the blood and provide a certain degree of coronary protection. Polyunsaturated fats include safflower, soybean, sunflower, corn, cottonseed and sesame oils. Monounsaturated oils include olive, canola, peanut, avocado and nut oils. (In general, the more liquid a fat becomes at room temperature, the less saturated it is.)

Monounsaturated fats deserve special mention. Studies in the United States and Canada indicate that while polyunsaturated oils reduce all cholesterol, protective HDL as well as harmful LDL, monounsaturated oil reduces LDL only. For this reason, olive oil and canola oil in particular may be instrumental in reducing the risk of coronary heart disease. This may explain the low incidence of heart disease among Mediterranean populations that use olive oil and Asian populations that use canola oil.

TOTAL FAT

Recently, however, the role of poly- and monounsaturated fats in maintaining good health has been called into question. Though "more healthful" than saturated fats, these oils should be used only in moderation. According to a study at the University of Southern California, the more fat of any kind a person eats, the more likely he or she is to develop fatty blockages in the coronary arteries.

While research on the role of fats and oils continues, the

consensus is clear. Choose polyunsaturated and especially monounsaturated fats and oils. But use all fats in moderation. Keep total calories from fat under 30% and calories from saturated under 10%.

THE REVERSIBILITY OF CORONARY HEART DISEASE

The prospect of reversing the process of coronary heart disease by lowering blood cholesterol level is not new. Over 50 years of animal studies on rhesus monkeys have consistently shown that cholesterol buildup in the arteries can be reversed, and a number of recent studies on humans have shown the same result. Among cardiac patients studied at the University of Southern California, reversal of the disease process took place in those who achieved a significant reduction in blood cholesterol (LDL under 130 mg/dl, HDL above 40 mg/dl). In a similar study at the University of Washington, Dr. Greg Brown reported reversal in 30% to 50% of his patients.

The most notable study involving diet and reversal is that of Dr. Dean Ornish of the Preventive Medicine Research Institute in Sausalito, California. The 48 men and women in this study all had arteries that were at least 40% clogged; in some, they were nearly 100% clogged. Dr. Ornish split the participants into two groups. All were counseled to follow standard medical recommendations such as quitting smoking and getting a half-hour of aerobic exercise three times a week. The control group was put on a diet that followed the recommendations of the American Heart Association—no more than 30% of calories from fat. The treatment group was put on a strict vegetarian diet of about 8% fat.

At the end of one year, 41 people remained in the study: 19 in the control group and 22 in the treatment group. In the control group, total cholesterol had dropped only 13 points and LDL cholesterol had dropped by 10 points. In 10 patients, the condition had worsened; 3 patients stayed the same: and 6 showed some improvement. In the treatment group, however, total cholesterol had dropped by 55 points and LDL cholesterol by 56 points. Eighteen patients showed improvement; 3 stayed about the same; and one who did not follow the regimen became worse.

According to Dr. Claude L'Enfant, director of the National Heart, Lung and Blood Institute, "This study is important because it shows that regression of coronary heart disease may be possible by making lifestyle changes—particularly those involving dietary fat."

A LAST WORD

Since virtually no family in America escapes coronary heart disease, it is only prudent to know the facts:

- Heart disease is the number one killer in the United States.
- When blood cholesterol goes up, so does the incidence of heart attacks; when it comes down, heart attack incidence also drops.
- A diet rich in saturated fat causes blood cholesterol to rise; a diet low in saturated fat causes it to fall.
- A diet rich in total fat increases the risk for heart attack; a diet low in total fat decreases heart attack risk.
- The lower your cholesterol count, the better. The national goal is to be under 200 mg/dl.
- The more HDL, the better protection from heart disease. Know your HDL count. At least 20% of total cholesterol in males should be HDL, and at least 22½% in females.
- To reduce LDL cholesterol, eat less saturated fat and control your weight; to increase HDL cholesterol, get more exercise.
- Lowering blood cholesterol can stop the progression of coronary heart disease and may even reverse it.

CHAPTER 5

DIETARY FAT AND CANCER

Across America, there is an impression that the "war on cancer" is being won. It is not. Despite the billions of dollars spent on research since President Nixon's administration, cancer incidence is on the rise. In 1985, there were 800,000 new cancer cases in the United States. Today, the number of people developing cancer is about one million. By the year 2050, according to estimates by the National Cancer Institute, the number of new cases per year will be 1.9 million.

The death rate from cancer has risen as well. In 1987 cancer claimed an estimated 476,700 lives, or about 22.4% of all deaths. Now it is expected to replace heart disease as the leading cause of death in the United States by the year 2000. A scientist at the Fred Hutchinson Cancer Research Center in Seattle told me recently that he had started out in cardiovascular research but switched to cancer because "cancer is a growth industry."

In actuality, "cancer" is not a single disease but comprises at least 100 different diseases. The causes of cancer are many and complex; however, the majority of cases can be attributed to just two environmental factors—smoking and diet. Tobacco is responsible for 30% of all cancer deaths in the United States. Diet is even more significant, causing some 35% of all cancer deaths.

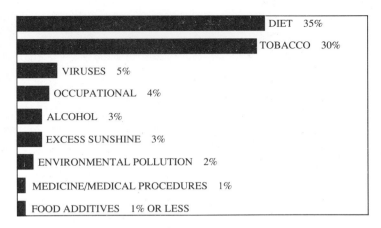

	DIET 35%
	TOBACCO 30%
VIRUSES 5%	
OCCUPATIONAL 4%	
ALCOHOL 3%	
EXCESS SUNSHINE 3%	
ENVIRONMENTAL POLLUTION 2%	
MEDICINE/MEDICAL PROCEDURES 1%	
FOOD ADDITIVES 1% OR LESS	

According to Dr. Oliver Alabaster, director of cancer research at George Washington University, "There is evidence that 60% of cancer in women and 40% of cancer in men is caused by diet. Because more than one-quarter of the population will eventually develop cancer, this means that about 60 million Americans might be affected. Of these, approximately 20 million cases might be prevented by making changes in our national diet." Says Dr. Bruce Ames of the University of California at Berkeley, "Toxic waste and alar may grab the headlines, but lowering dietary fat intake will do more to reduce cancer than eliminating pollutants."

More than any other dietary consideration, excessive dietary fat is linked to high cancer rates. This makes the high-fat U.S. diet, already damned for reasons of cardiac disease, a prime promoter of cancer risk. According to the National Research Council's 1989 Diet and Health Report, "The weight of evidence suggests that what we eat during our lifetime strongly influences the probability of developing certain cancers. A high-fat intake is causally associated with increased risk of cancers of the colon, prostate and breast. However, the evidence also suggests that a reduction of total fat intake is likely to decrease the risk of these cancers."

The diet-cancer link presents a mixed message. Cancer incidence and mortality are on the increase, and the high-fat U.S. diet is a primary risk, but it doesn't have to be that way. In a statement to the press concerning cancer risks, Margaret Heckler, former Secretary of Health and Human Services, said: "We now know that fully 80% of cancer cases are linked to lifestyle and environmental factors. The most important causes of cancer are the ones we can control ourselves." The key word, of course, is "control." How we eat has a direct impact on whether or not we develop certain cancers. But the choice is ours. So, to a great extent, we can exercise control over our cancer destiny.

THE NATURE OF CANCER

Cancer comes in many shapes and forms. It can affect the blood or the bones, the lungs, the skin or the intestines. All of the body's organs and tissues are susceptible. There are many types of cancer, yet what all have in common is that they result from cells growing wildly out of control.

The human body is made up of trillions of cells, each of which is designed to perform a specific function. Red blood cells, for example, carry oxygen to all other cells, while skin cells form a protective package for the whole body. Cells normally grow in an orderly fashion, reproducing only when necessary. In addition, healthy cells do not spread beyond their natural boundaries. (New muscle cells, for instance, do not spread to bone.) Cancer begins when the growth instructions to cells are disrupted. In such a case, cells divide in an uncontrollable way, multiply recklessly and, no longer recognizing their natural boundaries, spread to distant sites in the body to set up colonies.

A key to cancer development is DNA, an acid contained in every cell. Working like a computer chip, DNA "programs" certain cell behavior such as growth. In a fetus, for example, it will stimulate rapid cell growth; in later life, when such growth is no longer necessary or desirable, it will reprogram the cell to "shut down" growth. If, however, signals get mixed and DNA programs cells in later life to grow rapidly, the process can result in cancer.

Scientists believe that the development of cancer takes place in three stages: initiation, promotion and progression. In the initiation stage, cells are not cancerous; rather, they acquire the potential to become cancerous. Initiation takes place over a relatively short period of time and is irreversible. It occurs when a cancer-causing agent, or carcinogen, such as tobacco smoke or radiation, disturbs DNA within the cell, causing the character of the cell to change and providing it with the potential for uncontrolled growth. A number of agents can initiate cells, including chemical carcinogens (e.g., those in asbestos or air pollution), specific viruses, radiation and hormones (particularly estrogen). Exposure to these agents does not mean that cancer will result, but the risk does go up with the amount of exposure.

The disease germinates in the second stage, called promotion, when initiated cells begin to radically change character as a result of contact with one of the many possible cancer promoters. Such promoters, which exert their effects over a long period of time, stimulate development of the disease by causing actual growth in initiated cells. Normally, cells are uniform and line up in neat rows. When initiated cells begin to "transform" into cancer cells, this orderly pattern is completely disrupted. Some cells get larger, others become smaller. Not all abnormal growths are cancerous. Benign cells, such as those found in a harmless freckle, divide unnecessarily but do not spread beyond their natural boundaries. Malignant cells, by contrast, do not recognize the rules of cellular organization. After dividing, they invade adjacent tissues and spread to distant sites. This heralds the progression stage, the last in the cancer process.

Malignant cells in progression are prolific, dangerous and lethal. As long as nutrients are available, they will multiply wildly and endlessly, requiring an ever increasing share of the body's food, oxygen and water. Tumors form when malignant cells clump together into a small, expanding mass. As cells proliferate rapidly, the mass enlarges and a "domino" effect starts to take place as malignant cells invade surrounding tissues. Soon these tissues are destroyed. When health professionals speak of a "primary" tumor, they mean the original tumor mass, generally referred to by its location—lung, breast, colon, etc. "Secondary" tumors, called metastases, result when cancerous cells journey from the original tumor to distant sites in the body, usually through the blood or lymphatic system. If metastases are widespread to other organs and sites, treatment usually becomes difficult, if not impossible. What begins as a limited excursion turns into a global war, overcoming all defense efforts. Tragedy is the result.

The key to controlling cancer is prevention. One of the first steps is to avoid triggers that initiate the process, such as nicotine and tar in cigarette smoke. However, there are other factors that are crucial in determining whether exposure to a cancer-causing agent will lead to disease. And none is more important than diet. According to Dr. Leonard A. Cohen of the American Health Foundation, "Dietary fat is one of the most important cancer promoters. It does not cause the cancerous process to take place in a breast, for example, but it can prompt initiated cells to proliferate."

THE IMPACT OF DIETARY FAT

It is often said that in medical research "there is no black and white, only shades of gray," and this is certainly true of cancer studies. Numerous global population studies and clinical laboratory trials, however, strongly suggest that a high-fat diet directly increases risk of colon, breast and prostate cancers. The 1982 report of the National Academy of Sciences' Committee on Diet, Nutrition and Cancer takes a direct stand: "Of all the dietary components studied, the evidence shows a *causal* relationship between total fat intake and the occurrence of these cancers."

The fat/cancer link is important because, after lung cancer, the second, third and fourth causes of cancer deaths in the United States are colon, breast and prostate cancers.

- Colon cancer is responsible for 51,000 deaths a year. Each year it is diagnosed in some 41,000 men and 49,000 women. Five years later, only about half this number are still alive. Many of the survivors have had a colectomy, surgery replacing their large bowel with a plastic sack outside the body to collect waste.
- One out of every 10 women develops breast cancer. Every 13 minutes another woman dies of the disease. And despite all efforts to better detect and treat it, breast cancer claims lives at the same rate today as in 1950.
- Prostate cancer, which accounts for more than 18% of all male cancer cases, is responsible for more than 25,000 deaths each year. Before 1900, prostate cancer was considered a rare disease. Today, as a result of our fatty diet, it is a major cause of cancer death in males.

Colon, breast and prostate cancer accounted for 39% of all new cancer cases and 27% of all cancer deaths in 1988. This is an enormous price to pay for high-fat eating habits.

THE SCIENTIFIC EVIDENCE

In particular, the connection between dietary fat intake and breast cancer is very strong. This link was first isolated over 40 years ago at the Michael Reese Hospital in Chicago, where Dr. Albert Tannenbaum showed that animals fed high levels of fat in their diet produced more breast cancer than animals fed a low-fat diet. In the late 1960s, Dr. Kenneth Carrol at the University of Western Ontario examined breast cancer rates in relation to diet patterns in more than 40 countries and found the same results as with test animals: those countries with high-fat intake (United States, Great Britain, Argentina) had an elevated rate of death from breast cancer; those with a low-fat diet pattern (Japan, Thailand, Ecuador) had just the opposite.

The impact of dietary fat consumption on the risk for breast cancer was studied in England, where researchers compiled a record of dietary habits over the 50-year period between 1928 and 1978. The record showed a steady rise in the fat content of the English diet from 1928 until World War II, when intake dropped sharply due to a shortage of meat, eggs and butter. Vegetables and whole grains became dietary staples. During this time, the rate of breast cancer dropped significantly. However, it shot up again in the postwar years, when fatty foods again became available.

The impact of fat intake on breast cancer risk within the same population was measured in the United States, a decidedly high-risk country with a national diet very rich in fat. Where the population deviated from the high-fat norm, cancer risk was lessened. For 20 years, Dr. R. L. Phillips of Loma Linda University followed 25,000 Seventh-Day Adventists, a bona fide low-fat group whose diet is primarily vegetarian. He found their breast cancer mortality rate was between one-half and two-thirds that of the overall U.S. rate. This demonstrates the dual nature of diet: it can increase or decrease cancer risk.

A recent study conducted by Dr. Paolo Toniolo of New York University Medical Center compared the diet of 250 women with breast cancer to that of 499 without breast cancer. All the women were from the same province in Italy. The cancer patients reported eating significantly more cheese, butter and milk. The study concluded that the risk of breast cancer is higher for:

- Women who get more than 36% of calories from fat;
- Women who get more than 13% of calories from saturated fat; and

- Women who get more than 8% of calories from animal protein.

"Our study is not conclusive," says Dr. Toniolo, "but it does support the recommendations made by the American Cancer Society, the National Academy of Sciences, the Surgeon General and others to reduce fat intake to below 30% of calories."

The same relationship is evident in international data on fat and prostate cancer. In the United States, an analysis of mortality rates from 1950 to 1969 revealed that more deaths from prostate cancer occurred in areas with high consumption of beef and dairy products. Other support for the link to fat comes from the findings of lower rates of prostate cancer among certain religious and ethnic groups who traditionally eat fewer fatty foods. Comparison of prostate cancer mortality rates of Japanese immigrants to the United States against those in Japan shows substantially higher mortality among Japanese-Americans. Recent studies in Japan show an increase in prostate cancer rate in Westernized areas such as Tokyo, where intake of dietary fat has gone up dramatically.

Finally, there is a broad body of research linking dietary fat to an increase in colon cancer. Again, as a population, Americans are at risk because of our fat-rich national diet. Yet pockets of low-fat populations prove that reducing risk is possible. Seventh-Day Adventists and Mormons, two low-fat groups, have far less colorectal cancer than the U.S. population at large. Furthermore, research shows that the pattern changes when a population moves from a low-fat country to a country where the consumption of dietary fat is considerably higher. One significant study tracked two groups of Japanese men and women. The first group lived in Japan and ate the traditionally low-fat Asian diet. After 20 years, their incidence of colon cancer was extremely low. The second group immigrated to the United States and adopted the high-fat American diet as their own. After 20 years, the Japanese in the United States developed colon cancer at the same rate as the rest of the population.

HOW DIETARY FAT INCREASES CANCER RISK

Unlike the risk of heart disease, which is increased by certain fats, cancer risk is tied to total fat. All dietary fats—saturated, polyunsaturated and monounsaturated—come into play. The richer the diet pattern in fat, the greater the potential for developing breast, colon and prostate cancers. Given a diet of almost 40% fat, it is not surprising that these cancers threaten health.

The U.S. diet contributes to cancer risk in three ways:

1. Dietary fat acts as a cancer promoter in cells.
2. Dietary fat contributes to overweight and obesity, an independent risk factor for certain cancers.
3. Foods rich in dietary fat often displace healthier foods in the diet pattern, such as fresh fruits, vegetables and whole grains.

Dietary Fat Is a Cancer Promoter

Laboratory studies show that breast cancer growth takes place when test animals are fed high-fat diets after—not before—exposure to chemical carcinogens. Fat also seems to facilitate the growth of breast cancer by its effect on female hormones. It is known that elevated levels of certain hormones, particularly estrogen, can overstimulate breast tissue and trigger cancer. For some reason, not totally understood, fatty diets tend to cause women to produce more estrogen, thus increasing breast cancer risk. Studies show that women who consume more than 36% of their calories as fat are approximately three times more likely to develop breast cancer as are women whose diets contain less than 28% fat.

The risk of colon cancer is elevated as well by an increase in dietary fat, which in turn increases production of bile acids in the large bowel. Excess bile can combine with bacteria, which are plentiful in the intestine, to produce cancer-causing chemicals. In addition, excess bile acids alone may promote tumor cell growth by injuring the lining of the large intestine.

International incidence and mortality data show a positive correlation of prostate cancer with per capita intake of dietary fat, especially from animal sources. The mechanism is not yet well understood, although many researchers hypothesize that fat may promote cell growth in the prostate. One thing is clear: in populations whose fat consumption rises, so does the incidence of prostate cancer.

Overweight and Cancer Risk

The relationship between a high-fat diet and overweight/obesity is covered in detail in Chapter 6. Suffice it to say here that being overweight is an independent risk factor for certain cancers. In a long-term study of 750,000 men and women by the American Cancer Society from 1959 to 1972, the rate of cancer was significantly higher among people 40% or more overweight. In men, this mainly involved cancer of the colon and rectum; in women, there were higher death rates from breast and endometrial cancers, as well as cancer of the gallbladder and cervix. The relationship of overweight to cancer risk is especially strong in postmenopausal women, who are at a much higher risk of developing breast and endometrial cancers. Researchers think the reason for this is that obesity tends to increase the production of estrogen, the female hormone that can enhance tumor growth at these sites.

Other research has shown a relationship between caloric intake and cancer risk. A study of 32 countries found a connection between total caloric intake and cancers of the colon (men) and breast (women). Another study, conducted in Hong Kong, showed twice the colorectal cancer in people with diets of 3,900 calories a day versus those with diets of 2,700 calories per day. Animal studies have also shown that those with restricted caloric intake after exposure to carcinogens develop fewer tumors than those with higher caloric intake.

Complex Carbohydrates and Fiber Reduce Cancer Risk

People whose diets are centered on fatty foods seldom take the time or make the effort to include fresh vegetables, fruits, legumes and whole grains in their diet. A benefit of these foods is that they are rich in fiber, vitamins and minerals that are associated with a lower cancer risk.

Fiber in the diet dramatically decreases the risk of colon cancer and other conditions, such as diverticulosis and diabetes. Some of the earliest research on fiber was conducted by Dr. Denis Burkitt, a British physician who worked in Africa from 1946 to 1966. He noted that the diet of many African tribes provided over 50 grams of fiber a day—more than two times the amount found on the affluent Western diet—and that these tribes had very low rates of colon cancer. Worldwide studies since the 1970s have corroborated Dr. Burkitt's observations. The National Cancer Institute, the American Cancer Society and the National Academy of Sciences all recommend a high-fiber diet—at least 25 to 35 grams per day—for the prevention of colon cancer. The average U.S. diet contains only 11 grams.

Fiber, or roughage, works to reduce cancer risk by moving food elements quickly through the intestines. In doing so, it shortens the time that cancer-promoting agents, such as dietary fat, are in the gastrointestinal tract. Current thinking is that the shorter the time any harmful elements are in the body, the less time they will have to do any damage. Fiber also absorbs and binds bile acids in the colon. These are the free-floating acids that can irritate the lining of the intestine and interact with intestinal bacteria, creating a positive atmosphere for cancer production. By moving bile acids out of the colon, fiber helps to prevent these dangers. This is also a theory for how cholesterol is removed from the body.

Along with dietary fiber, fruits and vegetables contain beta-carotene and vitamin C, which have been shown to reduce cancer risk. Beta-carotene is a member of the carotenoid family, a group of compounds that give red, yellow and orange fruits and vegetables their color. These compounds are converted by the body to vitamin A, which has been shown to reduce cancer risk. The National Cancer Institute recommends at least one serving daily of foods rich in beta-carotene. Dr. Paul La Chance of Rutgers University estimates that most Americans should be eating about four times more beta-carotene than is currently consumed.

Foods rich in vitamin C, shown to reduce cancer risk, include citrus fruits, strawberries and melons. In addition, laboratory studies have found that the risk for colon cancer is lowered by cruciferous vegetables such as broccoli, cabbage, kale, turnips, Brussels sprouts and cauliflower.

A LAST WORD

Cancer has grown to an epidemic proportion in the United States, so it is prudent to know the following facts:

- Cancer is the second leading cause of death in the United States. Cancer incidence and mortality are both on the rise.
- Thirty-five percent of all cancers are linked to diet. A fat-rich diet increases the risks for breast, colon and prostate cancers.
- Dietary fat acts as a promoter of cancerous growth in cells.
- Dietary fat also contributes to overweight/obesity, an independent risk factor for certain cancers.
- Fatty foods often displace foods rich in fiber, vitamins and minerals (fruits, vegetables, grains and legumes) that reduce cancer risk.
- Reducing total dietary fat intake reduces cancer risk.

CHAPTER 6

DIETARY FAT AND WEIGHT CONTROL

Says author Kim Chernin, "In this era, when inflation has assumed alarming proportions and the threat of nuclear war has become a serious danger, when violent crime is on the increase and unemployment a persistent social fate, 500 people are asked by the pollsters what they fear the most in the world and 190 answer that their greatest fear is 'getting fat.' "

American culture is, to put it mildly, preoccupied with weight. We describe a newborn by its weight and proudly announce the poundage along with gender and name. We are fascinated with the literal ups and downs of celebrity weight watchers like Oprah Winfrey and Elizabeth Taylor. We subscribe to magazines in which slim models, tummies as taut as army cots, epitomize the ideal human form. And every day millions of us use bathroom scales as part of the morning routine.

The obsession with weight in this country is readily demonstrated:

• A survey by *Better Homes and Gardens* revealed that

90% of the population, including small children, think they weigh too much.

- According to the National Center for Health Statistics, almost 70 million people are trying to lose weight (or at least not to gain it).
- A Gallup poll showed that 31% of U.S. women aged 19 to 39 diet at least once a month. Sixteen percent of this group consider themselves perpetual dieters.
- *HealthWeek*, a journal of the health care industry, reports that medically supervised fasting programs, unheard of a decade ago, now produce an estimated $1 billion in yearly revenue.

Despite an all-consuming interest in shedding weight (yearly revenues of the weight loss industry exceed $20 billion and are growing at the rate of $1 billion a year), the U.S. population currently ranks as one of the world's fattest. Data compiled by the National Institutes of Health show that over 40 million adults are overweight, which means they weigh more than the "ideal" weight for their height and gender. The typical adult male is 20 to 30 pounds overweight; the typical adult female, 15 to 30 pounds overweight. A more significant problem exists for the millions of people who are "overfat," that is, who carry too much body fat as a percentage of their total weight. According to the National Obesity Research Council, a male is considered obese when his body fat makes up more than 25% of his body weight; a female, when her body fat exceeds 30% of total body weight.

At the root of our concern is a seriously overweight population. Studies show that Americans tend to gain an average of one to two pounds each year from age 20 to 50. That may not seem like much, but a gain of one and a half pounds each year over that time frame would mean an extra 45 pounds by age 50. The prevalence of progressive fatness is clearly illustrated by a study in which couples were weighed on their wedding day and again on their 13th wedding anniversary. The brides put on an average of 23 pounds, while the grooms averaged an 18-pound gain.

And the problem is not just with adults. It is estimated that as many as four million children aged 6 to 11 are overweight. According to Drs. William Dietz and Steven Gortmaker of Harvard University, rates of obesity in children and adolescents went up an average of 45% between the 1960s and the early 1980s. The fattening of the United States is an issue that cuts across age differences.

If such studies and indices are not enough to demonstrate the scope of the problem, just look around. The country is filled with flabby adults, porky adolescents and chubby children, potato chips in one hand and a TV channel selector in the other. Dr. Ken Cooper sums it up succinctly: " . . . taken together, we are carrying well in excess of one billion pounds of extra weight. I hope that with a statistic like that, the country doesn't sink beneath the surface of the earth."

HEALTH CONSEQUENCES

"There are two reasons people don't like being overweight," says Dr. Rudolph Leibel of Rockefeller University in New York. "One is cosmetic, and while it's an individual's right to dislike his or her weight, that may not be the best reason to lose weight. The other is that being overweight poses health risks. The latter is a much more urgent reason for people to lose weight."

Medical research has illustrated that being overweight can constitute a serious health risk. Actuarial studies have shown that carrying as little as an extra five pounds can reduce longevity. According to NIH data, excessive body fat is clearly associated with an increased risk of heart disease, certain cancers, high blood pressure, respiratory problems, gallbladder disease, arthritis and gout.

The greater the degree of overweight, the higher the risk

for chronic disease. Cardiovascular disease in particular is impacted by excess weight. The NIH estimates that 25% of cardiovascular disease can be attributed to overweight. An eight-year study of 116,000 women aged 30 to 55 determined that being overweight by virtually any degree increases the risk of heart disease. Women who are mildly to moderately overweight (15% to 29% over their ideal weight), for example, have an 80% higher risk of heart disease. Says Dr. Charles H. Hennekens of Harvard University, "Obesity is right up there with cigarette smoking and heavy alcohol consumption as a major cause of excess morbidity and mortality in the United States."

The location of excess weight (or, more accurately, excess body fat) also seems to be important. Studies show that people with potbellies are three to five times as likely to suffer a heart attack as those who accumulate fat in other parts of the body. Abdominal fat, it seems, is more metabolically active and adds to cardiac risk. This may explain why men, who tend to accumulate extra fat in potbellies, are more susceptible to heart attack than females, who tend to accumulate extra fat in thighs and hips.

"OVERFAT" VS. "OVERWEIGHT"

For most of us, "overweight" is a misnomer. The real problem is not excess weight but too much body fat. The truth is we are "overfat."

This distinction is critical to understanding the problem (gaining excessive body fat) and the solution (losing excessive body fat), yet it runs contrary to general experience. Most people are concerned only with weight expressed in pounds, which can be measured and monitored easily. This is why the bathroom scale is often the final arbiter. If the scale reflects the gain of a few pounds, it's a disaster ranking with a major earthquake. Down a few pounds, and it's sweeter than winning a lottery. The problem with this view is that it overlooks the most important element: body fat.

The body is composed of lean body mass (muscle, bone, teeth, fluids) and body fat. The key element for health and appearance is body fat, but it can't be measured by a bathroom scale. The scale can reveal what you weigh in pounds, but it can't tell what makes up that weight. Not knowing how much of your weight is body fat is akin to evaluating your coronary risk without considering how much of your total cholesterol is harmful LDL. Some people are "overweight" simply because they weigh more than they "should" according to height/weight tables. But the excess weight may be muscle. A football player who stands six feet tall and, because of his weight-lifting regimen, has bulked up to 220 pounds could be considered seriously overweight. But his body is rippling with lean muscle and carries very little body fat. This man is in excellent physical condition. He may be "overweight," but he is certainly not "overfat."

Overweight, then, is simply an excess of body weight. It can be positive if the condition results from extra pounds of muscle; it is negative if it comes from excessive body fat. The fact is that the hated accouterments of excess weight—double chins, potbellies, bulging thighs—are really the result of too much body fat. A thick waist is filled out not with "weight" but with body fat. Thus the real problem is gaining excessive body fat, becoming "overfat," and losing excessive body fat is the true solution.

IDEAL WEIGHT

The most common measurement of "ideal," or most desirable, body weight has been the Metropolitan Life Insurance Company's height and weight table. Last revised in 1983, it provides a range of weight-for-height, with the midpoint considered the "ideal" weight for most people. In recent years, health experts have questioned the validity of these tables. One reason is that the data are based mostly on white, middle-aged males who have insurance. A similar guideline, issued by the Health and Human Services Department, provides ideal weight based on age and height. It has been criticized for providing a heavier range and suggesting that it is acceptable to gain pounds with the years.

The most glaring shortcoming of these tables is that they ignore body composition, the ratio of body fat to lean body mass. The simple truth is that what you weigh is far less important than how much of that weight is fat.

Ideal weight, say many health professionals, relates more to body composition than to pounds. According to Dr. David Parker, a physiologist, the ideal percentages of body fat for healthy adults are as follows:

Age	Males	Females
16–19	15%	19%
20–29	16	20
30–39	17	21
40–49	18	22
50–59	19	23
60+	20	24

"These percentages apply to the average person," says Dr. Parker. "Athletes and those who exercise regularly should be 2% or 3% less than the table represents."

There is a significant disparity between ideal and actual body fat percentages in the U.S. population. While the ideal range for males is 15% to 20% (depending on age), adult males average about 23%. The ideal range for females is 19% to 24%, but the average for adult women is 32%.

Body composition measurement is best taken in a clinical setting. The most commonly used techniques include skinfold measurement, electronic impedance and hydrostatic (underwater) weighing. Availability and cost are reasons so many people continue to rely on scales and height/weight charts to determine ideal weight, even though body fat percentage is a more important issue.

Fortunately, there is a simple formula for estimating ideal weight that relates both to pounds and to body fat content. According to Dr. Richard Freeman at the University of Wisconsin Medical School, it equates to body fat percentages of 15% to 19% in males and 19% to 23% in females. Ideal weight is calculated as follows:

1. Measure your height.
2. For males, the first 5 feet is equal to 105 pounds. Each additional inch is equal to an additional 6 pounds. (*Note:* If a man's wrist measurement is greater than 7 inches, he is considered large-boned and can add 10%).
3. For females, the first 5 feet is equal to 100 pounds. Each additional inch is equal to an additional 5 pounds. (*Note:* If a woman's wrist measurement is greater than 6 inches, she is considered large-boned and can add 10%.)

While this formula estimates a weight that is "ideal," some researchers feel that it is more accurate for younger than for older people. "It works well for teenagers," says Dr. George Bray of Louisiana State University, "but it may set up an ideal weight that is very difficult to achieve for mature, non-athletic adults."

The use of the formula in this book has less to do with establishing an ideal weight per se than it does with estimating a personal fat budget based on scientifically sound information. (Fat budgeting will be discussed in Chapter 9.) Understand that the formula is "ideal," but don't get hung up on it as an absolute best weight for you.

GENETICS AND "OVERFAT"

Developing excess body fat involves more than just overeating and underexercising. There is strong evidence today that genetics and heredity impact metabolism and, in some people, predispose obesity. Studies of populations show a strong inheritance factor in overweight: fat parents tend to produce fat children. If both parents are overweight, there is an 80% chance that the child will also be overweight. If only one parent is overweight, the chance of having a fat child drops to about 50%. And if both parents are of average weight, there is less than a 15% chance of producing an overweight child. Genetic predisposition to obesity is illustrated in a study on twins who were raised apart. Conducted by Dr. Albert Stunkard of the University of Pennsylvania, this study showed that pairs of adult identical twins who had been raised in different families were just as similar in body fat level as pairs raised together. This finding suggests that heredity is at least as important as environmental factors in determining weight differences among individuals.

Other people may have a relatively stable adult weight as a result of genetic factors. According to Dr. Gilbert Leveille, this "setpoint" weight is the weight at which the body is comfortable. The natural setpoint weight may put an individual 10 or 20 pounds overweight in relation to the height/weight charts. Having chosen a setpoint weight, the body works tirelessly to defend it by controlling appetite. In other words, a person may be programmed genetically for a certain weight. So, if too few calories are eaten, the body may respond by decreasing metabolism. By reducing its idling speed, in some instances by 15% to 25%, the body becomes more energy-efficient and weight loss is harder to achieve. If weight is lost, the body may strive to regain the setpoint weight.

For most of us, genetic makeup may not be the cause of the problem. Indeed, a study at the Medical College of Wisconsin in Milwaukee found that genetics may account for only 12% of people with excessive body fat. According to Dr. Thomas Wadden of the University of Pennsylvania School of Medicine, the steady increase in percentage of overweight and obese Americans during the 20th century shows that environment exerts the most major influence. "Our gene pool isn't changing," he states. "Rather, it's that our environment now supports fatness. Because our society encourages people to eat more and more and to exercise less and less, those people who are genetically predisposed to become fat will do so. For every dollar spent by the Surgeon General and researchers to prevent and treat obesity, a hundred dollars is spent by the food industry to lull people into eating more fattening foods. We're being fattened up by the food industry and slimmed down by the billion-dollar diet-and-exercise industry. That's great for the capitalistic system, but it's not so great for the consumer."

In the final analysis, genetic baggage does not guarantee a person to be overfat. However, when genetics combines with pro-fat cultural influences and a "fat tooth" disposition, an overfat condition is invariably the result.

THE IMPACT OF DIETARY FAT

Of all the cultural influences contributing to an overfat condition, none is more important than the excessive amount of dietary fat found in the U.S. diet. The key word is "excessive."

It should be clearly understood that there is nothing inherently wrong with dietary fat. Like proteins and carbohydrates, it is a component of foods and provides a source of energy (calories) to fuel the body. When more calories are taken in than the body can use immediately, the extra is stored as body fat. It accumulates primarily under the skin and around the internal organs, and is available to the body as a fuel reserve. In effect, stored fat becomes a "fuel tank" for the body, and fuel (fat) is drawn off and used as needed.

As long as energy input (calories consumed) is in balance with energy expenditure (calories burned in exercise, physical activity and basic bodily functions), excess fat does not accumulate. But because dietary fat is so calorically rich (at 9 calories a gram, it contains twice as many calories as carbohydrates and proteins), and because so much of the national diet is made up of dietary fat, it's relatively easy for most of us to overconsume calories. When 3,500 extra calories have accumulated, one pound of body fat has been created. It will take an energy expenditure of 3,500 calories to burn this pound of fuel. Unfortunately, the ability of the body to store fat is virtually limitless.

It is not easy to put on one pound of fat in a single day. In order to increase your intake by 3,500 calories, you'd have to consume eight McDonald's Quarter-Pounders, or 16 pieces of Domino's pepperoni pizza, or a case of beer. Theoretically, this would cause a person to gain one pound of fat (although studies on twins show that because of genetic metabolic differences, some people might be able to handle these extra calories while others cannot). The point is that, for most of us, gaining extra body fat is not accomplished in a short time. A few extra calories coming in, a few less going out, over time is what causes body fat percentage to creep up. As few as 50 extra calories a day, a single chocolate-chip cookie, can add 350 calories a week, or a total of 18,200 in a year. That's equal to a gain of 5 pounds of body fat, or 52 pounds in a decade.

Of course, it's possible to gain body fat by overeating any type of food. Enough fruit, pasta or carrots, and you could become overfat. But the principal problem in the United States is fatty foods.

Dietary Fat Is Calorically Dense

Because of its chemical nature, dietary fat is a more concentrated source of calories than other foods. One teaspoon of fat has 45 calories; the same amount of protein or carbohydrates has just 20 calories. This means that the quantity of food eaten may be less important than its content. High-fat foods are calorically dense, which means they pack a lot of calories into a small amount of food. A good example is M&M's peanut candies. A small package contains 250 calories and is 47% fat. It's not a lot of food (actually only 1.74 ounces), but it contains a king-size amount of calories because it's so rich in fat. As a rule of thumb, "high-fat" equals "high-calorie." In addition, dietary fat contains little water or fiber and takes up less volume than other foods, so you can eat a lot of it without feeling full.

The opposite is true of calorically light foods such as apples. An entire pound of apples contains only 242 calories—less than a small bag of peanut M&M's. Apples are low in fat and therefore low in calories. And, because apples are a bulky food, high in water and fiber, satiety is achieved long before overeating occurs.

Research shows that food selection plays an important role in weight control. One study measured the amount and caloric density of foods selected by two groups. The first group ate a diet low in fat and rich in high-carbohydrate, high-fiber foods; the second group ate a diet rich in fat. The second group actually ate 13% less volume than the first group but took in 56% more calories because their diet was high in fat and therefore calorically dense. As a result, the second group gained weight. The first group ate more food but lost weight.

Similar results were found in a study by Dr. Elliott Danforth, Jr., at the University of Vermont. Adult males fed excessive calories in a mixture of fat and carbohydrate took seven months to gain about 30 pounds, while men fed fewer calories exclusively as fat gained 30 pounds in only three months. The plain truth is that it's easier to gain weight from foods rich in dietary fat than from high-carbohydrate foods. Fat, it seems, is more fattening than carbohydrate.

Dietary Fat Turns into Body Fat

Anything eaten in abundance can turn into body fat. However, there is evidence that dietary fat converts very efficiently to body fat, making fatty foods a primary contributor to an "overfat" condition. For many years, scientific researchers thought that "a calorie is a calorie is a calorie." A growing body of evidence now suggests that once a calorie is eaten, this simple rule of dieting dogma doesn't always hold true. Says Dr. Eric Jequier of the University of Lausanne in Switzerland, "There is a marked difference in the body's response to fat and carbohydrate feeding."

When calories are consumed, some are utilized immediately by the body as fuel. Those not used right away are converted to body fat and stored for future use. The process of converting calories to body fat takes energy, and some of the calories being converted are used to produce that energy. This represents the "handling costs" of turning calories into stored fuel.

Not all foods call for the same amount of energy in the conversion process, so not all have the same "handling costs." Research conducted by Dr. Jean-Pierre Flatt of the University of Massachusetts Medical School indicates that almost one-fourth (23%) of the calories found in carbohydrates are burned off when they are converted to fat. So, of 100 calories processed, only 77 are available to be stored as body fat. But dietary fat uses just 3 calories in energy to process 100 calories into body fat. "This means 97% of all fat calories are converted to body fat," says Dr. Robert E. T. Stark, president of the American Society of Bariatric Physicians, specialists in treating overweight people. "On the other hand, you'd have to eat a tremendous amount of carbohydrates for any to be converted into body fat. The body has marvelous mechanisms to take care of carbohydrates and proteins." What it boils down to is that a fat calorie has a greater potential for increasing body fat than has a carbohydrate calorie. Says Dr. Danforth, "Fat is more fattening, calorie for calorie, than carbohydrate."

Not only is it "expensive" to convert carbohydrates into fat, but the body seems reluctant to do it. Studies show that a person could eat 2,000 calories of carbohydrates in just one meal without gaining an ounce of body fat. That is the amount of carbohydrate present in four to five pounds of bread, cereal and fruit. But fat is a different story. Research has shown that even on relatively low-calorie diets (1,500 calories per day), people can become obese if 50% of those calories come from fat. According to Dr. Flatt, "Only when people eat massive amounts of carbohydrates does it get converted into body fat. But it is not the same for dietary fat."

The impact of this phenomenon is evident in a study of overfat women conducted at Laval University in Quebec, Canada. At first only exercise was used as a reducing tool, but soon body-fat loss leveled off. However, when the women began to eat a low-fat diet and to exercise as well, the reduction in body fat was spectacular. While a low-fat diet is not a magic wand that will eradicate serious obesity, it can go a long way in helping. As one researcher commented, "If a formerly obese woman eats 1,500 calories of fat, she's sunk. But if she eats 200 calories of protein, 100 calories of fat and 1,200 calories of carbohydrate, she has a chance to keep the excess body fat off."

DIETS DON'T WORK

Every year, hundreds of gimmicks for rapid weight loss are sold to an unwary public. The desire to lose weight quickly and easily has created a market for a myriad of questionable products and programs ranging from "fat-burning" diets and "magic" powders for increasing metabolism to plastic body wraps for making inches disappear effortlessly. These so-called cures, which fluctuate in popularity like skirt lengths in *Vogue*, promise instant results. None delivers a permanent solution.

Of all the gimmicks, crash diets are by far the most popular. "One third of the world is on a diet. Another third just fell off a diet. And the remaining third is going on one next Monday." So says columnist Erma Bombeck, and statistics say she's right. But chronic "off-and-on" dieting, called the "yo-yo syndrome," doesn't work. Data show that 97% of dieters not only regain the lost weight within one year but actually put on extra weight. The cruel truth is that chronic dieting is ineffective. According to experts such as Dr. Kelly Brownell, "yo-yo" dieters find it harder to lose weight over time. In a study using laboratory rats, he found that after losing weight on a diet and then regaining it, the rats took twice as long to lose the weight a second time. "This indicates that chronic dieting can slow the metabolic rate as a protection against perceived starvation," says Dr. Brownell. "The more often you diet, the more your body resists shedding weight." This seems to be particularly true when caloric intake falls to under 1,200 calories a day for men and 900 calories a day for women. The result is that chronic dieting can actually produce the opposite of the desired effect by making the dieter even fatter!

In addition, there is evidence that "yo-yo" dieting may actually increase "fat tooth" cravings. Laboratory animals forced to lose weight, then to regain it, altered their dietary pattern to increase fat intake. The act of cyclical dieting by itself, it seems, may increase the desire for fat, or at least the propensity for choosing fatty foods.

And finally, the instant "results" of crash diets (losses of 10 or more pounds in a single week) must be questioned. Pounds may be down, but the real question is: What has been lost? According to the American Medical Association, crash diets produce a loss of fluid and muscle, but virtually no loss of body fat. Many diets, particularly those low in carbohydrates, are merely short-term diuretics. At some point, both fluid and weight will reappear. To make matters worse, very low-calorie diets may result in the consumption of muscle tissue as fuel—including that of the heart, brain, liver, lungs and kidneys. Since muscle burns fat, the more muscle you have, the more fat your body can burn. A person with a lot of muscle is like a car with a large engine. It guzzles fuel—gasoline in the case of the car, body fat in the case of the person. This is why fit people can eat more than out-of-shape people and not gain body fat. On the other hand, a body with little muscle operates very efficiently and may never draw on fuel storage. So, by going on crash diets and losing muscle, people penalize their own ability to burn body fat.

WHAT IS THE SOLUTION?

Permanent reduction of excessive body fat takes place on a slow, steady basis over a period of time, and involves three key steps:

1. Reduce dietary fat in order to moderate caloric intake.
2. Increase high-carbohydrate, high-fiber foods as a low-calorie means to satisfy appetite.
3. Increase exercise in order to burn calories, stoke metabolism and reduce "fat tooth" cravings.

Remember, one pound of body fat represents the storage of 3,500 extra calories. That same amount must come out of your reserve tank (fat storage) in order for one pound of body fat to be lost. This will not happen overnight. After all, you didn't gain a pound of body fat in one day, so you can't expect to lose it that quickly.

Reducing dietary fat, the most concentrated form of calories, can easily result in lower-calorie meals. This is accomplished by establishing a personal fat budget (see Chapter 9) and by making smarter dietary choices. For example, just a tablespoon of salad dressing, which can be as high as 90% fat, generally has between 60 and 80 calories. But by using less dressing, or a diet dressing, calories are saved. Drinking skim milk instead of whole milk will save 60 calories per cup; three cups a day saves 180 calories. Using plain non-fat yogurt in place of sour cream on a baked potato saves 360 calories per cup. What it comes down to is that over the course of the day you simply spread a little less butter or margarine on your morning toast, mix a little less mayonnaise into the tuna, and coat your salad lightly with dressing. Small dietary changes to reduce fat can be very productive.

It's the same with exercise. You don't have to run the Boston Marathon or compete in the Tour de France. Moderate exercise can be very effective. For example, a 150-pound person can burn 250 calories with just 42 minutes of brisk walking or 22 minutes of jogging.

The fact is that losing body fat permanently is simple. Not easy, but simple. And the reduction of body fat, changing the condition of being "overfat," is the only true solution to the overweight problem.

A LAST WORD

The U.S. population is carrying more than 1.5 billion pounds of excess weight. For most of us, the real problem is being "overfat," that is, carrying too much body fat. Remember:

- Excess body fat is a health risk, particularly for coronary heart disease, cancer, stroke and diabetes.
- Know how to calculate your ideal weight. Don't rely on height/weight tables.
- Excessive dietary fat produces an "overfat" condition because dietary fat is calorically dense and is easily converted into body fat.
- Chronic dieting doesn't work. It can set you up to gain weight by diminishing metabolism and increasing "fat tooth" cravings.
- It takes a negative energy balance of 3,500 calories to lose a pound of body fat. This is accomplished by reducing caloric intake (trimming fat from the diet) and increasing caloric output (exercise).

PART II

HOW TO BEAT THE ODDS IN A PRO-FAT ENVIRONMENT

CHAPTER 7

==========

BASIC PRINCIPLES TO CONTROL DIETARY FAT

==========

The previous chapters have dealt with two of the strongest influences on dietary decisions—an inherent "fat tooth" craving and an environment that fosters the selection of fatty foods. Together, these factors have helped to create a diet pattern so rich in fat that it undermines health.

Americans are becoming more and more aware of the need to lower dietary fat, yet the ability to do so has eluded many people. According to Dr. Nancy Wellman, president of the American Dietetic Association, "Many of us try to reduce fat in our diets, but our lifestyle overrides our good intentions. Demographic changes, the number of meals eaten away from home, the convenience pull, nutritional naiveté, and plain confusion confound our attempt."

And, it seems, this direction will not be changed in the near future. Experts predict that the following trends and developments will occur in the United States over the next decade:

- Health-conscious people will continue to substitute more "good fats" (unsaturated fats such as canola, safflower and olive oils) for "bad fats" (saturated fats such as butter, palm oil, coconut oil and lard), but the overall fat content of the U.S. diet will stay too high.
- The dominant foods of the decade will be snack foods, frozen foods, plastic-wrapped preprepared foods, and microwavable foods.
- The deli and bakery sections of supermarkets will expand.
- More foods, particularly meats, will be sold fully prepared. Some fresh fish will be available in grocery stores, but most will be sold as "ready to heat and eat."
- Half of U.S. kitchens will have two or more microwave ovens to make it easier to "grab, zap and gulp" our food.
- Fast-food restaurants will accept credit cards.
- Fast-food restaurants won't be fast enough for some of us. There will be more microwavable fast foods for home consumption.

So the bad news is, we live in a pro-fat environment that makes it easy to satisfy our "fat tooth" cravings, and this environment may promote even more fatty foods in the future. The good news is, it doesn't have to be that way. We can control our environment and create new dietary habits that will mitigate rather than support the "fat tooth."

A New Outlook

Of all the things that are critical to making lifestyle changes, perhaps none is more important than a positive mental attitude. This is a mind-set in which one accepts responsibility for and control over one's behavior. It is a mental resolve, a commitment to succeed. Positive mental attitude provides a perspective that centers on what can be done rather than on what cannot be done. It concentrates more on why a person wants to change than on what has to change. Most important, it creates an outlook that makes the process a positive experience where change is seen as something being gained, not something being lost.

This attitude also recognizes the possibility of setbacks, but it sees them as learning experiences rather then as "failures" or "mistakes." As Malcolm S. Forbes said, "Failure is success if we learn from it." Success, not failure, should be the focus. During his career in the major leagues, Babe Ruth was the definitive home-run hitter. He hit 714 of them. He also struck out 1,330 times, so he just as easily could have been labeled as strikeout king, but he focused on his successes, not his failures, and that's why he's remembered as the home-run king. This also applies to fighting fat cravings. Succumbing to a chocolate doughnut that causes you to exceed your fat budget does not mean you "blew it" and your entire effort is ruined. Instead, see it for what it really is: a temporary setback to your normal, healthy eating pattern.

Two other points should be understood by anyone who wants to modify dietary habits (or any behavioral habit):

- Significant change is not the result of a single quantum leap. Rather, it comes with the accumulation of small changes that add up to one large change.
- Permanent change takes place over time. It cannot be hurried. It is an evolutionary, not revolutionary process.

Many times, failure is the result of action taken too quickly. In the heat of the post-decision moment ("This time I *will* lose those 10 pounds!"), there is a rush of activity. Cupboards are cleared, new recipe books are purchased, and the entire family is given a pep talk. But often this takes place without a sense of focused direction. As one friend described his wife's efforts, "She's all over the place, like a ping-pong ball in a boxcar." The important thing is not the speed or degree of change, but the continuance of it—not quick results, but permanent change. Modifying deeply ingrained habits takes a plan and a goal. In other words, it takes proper organization.

A PLAN OF ACTION

Outlined below is a simple, effective, do-it-yourself (and at-your-own-speed) approach to lowering dietary fat without deprivation or prohibition. It considers where you are, where you want to be, how you will go from the former to the latter, and how long it will take. Above all, it considers what is realistic for you.

1. Exercise to Curb the "Fat Tooth"

The role of regular exercise in promoting physical fitness (particularly stamina, strength and flexibility) is well understood today. Research shows it is a key to lowering cholesterol, reducing body fat and controlling weight. But exercise offers even more. Studies now illustrate that it is related to positive dietary changes. Indeed, people who exercise regularly tend to eat less dietary fat and more complex carbohydrates and fiber. Some experts have hypothesized that a fit body "needs" certain foods for optimal performance, and this need is reflected in food choices. Others believe that because exercise reduces stress, people who exercise are more in control of their lives and do not overindulge in fatty foods (ice cream, chocolate, pastries) as a stress response. And finally, there is evidence that exercise may neutralize the brain chemicals responsible for "fat tooth" cravings.

Exercise is a key component of dietary change. Fortunately, an effective exercise program is easy to start, provides a degree of immediate accomplishment and can be moderate. You don't have to run a marathon or experience pain in order to gain benefits from exercise.

2. Construct a Personal Fat Budget

A realistic plan for dietary change must be as flexible as our modern lifestyle and must emphasize freedom of choice. This can be accomplished by constructing a personal fat budget, that is, by calculating how many grams of fat you should eat each day for ideal weight. Once this is established, you can spend the budget any way you want. With this approach, no food is "good" or "bad." Obviously, even within the fat budget, better choices exist. Canola oil, low in saturated fat, is a better choice than butter, high in saturated fat. Ultimately, however, you have the freedom to choose foods so that you can maintain your daily budget. In doing so, not only are you in control of food choices, but you also know that no more than 30% of your calories will come from fat.

3. Make Smarter Choices

The goal is to eat less fat. But this is not easily accomplished in our modern society. The world we live in is not perfect, nutritionally or otherwise. Constructing a personal fat budget is a necessary first step. The next is learning how to use that budget to make smarter food choices in the real world. For example, fast food may be a dietary disaster, but it's part of our culture. Chances are, at some time you'll end up at a McDonald's. What do you do? Using your fat budget as a guide, you can interpret product information to make smarter, more informed decisions. The more you know about your options before you pass through the Golden Arches, the better your decisions will be. And that is what good nutrition is all about: making the wisest possible food choices. In the final analysis, nutrition and health information is meaningless without the ability to apply it in a practical way.

CHAPTER 8

EXERCISE TO CURB THE "FAT TOOTH"

The first basic principle recognizes the positive influence of regular exercise on dietary control. Instituting a program of physical activity makes sense, since regular exercise is one of the most important components of a healthy lifestyle. Says Dr. Robert Butler, former director of the National Institute on Aging, "If exercise could be packaged into a pill, it would be the single most widely prescribed—and beneficial—medicine in the nation." Many of the benefits of regular exercise are understood by the public. Even hard-line "couch potatoes" concede that exercise keeps the heart and lungs functioning well, promotes "good" HDL cholesterol, lowers blood pressure, reduces body fat, and improves energy and vitality.

Unfortunately, simply understanding that exercise benefits health has not caused many of us to swing into action. On the one hand, we know that exercise is good. Indeed, polls conducted by the Harris and Gallup organizations and by *American Health* magazine showed health benefits to be the chief reason that people exercise. On the other hand, most of us don't exercise regularly. Data compiled by the

U.S. Public Health Service indicate that less than 20% of adults exercise enough to realize health benefits, another 40% exercise only on an irregular basis, and the remaining 40% are completely sedentary.

What may not be so well understood is the role of exercise in achieving dietary change. Most books that counsel dietary changes acknowledge the importance of exercise in a healthy lifestyle. But because food choices and eating habits are emphasized, there sometimes is a tendency to tack on a chapter about exercise at the back of the book as a kind of addendum to all the good nutritional stuff. This gives the mistaken impression that exercise, though important, is of secondary consideration—something to take up after dietary changes are made. On the contrary, exercise is the starting point for all dietary change. Exercise helps to bring about such change more easily and effectively because it influences eating habits in three ways: 1) it reduces "fat tooth" cravings; 2) it dissipates stress; and 3) it emphasizes the positive.

EXERCISE REDUCES "FAT TOOTH" CRAVINGS

Studies show that regular exercise may be instrumental in controlling dietary fat intake by offsetting "fat tooth" cravings. Scientists believe that endorphins, chemicals produced by the brain in response to exercise, could be the key. Acting as natural painkillers, endorphins generate a happy, self-satisfied attitude and are associated with feelings of increased self-esteem and control. People who exercise regularly tend to have a higher level of endorphins than those who exercise little or are sedentary, and this higher level is thought to affect "fat tooth" brain chemistry. The brain may actually be influenced by endorphins to inhibit or neutralize chemicals that promote fat intake, thereby reducing the desire for fatty foods. If this is the case, while brain chemistry may influence food preferences, exercise influences brain chemistry.

The effect of exercise on dietary fat intake has been shown in numerous studies. In a University of Pennsylvania study, laboratory rats that naturally chose a diet in which 35% to 40% of calories came from fat were forced to lose and regain weight. It was found that cyclical dieting (which may have an independent impact upon brain chemistry) was instrumental in moving these animals to select a diet with 50% to 60% of calories from fat. When the rats were exercised, however, their desire for fat decreased significantly to a diet with about 30% of calories from fat. Not only was their food selection lower in fat than after cyclical dieting, it was lower in fat than their natural inclination. It is still too soon to draw conclusions for human behavior, but such studies do indicate that exercise may play a critical role in reducing the craving for dietary fat.

EXERCISE DISSIPATES STRESS

In an environment where people are hurried and harried, anxious about what is to come and depressed over what already has come, nutrition is reduced to a low-priority item. The simple fact is that people under pressure feel a loss of control and often make poor lifestyle decisions, such as overeating, bingeing, or living on a diet of fast food, frozen meals and snacks.

Exercise, nature's own tranquilizer, may be the most effective method of dissipating stress and counteracting the influence of a "hurry-up" modern lifestyle. A University of Southern California study found that a 15-minute walk had a strong tranquilizing effect in reducing tension. Studies at Duke and Stanford universities have shown that regular exercise can moderate the aggressiveness and impatience of Type A behavior. Endorphins again seem to play the key role. According to the National Center for Health Statistics, frequent exercisers have higher levels of endorphins and consequently demonstrate more positive moods and less anxiety than those who exercise little or not at all. Says psychologist Dr. Thomas Steven, "Anxiety, depression, anger and other stressful emotions are banished through physical activity."

One of the results of dissipating stress is better control over eating habits. A calm, relaxed, de-stressed person is less likely to "pig out" on brownies or ice cream. A study at Case Western University of the dietary habits of sedentary versus physically active people clearly shows that active people choose to eat more healthful foods and fewer foods high in dietary fat. A similar study involving runners in the San Francisco area produced the same conclusion: the runners' diet contained far less fat than that of the sedentary participants. As clinical psychologist Dr. Kenneth R. Pelletier states, "When people take time out to exercise regularly, they're demonstrating a psychological stance that in itself is going to have them reacting differently to their job, their family, and their food choices." Thus exercise becomes a dominating influence over "fat tooth" behavior.

Says Dr. Judith Stern of the University of California at Davis, "Studies on the impact of endorphins on food choices so far have been small, so we're not certain how it works. But we have seen that exercise-induced endorphins can help people who eat too much fat due to the environment. The relaxing, de-stressing impact of increased endorphins seems to give people better control over food choices."

EXERCISE EMPHASIZES THE POSITIVE

One of the problems in changing to a healthful diet is that it usually involves giving up certain (often favorite) foods. In this respect, change can be a negative experience, particularly in the first few weeks. After a week or two of feeling deprived and frustrated, we decide the change has not been successfully made and return to our old way of eating. Exercise, however, can help turn a negative situation into a positive experience by emphasizing what we *can do* rather than what we *can't have*. Says Dr. Scott Weigle of the University of Washington Medical School, "Exercise serves as a positive distraction by giving people something to focus on besides food. In addition, because an exercise program is easy to start and progress can be made quickly, exercise often produces a feeling of success that carries over to other aspects of life—including making more healthful food choices. In this way, success with exercise breeds success with dietary changes."

OTHER BENEFITS OF EXERCISE

In addition to offsetting "fat tooth" cravings and providing a positive framework for making dietary changes, regular exercise provides a variety of health benefits.

EXERCISE INCREASES LONGEVITY

An eight-year study of 13,344 subjects, conducted at the Institute for Aerobics Research in Dallas, showed that regular exercise is associated with increased longevity by potentially conferring significant protection from a wide range of diseases, including cardiovascular disease and cancer. Participants in the study were divided into groups based on fitness: the "least fit" group comprised sedentary people; "medium fit," people who exercised moderately; and "most fit," those who exercised vigorously, including running up to 40 miles a week. Deaths were found to be sharply higher in the "least fit" category than in the "medium fit" and "most fit" groups.

This study is especially significant in a number of

respects. First, it included men and women. This is a change from earlier studies, which focused almost exclusively on men. Second, it strengthened evidence that exercise is not only beneficial for cardiovascular health but can also ward off cancer. For example, while no one is certain of the mechanisms involved, it may be that exercise increases bowel motility, a factor in avoiding colon cancer. And finally, the study showed that even a minimal amount of exercise—a brisk half-hour walk once a day to produce "medium fitness"—provides significant protection. Says Dr. Carl Caspersen at the federal Centers for Disease Control in Atlanta, "You don't have to be a marathoner to greatly reduce your mortality. Research shows that people who exercise just a little bit still tend to live longer."

EXERCISE INCREASES HDL CHOLESTEROL

There is much evidence that physical activity is effective in reducing risk of cardiovascular disease. A major study conducted by Dr. Ralph Paffenbarger of the Stanford University Medical School traced the health histories of more than 17,000 alumni of Harvard University, dividing the subjects into three groups:

- Those who burned fewer than 500 calories in exercise every week;
- Those who burned between 500 and 2,000 calories; and
- Those who burned more than 2,000 calories.

Dr. Paffenbarger found that those who were active (i.e., those who burned more than 500 calories a week) reduced their risk of heart attack by 35% and lived about 30 months longer than their sedentary classmates. Interestingly, peak benefits came to those who burned 2,000 to 3,500 calories a week (it takes approximately 20 miles of brisk walking to burn 2,000 calories), while there was no appreciable increase in benefits for those who burned more than 3,500 calories. Regular, moderate exercise was therefore considered optimum.

The link between exercise and cardiac health is well established. Some experts attribute reduced coronary risk to a strengthening of the heart muscle. Others point to an improvement in blood flow, which in turn reduces clotting, lowers blood pressure and limits artery blockage. Certainly one of the most important aspects is the impact of exercise on cholesterol. Exercise may increase HDLs and at the same time reduce LDLs. Fortunately, you don't have to run great distances or do aerobic dance three hours a day to change the makeup of your cholesterol. The recommendations of Dr. Ken Cooper call for a moderate level of aerobic exercise—a 2-mile, 30-minute walk, for example—three times a week.

EXERCISE REDUCES BODY FAT

Medical experts agree that physical activity is fundamental in effective body-fat reduction. This is important to understand because excess body fat is at the root of the so-called overweight problem.

Excessive body fat cannot be dieted away. Simply reducing caloric intake by dieting doesn't produce lasting results. "The best reason not to diet is simple: Diets don't work. Experience and statistics show that the vast majority of people who lose weight on a diet will gain it back almost as quickly," says Dr. Evette Hackman. To be sure, low-fat eating habits are necessary, but they work best in concert with physical activity.

Exercise burns calories (in the form of body fat) for energy. In the chart that follows, the number of calories burned per minute is given for different types of exercise. Obviously, the more you weigh, the greater the number of calories burned.

Activity (average intensity)	Calories Burned per Minute at a Weight of:					
	120	140	160	180	200	220
Aerobic dance/exercise	5.7	6.6	7.5	8.5	9.4	10.3
Calisthenics, ice/roller skating, soccer, downhill skiing	4.7	5.5	6.3	7.1	7.8	8.6
Jump rope	9.4	10.9	12.5	14.0	15.6	17.1
Cross-country skiing, swimming	6.6	7.7	8.8	9.8	10.9	12.0
Handball, racquetball, squash, tennis (singles)	7.5	8.8	10.0	11.2	12.5	13.7
Walking (4 mph)	4.7	5.5	6.3	7.1	7.8	8.6
Jogging (11-minute mile)	8.4	9.8	11.2	12.6	14.0	15.4
Bicycling (13 mph)	9.1	10.5	11.9	13.3	14.7	16.1

Source: American College of Sports Medicine.

If burning calories directly were the only benefit, exercise would not be a very efficient way to reduce body fat. The fact is that because body fat is such a concentrated form of energy, it takes a long time to burn 3,500 calories—about one pound of body fat. A 150-pound person, for example, would have to walk more than 9 hours at an aerobic pace (4 mph) to do so. Fortunately, exercise does more than burn calories directly. It also raises the metabolic rate, or the rate at which calories are used for normal body functions such as breathing and digestion. Researchers have shown that the body continues to burn calories at a higher rate for a period of up to 12 hours after exercise. This may seem a small thing, but it can add up to a big difference. As stated by Dr. Jack Wilmore of the University of Texas, "If exercising regularly changes your metabolism even slightly, say 100 extra calories a day burned, that can add up to 10 pounds of weight lost in a year."

And finally, exercise creates muscle, and muscle is what burns fat. Says Georgia Kostas, R.D., of the Cooper Clinic, "The more muscle you have, the easier it is to burn fat. Fat is the fuel, but muscle is the engine."

AEROBIC EXERCISE IS BEST

While anything that increases overall daily activity level is beneficial, even gardening, using stairs at the office or parking at the far end of the lot, aerobic activities are best for calorie burning, cardiac fitness and sustained endorphin production. Aerobic exercise is simply exercise that makes the muscles work hard—but not so hard that the heart and lungs cannot keep up with the oxygen demand. Some of the best aerobic exercises include:

Brisk walking	Running in place
Cycling (indoor)	Cross-country skiing
Rowing (indoor)	Swimming
Skipping rope	Stair machine
Jogging	

There is also a group of activities that meet the aerobic criteria if performed at a continual vigorous pace for a period of time. These include:

Aerobic dance/Aerobicize	Soccer
Basketball	Tennis (singles)
Cycling (outdoor)	Hiking
Rowing (outdoor)	Skating (ice or roller)
Handball/squash/racquetball	

In order for an exercise to be aerobic, it must meet the F.I.T. criteria: frequency, intensity and time.

Frequency

According to the American College of Sports Medicine, exercise from three to five days a week, preferably on alternate days, for optimal fitness conditioning. People who want to lose excess body fat should exercise daily. However, anyone who exercises more than five days a week should be sure to use a non-jarring activity, such as walking or swimming, to minimize strain and other injuries.

Intensity

How hard you exercise is an important determinant of effectiveness. Exercise that is too light (casual walking, golf) or too heavy (sprinting) is not as effective as moderate exercise. Intensity is determined by exercise heart rate, the point where the pulse should be during exercise.

The pulse rate, of course, indicates how many heartbeats it takes to meet the blood circulation needs of the body. At rest, it might be 70 or so beats per minute; during a brisk jog, it might be twice that number. Aerobic exercise calls for the pulse rate to be elevated and maintained within certain parameters called the "target zone," a function of maximum heart rate (MHR)—the maximum number of heartbeats per minute the heart is designed to beat. MHR is determined by age, not by level of fitness. A 50-year-old fit person, for example, will always have a lower MHR than a sedentary 30-year-old. The formula for estimating maximum heart rate is as follows:

$$220$$
$$\underline{-\ Age}$$
$$=\ \text{Maximum heart rate}$$

So, in the case of a 50-year-old, MHR is approximately 170 beats per minute.

No one should exercise at maximum heart rate. The pulse should fall within the "target zone," which is defined as between 70% and 85% of MHR. The 50-year-old in the above example has a "target zone" between 119 (70%) and 145 (85%) beats per minute. There is some evidence that cardiovascular conditioning and fat-burning are most effective at the lower end of the "target zone." Says Dr. Victor F. Froelicher of the Long Beach Veterans Administration

Medical Center, "Less intense activities such as walking or low-impact aerobics are very effective." Use the following guide to establish your own target zone.

GUIDE TO TARGET EXERCISE RATE

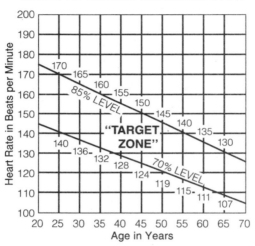

Source: American College of Sports Medicine.

To determine if you are within the zone, learn to count your pulse immediately upon stopping your exercise. With the first three fingers, find your pulse on the wrist, neck or chest and count for six seconds. Be sure to count the first beat as zero. Then multiply by 10 to calculate your rate per minute. If your pulse rate is below the zone, you need to increase effort; if it is above, you need to decrease effort.

Time

It is necessary to keep your pulse in the "target zone" for a minimum of 20 continuous minutes in order to promote cardiovascular fitness. This is the minimum amount of time you should spend on nonstop exercising. An ideal duration would be between 30 minutes and one hour. Remember, warm-up and cool-down activities such as stretching are not part of the 20-minute minimum since they do not take place within the "target zone."

A LAST WORD

The benefits of regular exercise are numerous in terms of longevity, reduced cardiac risk, and reduced body fat. It may be, however, that no benefit is more important than the positive influence of exercise on the food selection process. Simply put, people who exercise regularly choose to eat less dietary fat.

Make exercise the first step in your reducing dietary fat intake. But before you take any action, remember to:

- Get an okay from your doctor, particularly if you are severely overweight, are over 35 years old, have a family history of heart disease or one or more coronary risk factors (high blood pressure, smoking, elevated cholesterol, or haven't had a checkup recently).
- Select an activity that you find enjoyable. If you hate jogging, don't do it. Try brisk walking or aerobic dance. Keep looking until you find an activity that suits you.
- Exercise with other people. Walking daily with a friend can provide a sense of commitment that may not be there when you exercise alone.
- Learn how to take an exercise pulse and determine your "target zone." Listen to your body: if it hurts, stop the activity. Never "go for the burn."
- Wear the right footwear and clothing. They will affect your comfort and performance.
- Take time to warm up and cool down. Gentle stretching before and after exercise reduces muscle soreness and injury. Always start your exercise routine slowly, gradually moving into your "target zone," and end with a gentle slowing down.
- Build your fitness gradually. Don't try to undo years of sedentary habits in the first week of exercise.

- Keep an exercise diary. It will help you schedule exercise in advance and will provide you with great satisfaction as the miles and minutes accumulate.
- Most important, have fun. Make exercise a positive part of your daily activities. See it as an area of your life where you are in control.

CHAPTER 9

CONSTRUCT A PERSONAL FAT BUDGET

The second basic principle addresses the question: How much fat should you eat? According to the Surgeon General, the American Heart Association, the National Cancer Society and the National Institutes of Health, among others, the guidelines are quite clear:

- No more than 30% of total daily calories should come from fat.
- No more than 10% of total daily calories should come from saturated fat.

But what do these percentages mean?

"Often percentage of calories from fat is difficult to figure when balancing food choices for low-fat eating," says Dr. Hackman. "A better way is to use grams of fat as a measurement. So, if you want to know whether or not a particular food meets the 30% guideline, an easy rule of thumb is: no more than 3 grams of fat per 100 calories."

Estimating your maximum daily fat intake in grams creates a personal fat budget, based on scientifically sound information, that will tell you what you can "spend" on dietary fat each day and help you to make smarter food choices.

CALCULATE YOUR DAILY ALLOTMENT

The amount of fat allowed in your diet depends on how many calories you should eat, which in turn is a function of ideal body weight. Your fat budget can be calculated in three simple steps.

Step 1: Determine Your Ideal Weight

Ideal body weight is the most desirable weight for optimal health. However, as discussed in Chapter 6, a more accurate estimate for ideal weight is based on body-fat percentage, that is, how much of your weight is stored fat. Healthy body-fat percentages in males range from 15% to 20%, and in females from 19% to 24%, depending on age. The following chart presents an estimated ideal weight that corresponds to a healthy body-fat percentage.

Men		Women
Ideal Weight	Height	Ideal Weight
	4'11"	95
	5'0"	100
	5'1"	105
118	5'2"	110
124	5'3"	115
130	5'4"	120
136	5'5"	125
142	5'6"	130
148	5'7"	135
154	5'8"	140
160	5'9"	145
166	5'10"	150
172	5'11"	155
178	6'0"	160
184	6'1"	
190	6'2"	
196	6'3"	
202	6'4"	

Your ideal weight: _____

It should be noted that some experts believe these weights are best suited to younger people. Says Dr. George Bray, "An ideal weight of 125 pounds for a five-foot-five woman may be achievable for an 18-year-old, but it is difficult to achieve for an older woman. However, used as a scientific basis for creating a personal fat budget, these ideal weights have universal application."

Step 2: Determine Caloric Intake Needed to Sustain Ideal Weight

Once you've estimated your ideal weight, the next step is to determine how many calories you need daily to support that weight. Remember, calories are the fuel that runs your body. Eat too many, and the excess is stored as body fat. Too few, and your body may not have sufficient fuel to operate efficiently; it may even end up consuming muscle tissue for fuel. Either way, too many calories, or too few, will have a negative effect on your ideal weight.

According to the Food and Nutrition Board of the National Academy of Sciences–National Research Council, the amount of calories required to meet the energy needs of average healthy adults (15 to 75 years of age) range from 2,000 to 3,900 for males and from 1,200 to 3,000 for females. Precise requirements may vary, depending on basal metabolic rate, height, weight, frame size, body-fat percentage and, most important, level of activity. The more physically active you are, the more calories you need for fuel (another good reason to make exercise the first basic principle). The following formula suggests that active people could need more calories than the range recommended by the Food and Nutrition Board to sustain ideal weight. An "active" 100-pound woman who goes to an aerobics class four times a week, for example, needs about 15 calories per pound, or 1,500 calories a day, to sustain her weight. An "inactive" woman the same size would need 11 calories per pound, or 1,100 calories a day.

Level of Activity	Calories Needed per Pound per Day
Extremely inactive, or sedentary (*Example:* No aerobic exercise in the course of a week)	11
Moderately active, or light activity (*Example:* Aerobic exercise 2–3 times a week)	13
Active, moderate exercise and/or work (*Example:* Aerobic exercise 4–5 times a week)	15
Extremely active, heavy exercise and/or work (*Example:* Aerobic exercise 6–7 times a week)	18

Your level of activity: _____

By combining the ideal weight formula with the above guidelines, it is possible to estimate by sex the calories needed to sustain ideal weight.

CALORIES NEEDED DAILY BY MEN TO SUSTAIN WEIGHT

Height	Ideal Weight	Extremely Inactive	Moderately Active	Active	Extremely Active
5'2"	118	1,298	1,534	1,770	2,124
5'3"	124	1,364	1,612	1,860	2,232
5'4"	130	1,430	1,690	1,950	2,340
5'5"	136	1,496	1,768	2,040	2,448
5'6"	142	1,562	1,846	2,130	2,556
5'7"	148	1,628	1,924	2,220	2,664
5'8"	154	1,694	2,002	2,310	2,772
5'9"	160	1,760	2,080	2,400	2,880
5'10"	166	1,826	2,158	2,490	2,988
5'11"	172	1,892	2,236	2,580	3,096
6'0"	178	1,958	2,314	2,670	3,204
6'1"	184	2,024	2,392	2,760	3,312
6'2"	190	2,090	2,470	2,850	3,420
6'3"	196	2,156	2,548	2,940	3,528
6'4"	202	2,222	2,626	3,030	3,636

CALORIES NEEDED DAILY BY WOMEN
TO SUSTAIN WEIGHT

Height	Ideal Weight	Extremely Inactive	Moderately Active	Active	Extremely Active
4'11"	95	1,045	1,235	1,425	1,710
5'0"	100	1,100	1,300	1,500	1,800
5'1"	105	1,155	1,365	1,575	1,890
5'2"	110	1,210	1,430	1,650	1,980
5'3"	115	1,265	1,495	1,725	2,070
5'4"	120	1,320	1,560	1,800	2,160
5'5"	125	1,375	1,625	1,875	2,250
5'6"	130	1,430	1,690	1,950	2,340
5'7"	135	1,485	1,755	2,025	2,430
5'8"	140	1,540	1,820	2,100	2,520
5'9"	145	1,595	1,885	2,175	2,610
5'10"	150	1,650	1,950	2,250	2,700
5'11"	155	1,705	2,015	2,325	2,790
6'0"	160	1,760	2,080	2,400	2,880

Find your ideal weight on either of the above charts. Then, estimating your activity level, find the number of calories you need daily to sustain your ideal weight.

Total calories needed per pound per day: _____

You may be surprised by the number of calories you need each day, particularly if you're an active person. Remember, if the calorie intake falls too low (generally under 1,200 calories per day for males and under 900 calories per day for females), a drop in metabolism can occur and this could make weight loss very difficult to achieve. On the other hand, if you want to be at your ideal weight, you must eat for that weight.

"What it boils down to," says Dr. William Rumper of the USDA's Human Nutrition Research Center, "is that if you start out at 200 pounds and want to weigh 160, you have to eat like a 160-pound person."

Step 3: Figure Your Fat Allotment

Now that you've determined the total number of calories you need each day to sustain your ideal weight, you can calculate how many of those calories should come from fat. This calculation, in effect, will establish your budget.

The guideline here is that no more than 30% of total daily calories should come from fat. Start by multiplying your daily caloric need by 30% to find the maximum number of fat-calories per day in your budget. (Multiply daily calories by 10% for saturated fat.) For example, a man who is five-foot-nine might have an ideal weight of 160 pounds. Let's say he's "moderately active," which means he needs about 2,080 calories daily to sustain that weight. At a 30% diet, no more than 624 of his total calories should come from fat $(2.080 \times .30 = 624)$. And no more than 208 calories should come from saturated fat $(2,080 \times .10 = 208)$.

Your daily fat-calorie budget: _____

Next, translate fat-calories into grams of fat. Remember, one gram of fat contains nine calories. So, all you have to do is divide the number of fat-calories in your budget by 9 to convert them into grams. The man in the above example has a total fat budget of 624 calories. This equates to 69 grams of fat $(624 \div 9 = 69)$. The same calculation is used to determine grams of saturated fat. In the example given above, the man's saturated fat budget should be about 23 grams $(208 \div 9 = 23)$.

Your daily fat-grams budget: _____

Check the chart on the following page to estimate your fat-calorie budget based on the guideline of no more than 30% of calories from fat and no more than 10% of calories from saturated fat.

Total Calories per Day	Total Fat Calories per Day	Total Grams of Fat per Day	Total Saturated Fat Calories per Day	Total Grams of Saturated Fat per Day
1,000	300	33	100	11
1,200	360	40	120	13
1,400	420	46	140	15
1,600	480	53	160	18
1,800	540	60	180	20
2,000	600	66	200	22
2,200	660	73	220	24
2,400	720	80	240	26
2,600	780	86	260	29
2,800	840	93	280	31
3,000	900	100	300	33
3,200	960	106	320	35
3,400	1,020	113	340	38
3,600	1,080	120	360	40
3,800	1,140	126	380	42

The fat allotment establishes a dietary criterion specifically for you. This is important because it gives you a guideline against which to measure your food choices. But remember, it's just that—a guideline. I disagree with the dietary experts who recommend a rigid fat allotment. If you're too busy weighing and calculating, if you turn your kitchen into a chemistry lab, you'll never be able to enjoy your food. And when that happens, boredom and feelings of deprivation surface and healthy eating goes out the window.

Suppose your daily budget calls for 2,200 total calories and 73 grams of fat, with no more than 24 grams from saturated fat, and you've stopped at a Burger King for lunch. Your first choice is a Double Beef Whopper with Cheese, French fries and a chocolate shake. What does this do to your fat and calorie budget?

	Calories	Total Fat		Saturated Fat	
		Calories	Grams	Calories	Grams
Double Beef Whopper with Cheese	970	576	64	243	27
French Fries, regular	227	117	13	63	7
Chocolate Shake (10 fl. oz.)	374	99	11	63	7
Grand total	1,571	792	88	369	41

This fast-food lunch takes up 71% of your allotted calories, which is bad enough. But from the standpoint of fat intake, it's a disaster, providing 120% of your total fat allotment and 170% of your saturated fat allotment *for the entire day*. That's not to say there is never a time for a Double Whopper with Cheese. But a better choice, if you must have fast food, would be Wendy's Hamburger on a Multi-Grain Bun, Baked Potato with one pat of margarine, and Orange Juice, for a total of 584 calories (24% of your budget), 22.5 grams of fat (30% of your budget) and 5.5 grams of saturated fat (23% of your budget).

To see how fat budgeting can help you make smarter food choices, consider the following guide.

0 Grams

Corn flakes (1 oz.)	Broccoli (½ cup)	Green peas (½ cup)
Cream of wheat, cooked (½ cup)	Cabbage (½ cup)	Green pepper (½)
	Cantaloupe (¼)	Greens (½ cup)
Macaroni, plain or vegetable (½ cup)	Carrot (1)	Lettuce (½ cup)
	Cauliflower (½ cup)	Orange (1 medium)
Rice, white (½ cup)	Celery (1 stalk)	Orange juice (½ cup)
Rice, wild (½ cup)	Corn, frozen, cooked (½ cup)	Peaches (½ cup)
Sugar-frosted flakes (1 oz.)		Pears (½ cup)
	Fruit cocktail (½ cup)	Pineapple (½ cup)
	Grapefruit (½ medium)	Potato, baked (1 large)
Apple (1 medium)	Grapes (½ cup)	Prunes, dried, cooked
Applesauce (½ cup)	Green beans (½ cup)	(½ cup)

0 Grams

Prunes, dried,
  uncooked (¼ cup)
Raisins (¼ cup)
Snow peas (½ cup)
Spinach (½ cup)
Strawberries (½ cup)
Sweet potato, baked
  (½ medium)
Tomato juice (½ cup)
Tomato, fresh (1)
Tossed salad,
  without dressing
  (½ cup)
Watermelon (½ cup)
Zucchini (½ cup)

Black-eyed peas,
  dried, cooked
  (½ cup)

Egg, hard-cooked,
  white only (1 egg)
Pinto beans, dried,
  cooked (½ cup)

Milk, non-fat dry
  (1 cup)
Milk, skim (1 cup)
Yogurt, plain,
  non-fat
  (1 cup)

Angel food cake
  (¹/₁₂ cake)
Barbecue sauce
  (1 tbs.)
Beer (12 fl. oz.)
Catsup (1 tbs.)
Coffee (1 cup)

Gelatin, flavored
  (½ cup)
Honey (1 tsp.)
Iced tea (12 fl. oz.)
Jelly (1 tsp.)
Maple syrup (1 tbs.)
Pickle (1)
Popcorn,
  air-popped,
  unbuttered (1 cup)
Soft drink, cola,
  low-calorie
  (12 fl. oz.)
Soft drink, cola,
  regular (12 fl. oz.)
Sugar (1 tsp.)
Tea (1 cup)
Wine (3.5 fl. oz.)

1 Gram

Bagel, plain (½ bagel)
Bran flakes (1 oz.)
Bread, cracked wheat
  or whole wheat
  (1 slice)
Bread, pita (½)
Bread, pumpernickel
  or rye (1 slice)
Bread, white (1 slice)
Crackers, graham (2)
Crackers, rye (2)
Crackers, saltines (4)
Egg noodles, cooked
  (½ cup)
Hamburger bun (½)
Hard roll (½)
Hot dog bun (½)
Muffin, English,
  plain, toasted (½)
Oatmeal, instant,
  cooked (½ cup)

Raisin bran (1 oz.)
Rice, brown (½ cup)
Tortilla, corn (6″)

Banana (1 medium)
Corn on cob, fresh,
  cooked (1 ear)
Corn, canned, cream
  style (½ cup)
Pear (1 medium)
Winter squash, fresh,
  baked (½ cup)

Baked beans
  (½ cup)
Black-eyed peas,
  canned (½ cup)
Flounder/sole, baked
  (3 oz.)
Navy beans
  (½ cup)

Refried beans, canned
  (½ cup)
Shrimp, boiled
  (3 oz.)
Soup, chicken noodle,
  dehydrated (1 cup)

Cheese, cottage,
  1% low-fat (½ cup)
Yogurt, frozen, plain
  (½ cup)

French dressing,
  low-calorie
  (1 tbs.)
Gravy, beef, canned
  (¼ cup)
Mustard (1 tbs.)
Pretzels (1 oz.)

3 Grams

Biscuit, from mix or
refrigerated dough
(1)
Crackers, whole
wheat (2)
Dinner roll (1)
Pancake, plain or
buckwheat (4″)
Tortilla, flour (8″)
Waffle, frozen (4″)

Coleslaw (½ cup)
Sweet potato, candied
(½ medium)
Chicken, roasted,
without skin (3 oz.)

Halibut, baked (3 oz.)
Tuna, canned in
water (3 oz.)

Soup, chicken noodle,
canned (1 cup)
Soup, clam chowder,
with water (1 cup)
Soup, cream of
tomato, with water
(1 cup)

Buttermilk (1 cup)
Cheese, cottage,
2% low-fat,
(½ cup)

Cheese, Parmesan,
grated (1 tbs.)
Ice milk, (½ cup)
Milk, 1% (1 cup)
Yogurt, fruit-flavored,
low-fat (1 cup)

Coffee whitener,
non-dairy, liquid
(1 tbs.)
Half-and-half (1 tbs.)
Popcorn, oil-popped,
unbuttered
(1 cup)
Sour cream (1 tbs.)

5 Grams

Potatoes, French-
fried, oven-heated
(10 strips)
Potatoes, mashed
(½ cup)
Crackers, snack (4)
Croissant, plain (½)
Granola (1 oz.)
Muffin, blueberry
(1 small)
Muffin, bran (1 small)
Muffin, corn (1 small)

Bologna, turkey (1 oz.)
Burrito, bean (1)
Canadian bacon
(2 slices)
Chicken, fried,
flour-coated (3 oz.)
Chicken, roasted,
with skin (3 oz.)
Egg, fried (1)
Egg, hard-cooked (1)
Egg, scrambled (1)

Ham, 5% fat (3 oz.)
Pizza, cheese
(¼ of 12″)
Pork roast (3 oz.)
Roast beef, lean (3 oz.)
Salmon, canned, fish
and bones (3 oz.)
Soup, clam chowder,
with whole milk
(1 cup)
Soup, cream of
tomato, with whole
milk (1 cup)
Tofu (½ cup)
Tuna, canned in oil
(3 oz.)
Turkey (3 oz.)

Cheese, cottage,
creamed (½ cup)
Cheese, mozzarella
(1 oz.)
Cheese, mozzarella,
part skim (1 oz.)

Ice cream, hardened,
10% fat (½ cup)
Milk, 2% (1 cup)
Milk, chocolate, 2%
(1 cup)
Pudding, cooked or
instant (½ cup)
Yogurt, plain, low-fat
(1 cup)

Brownie, with nuts,
frosting (1 small)
Butter (1 tsp.)
Chocolate-chip
cookies (2 small)
French dressing,
regular (1 tbs.)
Granola bar, plain
(1 oz.)
Italian dressing
(1 tbs.)
Margarine (1 tsp.)
Popcorn, oil-popped,
buttered (1 cup)

10 Grams

Potatoes, French-
fried (10 strips)
Potatoes, hashed
brown (½ cup)
Waffle, homemade
(7″)

Bacon (3 slices)
Beef and vegetable
stew (1 cup)
Bologna, beef (1 oz.)
Burrito, bean and
meat (1)
Burrito, beef (1)
Chicken, fried,
batter-dipped (3 oz.)
Chili (1 cup)
Chow mein, chicken
(1 cup)
Fish sticks,
oven-heated (3 oz.)
Ham, 11% fat (3 oz.)
Hot dog, chicken (2 oz.)
Macaroni and cheese,
frozen, cooked
(1 cup)
McDonald's Egg
McMuffin (1)
Pizza, cheese and
pepperoni
(¼ of 12″)

Pizza, cheese, meat
and vegetables (¼
of 12″)
Salmon, baked (3 oz.)
Sausage, link (2)
Sausage, patty (1)
Shrimp, breaded and
fried (3 oz.)
Spaghetti with meat
balls, canned or
homemade (1 cup)
Steak, ribeye or
sirloin, broiled (3 oz.)
Steak, T-bone, broiled
(3 oz.)
Submarine sandwich,
with cold cuts and
cheese (3–4″ sub)
Taco Bell's bean
burrito or taco (1)
Tuna salad (½ cup)
Turkey sandwich, on
whole wheat (1)
Wendy's chili (9 oz.)

Cheese, American (1 oz.)
Cheese, brick (1 oz.)
Cheese, Cheddar (1 oz.)
Cheese, Monterey (1 oz.)
Cheese, Muenster
(1 oz.)

Cheese, Parmesan,
grated (1 oz.)
Cheese, Swiss (1 oz.)
Ice cream, premium,
hardened, 16% fat
(½ cup)
Ice cream, soft serve
(½ cup)
Milk, chocolate,
whole (1 cup)
Milk, whole (1 cup)
Milk shake (10 fl. oz.)

Chocolate cake
(1/16 cake)
Chocolate candy bar,
plain (1 oz.)
Chocolate candy bar,
with almonds (1 oz.)
Corn chips (1 oz.)
Cream cheese (1 oz.)
Doughnut, cake-type,
plain (1)
Mayonnaise (1 tbs.)
Oil and vinegar
dressing, home-
made (1 tbs.)
Pie, chocolate cream
(⅛ 9″ pie)
Potato chips (1 oz.)
Tortilla chips (1 oz.)

15 Grams

Avocado, sliced
(½ medium)

Arby's roast beef
sandwich (1)
Chef's salad, without
dressing (1½ cups)
Chop suey, beef and
pork (1 cup)

Ground sirloin/round,
broiled (3 oz.)
Hot dog, beef (2 oz.)
Kentucky Fried
Chicken's Original
Recipe Chicken
(3 oz.)
Lasagne, without
meat (2.5″ x 2.5″)

McDonald's Chicken
McNuggets
(6 pcs.)
Peanut butter (2 tbs.)
Peanut butter and
jelly sandwich, on
white bread (1)
Pork chop, broiled
(3 oz.)

15 Grams

Roast beef, fat (3 oz.)	Doughnut, yeast, glazed (1)	Sweet roll, cinnamon (1)
Roast beef sandwich, on bun (1)	Pie, apple (⅛ 9″ pie)	Sweet roll, fruit (1)
Wendy's single hamburger, plain (1)	Sunflower seeds, dry-roast (¼ cup)	

20 Grams

Avocado, puréed (½ cup)	Enchilada, cheese (1)	Macaroni and cheese, homemade (1 cup)
Bratwurst (3 oz.)	Enchilada, cheese and beef (1)	Quiche, without bacon (⅛ pie)
Burger King's Croissan'wich (1)	Ground beef, broiled (3 oz.)	Taco (1 small)
Cheeseburger, regular (1)	Italian sausage (3 oz.)	
Chicken stir-fry, with rice (1½ cups)	Kentucky Fried Chicken's Extra Crispy Chicken (3 oz.)	Cheesecake (¹/₁₂ cake)
Dairy Queen's chili dog (1)	Lasagne, with meat (2.5″ x 2.5″)	Peanuts, dry- or oil-roast (¼ cup)
		Sunflower seeds, oil-roast (¼ cup)

25 Grams

Burger King's Whaler (1)	Chicken salad (½ cup)	Spareribs (3 oz.)
Chicken pot pie, frozen, baked (1)	Fish sandwich (1)	Wendy's broccoli-and-cheese potato (1)
Chicken pot pie, homemade (¼ of 9″)	McDonald's Filet-O-Fish (1)	
	Polish sausage (3 oz.)	Pie, pecan (⅛ 9″ pie)
	Quiche, with bacon (⅛ pie)	

30 Grams

Fish sandwich, with cheese (1)	McDonald's biscuit with sausage (1)	Pizza Hut's supreme personal pan pizza (1)
McDonald's Big Mac (1)		

35 Grams

Arby's Roast Chicken Club (1)	Cheeseburger, large (1)	Wendy's Big Classic (1)
Burger King's Whopper (1)		

Source: National Dairy Council

The double influence of "fat tooth" cravings and a pro-fat environment on food selection will not be overcome by a casual approach. "I'll just stop eating ice cream at bedtime, and everything else will fall into place" is a great theory. Unfortunately, changing dietary habits isn't that simple. Reducing dietary fat comes about when scientifically sound information is applied in a realistic way. Your personal fat budget, based on ideal weight, is a tool for keeping track of your fat intake in the real world and for making smarter food choices. Budgeting doesn't call for "good" or "bad" foods. Indeed, all foods are acceptable and can be included, which provides you with maximum flexibility. It is your budget; you can spend it as you desire—as long as you stay within its limits. Saving or budgeting grams of fat for favorite foods or special occasions is perfectly acceptable. But by using your fat budget as a criterion against which to measure food choices, you have a better opportunity to lower fat intake while still including foods you enjoy.

Now let's recap your personal fat budget:

Your ideal weight _____

Daily calories needed to sustain that weight
    (based on activity level) _____

Daily total calories from fat
    (total calories × .30) _____

Daily total grams of fat
    (fat-calories ÷ 9) _____

GOING ON A BUDGET

Changing dietary habits starts with a conscious decision—in this case, to budget your intake of dietary fat. But simply making this decision does not guarantee success. Millions of people resolve to eat less fat, set out strongly to do so, yet end up failing. Changes usually work well at the start. Oatmeal replaces pop tarts, apples take the place of candy bars, and so on. But within a week or so, efforts typically become sporadic and begin to wane, and soon there is a return to the old, high-fat eating pattern. A tough lesson has been learned: it's one thing to alter food choices for a week, and quite another to change habits for a lifetime.

HABITS, NOT DIETS

Sandra Bergeson, in her *I Hate to Diet Dictionary*, defines "diet" as "the all-consuming obsession with the food you shouldn't have eaten yesterday, but did; the food you have eaten today, but shouldn't have; and the food you shouldn't eat tomorrow, but probably will."

This illustrates a major problem. We are often so obsessed about what we are eating immediately on our "diet" that we fail to recognize reality. In the world of advertising fantasies, you can change the way you eat for a week or two and be thin for a lifetime. In the real world, this concept is a sham. Diets don't work. They offer a quick fix with temporary results. Invariably, they fail because they do not address fundamental habits.

It must be understood that high-fat eating habits cannot be changed with a one-week diet that bans all cakes and cookies. At the end of the week, nothing will really have been accomplished. You'll still crave fat and live in a pro-fat environment. And now, off the diet, cakes and cookies will be available to you, and a binge could result. The roller-coaster ride of being "on," then "off" a diet is completely ineffective. Controlling fat intake results instead from a change in eating style, based on informed food choices, that you can practice over your lifetime.

Too often, people attempt to change everything at once, become discouraged, and end up accomplishing nothing. A more effective way is to institute small changes over a period of time. One successful change each week equals 52 successes per year. For example, if you're a person who eats fast food often, snacks on cookies and pies, and loves ice cream, it's unrealistic to expect that you'll immediately abstain from all of these high-fat foods. It might work for a week or so, but then the "fat tooth" craving kicks in and total reversal takes place. The result: initial success, long-term failure.

It makes more sense to focus on one area only, establish a firm foundation of change, and build on it gradually. In this case, it might be better to start by limiting fast food to twice a week and by making fast-food choices within your fat budget. While working on this problem, you should not feel pressured to make other dietary changes. Only when you've adjusted to the changes concerning fast food should you make changes with other foods. This perspective provides a sense of timing that removes the pressure for quick and total change. After all, individuals are different and will not make the same changes at the same time. And that's okay. Dietary change is not a competition or a race. Steady progress should be the name of the game.

FAT BUDGET TECHNIQUES

Using your personal fat budget to make smarter food choices is easier when you employ the following three important techniques.

Determine Where You Are Now

Now that you know how many grams of fat are in your daily budget, it's time to count up your fat. What are your food preferences right now? And how fat are they? If you could rely on memory, it would be easy to identify frequently eaten fatty foods. But we often forget (or choose to forget) what we eat. As one chronic dieter told me, "I count calories when I sit down to eat. But the food I eat when I'm walking through a mall or clearing the dinner dishes, those are standing calories—and standing calories don't count!"

The best way to monitor your present eating habits is to keep a record of your daily food intake. Health professionals usually recommend a three-day record. Simply write down everything you eat during that time. Have a gumdrop? Put it in the record! Be sure to include foods such as salad dressings, butter or margarine, and coffee creamer. Keeping a food record may seem like a hassle, but it's the only way to get a look at your real food habits.

It's important not to change anything during this time. Don't start a diet or "be good." Just eat as you normally do, and record everything eaten when it is eaten. By the end of three days, your food record will tell you what and when you eat. It may even give you some insight into *why* you eat. Most important, as shown in the sample food record on the facing page, it will reveal high-fat habits that need to be changed. No one food choice in the sample record would break the fat budget for the day. In combination, however, the choices add up to a high-fat disaster, and the record makes this easily understood.

Keep track of your fat intake on the food record and compare it with your budget. This is not so much to keep a running total as to identify favorite foods that are high in fat. Many food product labels provide fat content in grams. Be sure to take "serving size" into consideration. For foods with no nutritional labels, refer to a guide such as *The Complete Book of Food Counts* by Corinne Netzer.

Make Food Palatability a Priority

If experience regarding food behavior has taught us anything, it is this: people will eat healthy, low-fat food only when it tastes good. Most people will not trade taste for health. That's the reason some heart patients sneak a Big Mac; that's why many patrons of weight loss programs, fresh off an expensive week of dieting, will undo everything with a pint of Ben & Jerry's finest.

Lettuce and carrots may be healthier for us, but they won't offset the craving for a sirloin steak or a wedge of Brie. Better food selection comes about when we shed the concept that healthy food must be boring. Nothing is farther

SAMPLE FOOD RECORD

Day of Week: Tuesday

When	Where	With Whom	Food Eaten	Fat Budget: Calories	65 grams Grams of Fat
7:30 A.M.	Kitchen	Family	Orange juice (½ cup)	55	0
			Egg fried in margarine	83	6
			Bacon (3 strips)	109	9
			Wheat toast (2 slices)	140	
			w/ margarine (1 Tbs.)	100	11
			Coffee w/ Half & Half (2 Tbs.)	40	4
10:00 A.M.	Office	Co-worker	Jelly doughnut	226	9
			Coffee w/ Half & Half (2 Tbs.)	40	4
Noon	Burger King	Alone	Cheeseburger	317	15
			French fries (regular)	227	13
			Chocolate shake	320	12
6:30 P.M.	Kitchen	Family	Lamb chops (2)	510	42
			Baked potato	145	0
			w/ Sour cream (2 Tbs.)	50	6
			Green salad	15	0
			w/Blue cheese dressing (2 Tbs.)	154	16
			Glass of white wine	70	0
9:00 P.M.	Den	Kids	French Vanilla Ice Cream, Ben & Jerry's (½ cup)	267	17
			TOTAL	2868	166

from the truth. A low-fat dietary pattern can involve foods that are tasty, attractive and appealing. The trick is to make low-fat foods so satisfying that high-fat foods are not missed. Would you yearn for prime rib, for example, if you were served hickory-smoked salmon, Cajun turkey breast or seafood fettuccine? That is why we've included over 200 real-life recipes here (and over 650 in *Don't Eat Your Heart Out Cookbook* and *Choices for a Healthy Heart*).

One of the key concepts in fat budgeting is to understand that you can modify your favorite meals without sacrificing taste. Studies show that most American families prepare a dozen recipes 80% of the time. The greatest opportunity, then, is to modify these 12 recipes. In doing so, you get the best of both worlds—familiar, favorite foods that conform to your personal fat budget.

Learn to Read Food Labels

Fresh, whole foods are the best choices for controlling your personal fat budget. Because of the on-the-run nature of modern life, however, it's unrealistic to think you'll never eat packaged foods. Virtually everyone in the United States, even the most serious anti-fat activist, at some time eats food from a box or a can. Unfortunately, packaged foods lend themselves to hidden fat, so knowing their fat content is critical to making informed choices. For this reason, it is essential to know how to read food labels.

Under the present labeling law, nutrition information is required on packaged foods only when a claim is made about nutrition content or when the product is fortified with vitamins, minerals or protein. This covers about 30% of FDA-regulated foods. Another 30% display nutrition information anyway. But that leaves 40% with no nutritional data. Some even lack ingredients lists, so we have no clue as to what's in the food. This often means that we end up relying on advertising for information on fat.

Watch out for "low-fat" hype. Food advertising is generally more hype than truthful information. Nowhere is this problem worse than in the promotion of "low-fat" foods. Contrary to advertising claims, many such foods are actually rich in fat. Take ground beef labeled "20% fat," for example. It certainly appears to be low in fat, well below the 30% guideline. All well and good, except that "20%" refers to the weight of fat in the package; that is, fat constitutes 20% of total weight. But the body doesn't care what fat weighs. It is more concerned with how many calories fat produces. The truth is that almost 60% of calories in ground beef are derived from fat. So, instead of meeting the guideline, it contains about twice the amount of fat recommended.

Many food processors advertise fat content by percentage of weight as a clever way to deceive customers about the true fat content of the product. The information may be technically correct according to the letter of the labeling law, but it certainly violates the spirit. When weight is the measurement used, most foods will look deceptively low in fat. Even hot dogs and sausages can meet this test. Because about half the weight of a hot dog is water, the fat content is just about 30% by weight. But fat actually supplies over 80% of the calories! The same is true of a luncheon meat labeled "93% fat-free." What this means, of course, is that fat makes up 7% of the weight, but the percentage of calories from fat is much higher. This is one reason for using grams of fat in your personal fat budget.

Food Item	Calories	% of Calories from Fat	Grams of Fat
Butterball turkey bologna, 1-oz. slice, "80% fat free"	70	77%	6
Lean Supreme chopped ham, 1-oz. slice, "94% fat free"	35	51	2
Louis Rich turkey cotto salami, 1-oz. slice, "86% fat free"	52	64	3.75

Source: Individual food companies.

Terms such as "low-fat" and "lean" have little to do with reality. For example, 92% of calories in Kraft Philadelphia Brand Cream Cheese come from fat. It is recognized as a high-fat food. But Kraft Neufchatel Cream Cheese is promoted as a "low-fat" alternative, even though 79% of its calories come from fat. How can a food that is four-fifths fat be "low-fat"? It can't! It may be lower in fat than the original product, but it's not low in fat.

And what does the term "light" or "lite" mean? Apparently, a number of things. To Bertoli, producer of "extra light" olive oil, it means that this oil has a milder taste—but no fewer calories or less fat. To Sara Lee, the "light" in French Light Cheesecake means a lighter, creamier texture. Indeed, this "light" cheesecake actually contains more fat and calories than the Sara Lee Original Cream Cheesecake. There is even a "light" mineral water from Brazil. The importer claims it has a "light taste" because it contains fewer minerals than other bottled waters.

Foods advertised as containing "no cholesterol" can also pose a problem. Since most people perceive cholesterol as a risk for heart disease, it's natural to avoid cholesterol-rich foods. Some food manufacturers have used the concern about cholesterol to boost their sales. Canned vegetable shortenings, for example, may carry a "no cholesterol" label. This is accurate but misleading. Vegetable foods do not contain cholesterol, only animal foods do, so by its very nature vegetable shortening is cholesterol-free. But it's not fat-free! And in many instances the fat contained may be palm oil or coconut oil, both of which raise cholesterol. The "no cholesterol" designation does not ensure that the food has a low fat content or, for that matter, is a healthy choice.

Count grams of fat. The labeling law may undergo changes in the future to give more people access to needed nutritional information. But for now you have to work with labels as they are. Counting grams of fat is the easiest way to use food label information to support your fat-budgeting efforts. This is easily done by referring to the nutritional data on the food label. For example, the following data are found on a carton of whole milk:

Serving size:	1 cup
Servings per container:	4
Calories:	150
Protein:	8 grams
Carbohydrate:	11 grams
Fat:	8 grams
Sodium:	125 milligrams

The label provides two important pieces of information: number of calories per serving, and grams of fat. It shows that a one-cup serving contains 150 calories and 8 grams of fat.

The first step is to determine the number of grams of fat in a serving. Earlier in this chapter, you learned how to calculate your fat budget, the maximum number of grams of fat you should average in a day. This budget is a product of the calories needed to maintain your ideal weight. Let's suppose you need 2,000 calories a day. No more than 30% (or 600 calories) should come from fat. By dividing the allotted fat calories by 9, you'll have your fat budget expressed in grams—in this case, 67 grams per day. Once this is known, you can determine from the label whether or not the food will break your fat budget. A good rule of thumb is that there should be no more than 3 grams of fat per 100 calories.

Make comparisons of similar products to determine their respective impact on your fat budget. Labels on cheese, for example, show that a one-ounce serving of Cheddar has 9 grams of fat, while Parmesan has 7 grams and part-skim mozzarella has just 4 grams. Or let's assume you'd like a snack and you're eying two Hostess Suzy Q's. How much fat is involved? About 20 grams, or almost one-third of your 67-gram fat allotment for the day. A fresh peach, which contains .1 gram of fat, would be a better choice. Because of the difference in fat content, the Suzy Q's total 480 calories and the peach just 37. Or put it this way: you could have 13 peaches if you wanted to consume 480 calories. Even if you could eat all 13, they would provide you with less than 2 grams of fat.

It is not that Suzy Q's should be off-limits forever. In a realistic low-fat diet, no single food is forbidden. But if you have a fat budget of 67 grams, and you choose one food with 20 grams of fat, your choices for the rest of the day are very restricted. If you eat something high in fat, balance it out with low-fat foods at other meals to keep within your budget for the day. The trick is not to eat too many high-fat foods.

A second way to use label information is to calculate the percentage of calories from fat. If the label provides calories and grams of fat per serving, it's easy to estimate this percentage.

1. Determine calories and grams of fat per serving from the label. The whole-milk label on page 133 shows that a one-cup serving contains 150 calories and 8 grams of fat.

2. To find the number of calories supplied by fat, multiply the number of grams of fat by 9. That's because there are 9 calories in one gram of fat. This calculation ($9 \times 8 = 72$) tells you that one cup of milk contains 72 calories from fat.

3. To find the percentage of calories from fat, divide the outcome of step 2 by the total number of calories in the product. This calculation ($72 \div 150 = .48$) tells you that 48% of the calories come from fat.

Remember, the object is to develop a diet pattern that supplies no more than 30% of calories from fat. At first glance, it might seem that you could never drink whole milk, which is considerably more than 30% fat. It doesn't work that way. Foods greater than 30% fat can be included if balanced by sufficient low-fat foods to produce an overall diet pattern of less than 30% fat. The key is looking at how all the foods eaten in a day fit together.

Plan for Change

Your food record will reveal present food habits, and your budget will provide fat and calorie goals. Getting from one to the other means changing food habits. This often seems easy at first. Almost anyone can replace a Danish pastry with an apple—for a week! The challenge is how to make the change stick, to make it a permanent part of your daily life, so that low-fat eating becomes the norm rather than the exception.

It is difficult enough in our fast-paced modern society simply to prepare food, much less to prepare food that is low in fat and also tastes good. If it's five o'clock in the afternoon and you're at the store shopping for dinner to be served at six, you may be too pressed to think of low-fat alternatives. It's very easy then to choose old, familiar, high-fat favorites—hot dogs, frozen meals, fast food. Or, if you're headed out to lunch and have just 30 minutes to eat, that isn't the time to begin thinking about healthy choices. Chances are, you'll end up with a high-fat deli sandwich, coleslaw and potato chips. Breaking the high-fat habit is too difficult to accomplish if it's approached in an "as-you-go" fashion. Habits change when you make a plan to change them.

Planning is essential for the success of most endeavors. Few people, for example, create economic security in retirement without a financial plan. The plan may call for them to put money aside year after year. Then, when they reach a certain age, their "nest egg" is as ready for retirement as they are. It's the same in sports. No manager or coach would enter a contest without a game plan. Baseball pitchers study films of opposing teams so they can plan how to pitch to certain hitters; without planning, the strongest arm would be wasted.

The process of meal planning is really nothing more than preselecting foods that appeal to you and meet your calorie/ fat criterion. By planning, you ensure the exclusion of high-fat foods and the inclusion of low-fat foods, and minimize the selections left to chance. Experience shows that if you don't plan ahead to trade your Danish pastry for an apple, it won't happen. There is nothing magical about meal planning; it is simply a tool for success. Many prominent weight loss programs include meal planning as an integral part of their approach. They plan what you will eat, you follow the plan, and success is often the result. You have the same opportunity to do this for yourself.

Start by examining your food record. It will help you to identify areas that need to be changed. If it indicates you like ice cream as an evening snack, plan to have popcorn instead. You'll still have your snack, so you won't feel deprived, but it will contain less fat and fewer calories. Plan for reasonable changes: if they're too drastic, you might feel deprived and lose your resolve. If you usually eat a breakfast of bacon and eggs three or four times a week, don't eliminate it from your meal plan. Instead, reduce it to one day a week. Perhaps Saturday is designated as "bacon and eggs" morning. You can look forward all week to enjoying that special breakfast. Then concentrate on making better breakfast choices for the other six days of the week.

The meal-planning process is easier if you carry a list of foods and meals to choose from. If you're behind schedule when you're shopping for dinner, or have just a few minutes for a restaurant lunch, you can refer to the list for suggestions. This is how it works for me: I'm usually running late in the morning. The last thing I want to do is think about healthful food. To be sure, I do want my breakfast to be low in fat, appetizing and satisfying. (Don't overlook "satisfying," or you'll be hungry at midmorning and may resort to a doughnut for satisfaction). But I don't want to spend a lot of time and effort on the meal. So I have a list of quick and easy "no-think" breakfasts from which to choose:

- Hot oatmeal with fresh strawberries and sliced bananas
- Toasted English muffin with raspberry jam and one-half cantaloupe
- Whole-grain toast with blackberry jam and sliced peaches
- Cold cereal (nutri-grain, all-bran) with sliced bananas
- Non-fat yogurt with fresh blueberries

If I'm really hungry, I'll choose one of the heartier breakfasts on my list:

- Scrambled eggs (Egg Beaters) with tomato salsa, English muffin with strawberry jam, Granny Smith apple
- Smoked salmon with onion and tomato on toasted bagel, green grapes
- Sesame seed waffles with maple syrup, sliced oranges

I might not have a lot of time for making breakfast choices, but I know that my choices will be smart if I stay with my list. This same approach works for other meals, including restaurant meals.

Another approach used in our home involves planning for dinner, our main meal. Chances are, there will be little time during the day to plan a healthful one. In the likely scenario my wife and I arrive home from the office at 5:30 P.M. and have to prepare dinner for the family and serve it by 6:00 so we can be at a school conference at 7:30. There is no time for pondering healthful food decisions that also meet everyone's needs. We attempt to solve this problem with flexible planning that calls for certain types of foods on specific nights.

The following is an example of a general plan that covers our meals for one week:

Day	Type of Food
Monday	Soups, stews, pasta
Tuesday	Poultry
Wednesday	Main meal salads
Thursday	Seafood
Friday	Pizza, casseroles, chili
Saturday	Take-out, restaurants
Sunday	Meat

We can choose from a variety of recipes for each of the categories. On Tuesday, poultry night, we might have chicken tostados, hot-and-spicy Cajun turkey, or King Pao chicken. Each recipe is quickly and easily made, and conforms to our fat budget. We do not treat this as a hard-and-fast rule, but use it as a general guide to help us more easily make smarter food choices. The plan has to be elastic. If the day has totally gotten away, or if plans for the evening change, we might eat out or have a healthful frozen meal. The plan also recognizes that not everyone in the family has the same nutritional needs. My wife and I might be satisfied with pasta salad as a main meal, but not my football-playing son. Obviously, no one wants to cook a number of different meals (although statistics show that many American families cook hamburgers for the children and Lean Cuisine for adults), so we simply add a pan-fried chicken breast to the meal for him.

Meal planning should be realistic and flexible, and should reflect your family's tastes and needs. By considering these factors in a plan, you optimize the opportunity to prepare and serve foods that are easy, quick, appetizing and satisfying, yet allow you to stay safely within your fat and calorie budget.

A LAST WORD

Fat budgeting provides you with a simple, effective approach to managing dietary fat intake without deprivation or prohibition. It emphasizes freedom of choice, so no food is "good" or "bad." Instead, your fat budget provides a criterion against which to measure food choices. By doing so, it puts the control in your hands for balancing good food and good health.

Think in terms of balancing your checkbook. If your fat budget is 65 grams a day, for example, you start with that amount in your "account" each morning. As you make your food choices throughout the day, you "spend" your budget. Here is an example:

	Fat-Grams in Budget	
Food Choices	Grams Spent	Balance
Starting balance		65
Breakfast		
Oatmeal (⅓ cup)	0	65
Banana	0	65
Skim milk (½ cup)	.5	64.5
Whole-wheat toast (2 slices)	2	62.5
w/ margarine (1 pat)	4	58.5
Coffee w/ whole milk (2 Tbs.)	1	57.5
Midmorning snack		
Apple	0	57.5
Lunch		
Arby's Chicken Fajita Pita	7.5	50
Tossed salad	0	50
w/ lo-cal dressing (2 Tbs.)	2	48
Coke	0	48
Dinner		
Grilled salmon fillet	10.5	37.5
Rice pilaf	0	37.5
Snow peas	0	37.5
Tossed salad	0	37.5
w/ lo-cal dressing (2 Tbs.)	2	35.5
Coffee w/ whole milk (2 Tbs.)	1	34.5

Food Choices	Fat-Grams in Budget	
	Grams Spent	Balance
Evening snack		
Oreo cookies (3)	6	28.5
Skim milk (1 cup)	1	27.5
Total fat-grams spent	37.5	
Ending balance		27.5

In the above example, a balance of low-fat and good taste was achieved. This type of calculation won't be needed forever, but in the beginning it's a very helpful tool in actively managing your fat intake and still allowing for favorite foods.

Changing dietary habits, even with a fat budget, is not automatic. Budgeting techniques will help you to make meaningful dietary changes that stick and to make them as simply and easily as possible. These techniques can help you to manage your fat budget and, over time, create new habits. Remember this:

- Learn how to construct your personal fat budget:

  —Determine your ideal weight.
  —Determine how many calories you need to sustain that weight (based on physical activity).
  —Determine maximum calories from fat per day (total calories × 30%).
  —Determine maximum grams of fat per day (fat calories ÷ 9).

- Keep a food record for three days to determine your present food habits and fat intake. Compare it with your personal fat budget. Use it to identify problem areas.
- Read food labels. Use the information to keep your fat budget in the black.

- Use planning techniques such as lists of "no think" meals to help you make smart food choices easily and quickly.
- Think in terms of changing food habits rather than going on a diet.
- Start with a positive mind-set. Concentrate on what you can have and do, not on what you can't have or do.
- Remember, small but smarter changes will significantly cut calories and fat, and will over time permanently alter dietary habits.
- Focus on how you spend your fat budget. Don't get hung up on "good" and "bad" foods.
- Look for ways to alter your favorite recipes to balance health and palatability. Low-fat food does not have to be boring or unappealing; it can be well-prepared and flavorful.

CHAPTER 10

MAKE SMARTER CHOICES

If we lived in a utopia where life was free and easy, and people sat around debating the merits of legumes, fat-restrictive diets might be something more than just a theory. But life in the real world is hurried and stressful, and virtually everyone is short on time. With less time for making food decisions, many people elect to eat what is readily available, that is, what is quick, easy and convenient. And many of the foods that fall into this category are high in dietary fat. If the options for dinner are limited to fast-food fried chicken, a frozen dinner of breaded fish fillet in butter sauce, a deli take-out meal consisting of a pastrami sandwich with coleslaw, or a restaurant steak, there is little real opportunity to control fat intake.

The world we live in is not perfect, nutritionally or otherwise, but it's the only world we have. It is a fact that our environment promotes the consumption of dietary fat. There may be a lot of talk about healthy changes, but little, I think, will really be done in the next few years. Somehow I just do not see McDonald's announcing that Big Macs will no longer be served.

The real opportunity, then, is to learn how to operate

within this pro-fat environment to mitigate both "fat tooth" tendencies and environmental impact on the decision-making process. Fat budgeting and better information are the keys. The following sections examine how to use fat-budgeting with different food groups. The intent of this information is simple: to help you make smarter food choices in a world that fosters high-fat eating.

RED MEAT

Although its consumption has fallen slightly over the past 20 years, primarily as a response to cholesterol education, red meat continues to be a favorite food of Americans. And there's nothing wrong with that. If we make smart choices, red meat can be part of a healthy low-fat diet pattern.

There are, in fact, positive nutritional considerations about red meat. Three ounces of beef contains about 15% of the recommended dietary allowance for iron for women of childbearing years and about 25% of the RDA for men. Along with pork and lamb, beef is also an excellent source of the B vitamins. A three-ounce serving provides more than 40% of the RDA for vitamin B_{12}, a nutrient totally absent in plant food, as well as substantial amounts of B_1 (thiamin), B_2 (riboflavin), B_6 (niacin) and zinc. And it provides 40% of the RDA for protein for men, 50% of the RDA for women.

On the other hand, as a prime contributor to the high fat intake in the United States, red meat is a problem food. Essentially, Americans eat too much red meat (we average about 105 pounds of beef and pork per person yearly). In addition, the types of meat most frequently eaten are too high in fat. There is no way that current meat-eating habits square with the precepts of low-fat eating. Using your personal fat budget as a guideline, however, you can enjoy red meat and still control fat intake. You'll know very quickly whether or not your choice will break your budget.

Leaner Cuts

Fortunately, red meat is leaner than it was in the past. Ranchers are breeding leaner animals, feeding them more grass and less corn, and bringing them to market at a younger age. Also, meatpackers and retailers are trimming more external fat.

Selecting cuts is very important because butcher labels are not always helpful in identifying fat content. When information is provided at all, it generally speaks to the weight of fat but says nothing about the calories from fat. It's up to you to know which cuts of beef are the leanest. (Altogether, there are nine cuts, or parts of the animal that provide meat. "Beef loin" on the tag of a porterhouse steak, for instance, indicates that it came from the loin area of the steer.) As a rule, beef cuts labeled "loin" or "round" are the leanest choices. According to the Beef Council, the "Skinniest Six" cuts include:

Cut of Beef (3 oz.)	Total Calories	Grams of Fat	% of Calories from Fat
Top round, broiled	162	5.3	29%
Eye of round, roasted	155	5.5	32
Round tip, roasted	162	6.4	36
Sirloin, broiled	177	7.4	37
Top loin, broiled	172	7.6	40
Tenderloin, broiled	174	7.9	41

Source: USDA.

A three-ounce serving of these cuts would certainly not upset the personal fat budget for most people. For example, an active woman with an ideal weight of 120 pounds has a personal fat budget, based on 1,800 calories a day to sustain her weight, of 60 grams of fat per day. None of the above cuts would use up very much of her budget, nor would they upset her daily calorie goal. She could have sirloin steak for dinner (three ounces, not a slab) and still have more than 52 grams of fat to spend that day. And, even though sirloin steak exceeds the recommended daily goal of 30% fat, its impact on the percentage of fat from the meal can be reduced by accompanying it with low-fat foods.

On the other hand, choosing fatty cuts could be a budget-buster for this woman. Consider the following:

Cut of Beef (3 oz.)	Total Calories	Grams of Fat	% of Calories from Fat
Whole brisket, braised	300	22.5	68%
Prime rib, roasted	316	25.9	74
Short ribs, braised	400	35.7	80

Source: USDA.

If she dined on short-ribs, over half her fat budget would be consumed by this single choice. Staying within her budget would mean very restrictive food choices for the rest of the day. The choice of what to eat, of course, rests with each person. But by being conscious of the fat budget and by being knowledgable about leaner cuts, we can achieve the best of both worlds—red meat and a low-fat diet.

Because so many hamburgers are eaten in the United States, a point needs to be made: there is no such thing as a truly lean hamburger patty. Even extra-lean ground round has almost double the grams of fat as the same amount of the "Skinniest Six."

Food (3 oz., broiled)	Total Calories	Grams of Fat	% of Calories from Fat
Ground round, extra lean	217	13.9	57%
Ground round, lean	231	15.7	61
Hamburger	287	20.5	64

Source: USDA.

Grade also supplies some information about fat. In the traditional grading system, "Prime" contains the most fat, followed by "Choice" with moderate fat and "Select" with the least fat. The Select label indicates that the cut is almost 20% lower in calories and 33% lower in saturated fat than Prime. Be aware that to get the lowest amount of fat possible, you have to consider both cut and grade. Select beef from a fatty cut generally contains more fat than Choice beef from a leaner cut. Not all beef is graded, so you may have to "grade" it yourself on the basis of cut and appearance. Always check for marbeling, the fat that cannot be trimmed. The more uniform the appearance and the fewer flecks of white or yellow marbeling, the better. Lean beef has little marbeling.

And finally, trimming all visible fat from meat before cooking, a simple thing to do, produces a dramatic impact. A three-ounce T-bone steak that has been trimmed contains about 20 fewer grams of fat than the same size steak untrimmed. For many people, the trimmings alone constitute a great part of the fat budget.

As a rule, the leanest cuts for pork, lamb and veal are those labeled "loin" or "leg." Many cuts of pork, in particular, are leaner than in the past. However, contrary to industry advertising, pork is not a "white meat" and is not comparable to poultry in fat content. Some of the leanest cuts of pork, lamb and veal include:

Cut of Meat (3 oz.)	Total Calories	Grams of Fat	% of Calories from Fat
Canned ham, extra lean	102	3.9	34%
Pork tenderloin, broiled	141	4.1	26
Canadian bacon, grilled	156	7.2	42
Pork center loin, broiled	196	8.9	41
Fresh ham, whole, roasted	187	9.4	45
Lamb loin chop, broiled	159	6.3	36%
Lamb leg, roasted	175	8.1	42
Veal leg, pan-fried	120	7.6	57%
Veal cutlet, braised	183	9.0	44

Source: USDA.

As with beef, choosing leaner cuts of pork, lamb and veal—and eating them in moderation—will not upset most fat budgets. On the other hand, many high-fat choices will:

Cut of Meat (3 oz.)	Total Calories	Grams of Fat	% of Calories from Fat
Pork spareribs, braised	340	25.9	69%
Pork top loin, pan-fried	333	28.3	76
Lamb rib, roasted	306	24.9	73
Lamb blade, braised	294	21.0	64
Veal breast, braised	258	18.0	63
Veal rib, roasted	195	16.0	74

Source: USDA.

Cooking Methods

How you cook is as important as what you cook. The best cooking methods for red meat are those that allow fat to drip off, such as roasting, broiling, baking, grilling and stewing. Frying seals in fat. In general, the longer meat cooks, the more fat is lost, so medium and well done are preferable to rare. It's also a good idea to braise lean beef or use it in stews so that it doesn't end up too dry. Putting braised meat or stew in the refrigerator for a few hours overnight will help congeal the fat, which can then be removed before reheating. When using ground beef, sauté it in a nonstick pan and drain it on paper towels to de-fat the meat as much as possible. Be sure to pour off juices before adding other ingredients to browned meat. In general, less fatty cuts are also less tender. To enhance flavor and tenderness, marinate these cuts for a few hours before cooking.

Portion Control

There is no room in a low-fat diet for 12- or 16-ounce servings of red meat. Too large a portion even of a leaner choice, can produce excessive fat intake. But there's nothing wrong with eating three or four ounces of beef in which

35% or 40% of total calories are from fat. Since that amount of cooked lean beef often contains fewer than 200 calories, a small portion of the daily caloric intake, it's easy to offset the extra fat calories by eating other foods during the day that have fewer than 30% of their calories from fat.

One way to do this is to "stretch" the meat in chilis, casseroles and stir-fries. Don't just think "steaks, chops and burgers." In place of four steaks for four people, thinly slice one steak and cook it with crisp vegetables in a stir-fry. Or use one pound of extra-lean ground round to make a double batch of spaghetti sauce, then freeze what you do not use. Substitute grains and beans for part of the meat in many recipes. Using red meat as a condiment, instead of a main course, lets you enjoy its flavor without compromising your budget.

Don't overlook hearty soups. They're easy to prepare and well worth the effort. Beef stock, the basis for many soups, takes about two hours to cook. You can degrease the stock by chilling it in the refrigerator, then skimming off the fat that hardens on the surface. Add all types of tasty foods—beans, peas, pasta, rice, vegetables—to make a nutritious, flavorful, low-fat meal.

Watch Out For...

Cold cuts and sausages. The calories in these foods overwhelmingly come from fat, much of it saturated.

Over 60% Fat	Over 70% Fat	Over 80% Fat
Beer salami, pork	Bratwurst	Beer salami, beef
Bologna, turkey	Bologna, pork	Bockwurst
Corned beef	Hot dog, turkey	Bologna, beef
Hot dog, chicken	Ham, chopped	Liverwurst
Picnic loaf	Italian sausage	Hot dog, beef and
	Kielbasa sausage	pork
	Pastrami, beef	Knockwurst
	Salami	Pepperoni
	Sausage, smoked link	Polish sausage
	Summer sausage	Beef sausage stick
Source: USDA.		

The smartest choice by far is to avoid cold cuts and sausages. If you do eat them, make it on a *very* occasional basis and understand that there can be a wide range of difference in products. For example, "beef luncheon meat, thin-sliced" is 35 calories an ounce, while "beef luncheon meat, loaved" contains 87 calories per ounce. Obviously, a fair amount of fat has been added to the loaf. The same is true for bologna. Two slices of Oscar Mayer's sliced Lebanon Bologna contains 6.6 grams of fat. The same amount of Eckrich Thick Slice Bologna has 28 grams of fat—over four times as much!

The fattest cold cuts are the drier ones, such as pepperoni and hard salami, which run about 12 grams of fat per ounce. (In general, poultry versions of cold cuts are lower in fat and calories than their red meat counterparts. But remember, they are not "low fat," just lower in fat than the beef and pork versions.) Again, it's important to read food labels to determine how many grams of fat are contained in the product. Then you can make a decision as to whether or not you can "afford" the product in your budget.

Better choices for sandwich fillings include roasted turkey breast, roasted chicken breast, lean roast beef and lean ham. Many supermarkets now carry these items "fresh," rather than in processed, high-sodium varieties. In our home, nothing is as popular as sandwiches made from boneless, skinless breast of chicken. Three ounces contains less than 4 grams of fat. The breast is poached in two cups of boiling chicken broth for about 20 minutes, allowed to cool in the broth for another 10 minutes, and refrigerated. Cooking the chicken in broth gives it a rich, satisfying flavor.

Hot dogs, wieners, frankfurters, Italian and Polish sausage, knockwurst and the hundreds of other foods categorized as "sausage" are invariably high in fat. A single link of cooked Italian sausage, for example, contains about 275 calories and 22 grams of fat. Most sausages have 15 to 30 grams of fat. Chicken and turkey sausages are somewhat lower, but still too rich to be eaten other than as an exception. One thing you can do is check out specialty stores, which generally offer higher-quality sausages with less fat. Also, you can ask your butcher to make sausages with less fat. And finally, be realistic about portions. One link of Italian sausage can cover an entire pizza or flavor a double batch of spaghetti sauce. A little bit can provide flavor without loading the food with fat.

If you do choose to eat these foods, don't add to the problem by surrounding them with other high-fat foods. Remember, a tablespoon of regular mayonnaise, margarine or butter will add about 11 grams of fat to your sandwich. (The same amount of mustard has about one gram.) Add a slice of Swiss or American cheese, and you'll pick up another 8 or 9 grams of fat. Top it off with a half-cup of potato salad (6 to 9 grams of fat) or coleslaw (about 16 grams), and you'll take in enough grease to offset your budget for the week!

Frozen meals. Packaged beef dinners are typically among the fattest of the prepared meals, so it is important to make smart choices. Many come smothered in fatty sauces and surrounded by other high-fat foods. Swanson Home-Style Salisbury Steak in Gravy with Macaroni and Cheese, containing 410 calories and 32 grams of fat, is a good example. Fortunately, better choices exist:

Food Item (1 pkg.)	Total Calories	Grams of Fat	% of Calories from Fat
Healthy Choices Oriental			
Pepper Steak	270	5	17%
Lean Cuisine			
Herbed Lamb			
with Rice	280	8	26
Armour Dinner Classics			
Sirloin Roast	250	8	28

Source: Individual food companies.

The following frozen meals are considerably higher in fat content:

Food Item (1 pkg.)	Total Calories	Grams of Fat	% of Calories from Fat
Swanson Dinners Meat Loaf	430	22	46%
Armour Dinner Classics			
Veal Parmigiana	430	25	52
Stouffer's Dinner Supreme			
Beef Rib Tips Bour-			
guignonne	390	23	53

Source: Individual food producers.

Label-reading is, of course, very important. One glance at the grams of fat per serving will tell you whether or not the frozen meal will upset your fat budget. Remember to check out the number of servings in the package—sometimes more than one serving is contained. And finally, use the "no more than 3 grams of fat per 100 calories" rule as a guideline.

Restaurants. Dining out typically means being served fattier cuts of red meat, often covered with fat-laden sauce or gravy, and usually larger portions than you would eat at home. Ask for petite or smaller cuts, or share larger cuts with a friend. Consider ordering a beef appetizer as the main course. Make sure the meat is broiled, roasted or grilled with no added fat. In fast-food restaurants, a lean roast beef sandwich without cheese or fatty "special sauces" is actually a much better choice than a cheeseburger, fried chicken or fried fish. See Chapter 13 for additional tips on meeting the restaurant challenge.

POULTRY

In 1988, according to the USDA, 71% of U.S. households served chicken at least once every two weeks, and 34%

served turkey. In general, this is positive because most poultry is lower than red meat in fat and calories. Potentially, it offers a great opportunity for nutritious, delicious meals. In actuality, however, it often falls short because so much of it is eaten in high-fat forms, such as greasy fast-food chicken nuggets, fried chicken, and turkey hot dogs. So, as with red meat, you must make smart choices with poultry to help you manage your fat budget.

CHICKEN

Chicken has always been one of America's favorite foods, but in the past three decades its consumption has more than doubled to 50 pounds per person per year—slightly higher than annual pork consumption. Used in sandwiches, main dishes, stir fries, salads and soups, chicken offers a great opportunity to combine low-fat precepts with tasty food.

Leaner Choices

When buying chicken with an eye on your fat budget, remember this simple rule: *Choose a skinless white breast.* Unlike red meat, chicken flesh is not marbled with fat. Instead, fat is concentrated just underneath the skin, making chicken skin inordinately fat-rich. Removing the skin before cooking also removes most of the fat, making "skinless" the best buy. Some nutritionists maintain that skinning chicken before cooking isn't really necessary; the important thing is not to eat the skin. Be aware that a little bit of skin contains a tremendous amount of fat. Three ounces of roasted chicken skin, about the amount that covers a small breast, is equal in calories to 11½ ounces of roasted breast meat, almost three-quarters of a pound.

The same relationship exists between light (white) and dark meat. In general, light meat contains about one-third less fat than dark meat, so choose a breast over a drumstick or thigh.

Type of Chicken Meat (3 oz.)	Total Calories	Grams of Fat	% of Calories from Fat
Breast, light meat, skinless, roasted	140	3.0	19%
Breast, light meat, with skin, roasted	167	6.6	36
Thigh, dark meat, skinless, roasted	178	9.3	47
Thigh, dark meat, with skin, roasted	210	13.2	57

Source: USDA.

This illustrates the small amount of damage that skinless white breast meat can do to most people's fat budgets. For example, three ounces of the right chicken choice constitutes no more than 5% of a 60-gram personal budget, leaving someone on that budget with a lot of food options for the rest of the day.

There are a variety of chicken types available, and their fat content varies. Broilers, fryers and other small birds such as Cornish game hens generally are leaner than roasters and stewing chickens. Larger birds contain more fat. Chicken parts are very convenient, but pay attention to the label to know what you're buying. As with red meat, fat percentage relates to weight, not calories, so it can be misleading. Some valuable information can be found in label terminology, particularly in regard to processed products (which might contain dark meat, skin and fat as well as breast meat). According to the USDA, a product labeled "chicken breast," "chicken leg" or "chicken wing" contains both the poultry meat and the fatty skin. By law, up to 25% of ground chicken, for example, can be skin. But a product labeled "breast meat," "leg meat" or "wing meat" contains no skin or fat.

Food manufacturers have stampeded to cash in on the growing popularity of chicken. There are now dozens of chicken products on the market. Two of the most popular are marinated, ready-to-cook chicken parts and roasted chicken. Not all chicken products are as low in fat as a skinless breast, which is about 19% fat. For example, marinated, ready-to-cook chicken by George Mexican is 41% fat. Holly Farms thighs, roasted and ready to eat, are 69% fat. The message is clear: Read the product label to make smart choices.

Cooking Methods

How chicken is cooked can make a big difference. Frying a skinless breast or smothering it in fatty gravy will offset the innate leanness of chicken and play havoc with your fat budget. Always use cooking methods that allow fat to drip off, such as roasting, broiling, barbecuing, baking, steaming and stewing. Don't add fat when cooking. Frying flour-coated or batter-dipped chicken in oil, lard, vegetable shortening or butter can add about 3 grams of fat per ounce of meat. Instead, use a nonstick pan with non-fat wetting agents such as flavored vinegars, de-fatted broth or wine. Cooking sprays also work well.

Look for ways to be creative. Chicken breasts fried in a nonstick pan cook as quickly and easily as minute steaks. Skewered chicken is a great alternative to beef and lamb on the barbecue. Pound a breast flat, and you have a tasty substitute for veal piccata. Shredded chicken breast in particular makes a great substitute for hamburger in tacos, taco salad, ravioli, lasagne, chili and spring rolls. And don't overlook flavorful chicken broth. It is quickly made, easily de-fatted and, if reduced in cooking, incredibly rich-tasting. Add rice, pasta, beans and vegetables, and you have a nutritious, low-fat main meal.

Watch Out For...

Chicken franks and luncheon meats. These products may be lower in fat than their beef/pork counterparts, but they are not low-fat. Chicken franks generally contain about 8 to 11 grams of fat; one ounce of chicken bologna has about 8 grams of fat. And ground chicken typically contains skin, fat and dark meat as well as white breast-meat. If you're looking for sandwich fillings, a skinless breast—roasted, pan-fried (nonstick pan) or poached—is a much better choice.

Frozen meals. There is a wide range of chicken entrées and meals. Many frozen meals package chicken in a creamy sauce, producing a high-fat item. Others offer lean, skinless breasts, free of any added fat. Be sure to read labels for fat content and make smart choices. Examples of low-fat frozen meals include:

Food Item (1 pkg.)	Total Calories	Grams of Fat	% of Calories from Fat
Healthy Choices Chicken Oriental	220	2	8%
Lean Cuisine Chicken à l'Orange	270	5	17
Weight Watchers Imperial Chicken	220	5	20

Source: Individual food companies.

Following are examples of frozen meals that are not so low in fat:

Food Item (1 pkg.)	Total Calories	Grams of Fat	% of Calories from Fat
Le Menu Chicken à la King	490	23	42%
Swanson Dinners Fried Chicken	650	33	46
Swanson Hungry-Man Chicken Pot Pie	740	41	50

Source: Individual food companies.

Restaurants. Traditionally, restaurant chicken has been deep-fried with skin, often covered in a fatty gravy, and served with high-fat fries and coleslaw. Fortunately, today some healthier choices are available: skinless chicken breast that is baked, broiled, grilled or poached and served without fatty sauces. Chicken breast provençale, coq au vin and chicken cacciatore are good choices.

Most fast-food chicken has a high grease factor. Think what the following items would do to your personal fat budget:

Food Item	Total Calories	Grams of Fat	% of Calories from Fat
McDonald's			
Chicken McNuggets (6 pcs.)	323	20	56%
Kentucky Fried Chicken	371	26	63
Extra Crispy Thigh (1 pc.)			
Burger King	688	40	52
Specialty Chicken Sandwich			

Source: Individual food companies.

Happily, there are a few better choices. McDonald's Oriental Chicken Salad contains just 140 calories and 3.4 grams of fat, while Jack in the Box's Chicken Fajita Pita is 292 calories and 7.7 grams of fat. In the future, there will be more baked chicken available at fast-food outlets; for now, however, when you order fast-food chicken, be careful. For further tips, see Chapter 13.

TURKEY

The popularity of turkey has soared in response to its healthful reputation and is reflected in a sharp increase in sales. No longer reserved for the holidays, turkey is eaten throughout the year. While whole birds continue to be a favorite, turkey parts have become widely available. This has been a boon for turkey lovers, who can buy just the amount they need without having leftovers for a week. Turkey parts cook quickly and are good in a variety of recipes such as curries, stir fries, pot pies and tacos. Boneless breast cutlets are a great substitute for veal. Sliced turkey breast (roasted or microwaved) makes for a tasty sandwich and a smart alternative to fatty cold cuts. And turkey parts and bones make a flavorful broth to use as a base for hearty soups and stews.

Leaner Cuts

As with other meat, however, turkey has its downside. Not all turkey products are low in fat. The leanest choice is skinless white turkey breast. Since most of the fat in turkey is subcutaneous, removing skin means removing fat. Also, white meat contains less fat than dark, which means you can eat skinless white turkey breast without upsetting your fat budget.

Type of Turkey Meat (3 oz.)	Total Calories	Grams of Fat	% of Calories from Fat
Breast, light meat, skinless, roasted	133	2.7	18%
Breast, light meat, with skin, roasted	189	8.7	41
Thigh, dark meat, skinless, roasted	159	6.1	36
Thigh, dark meat, with skin, roasted	188	9.8	47

Source: USDA.

Skinless white turkey breast meat contains even less fat than its chicken counterpart. It is a very smart choice in balancing good food and reduced fat.

Cooking Methods

In general, turkey parts lend themselves to the same preparation methods used with chicken: roasting, broiling, grilling and microwaving. Do not choose self-basting turkey roasts, since the basting solution contains added fat (usually in the form of coconut oil, soybean oil, corn oil or butter) as well as added sugar and sodium.

Watch Out For...

Ground turkey. If only ground, skinless white breast went into ground turkey, this would be a very low-fat product. But commercial ground turkey typically includes fat, dark meat, and skin (the law allows up to 20% skin), as well as breast meat. Three ounces of ground turkey generally contains 191 calories and 11.1 grams of fat. You're better off grinding a skinless breast or cutlets in your own grinder, or having a butcher do it for you. That way, you know what you're getting. A few manufacturers do prepare their ground turkey without skin or added fat, so the key is to read the labels.

A similar problem exists with other turkey products. A turkey frank, for example, has about 8 grams of fat and is certainly not a low-fat product. Neither are most turkey cold cuts.

Frozen meals. Turkey frozen meals come in a range of fat content. Be sure to read labels carefully to identify those that are lower in fat. Following are some examples of leaner choices.

Food Item (1 pkg.)	Total Calories	Grams of Fat	% of Calories from Fat
Healthy Choices Breast of Turkey	270	5	16%
Budget Gourmet Slim Selects Glazed Turkey	270	5	16
Lean Cuisine Sliced Turkey Breast in Mushroom Sauce	220	5	20

Source: Individual food companies.

At the other extreme is Swanson Hungry-Man Turkey Pot Pie with 740 calories and 42 grams of fat. For some people, this would represent over half the fat budget for the day!

Restaurants. Full restaurant meals will often include both white and dark turkey meat, fatty gravy, and traditional accompaniments such as stuffing and mashed potatoes. Ask for white meat. If it comes with skin, trim it before eating. Look for lower-fat choices of other foods: rice pilaf, baked potato, vegetables and salad. A healthful turkey sandwich can be turned into a high-fat meal with cheese and mayonnaise. Skip the cheese altogether in favor of lettuce, tomatoes, onions, sprouts and cranberries. Go light on the mayonnaise, or ask for light mayonnaise. The best choice, of course, is to substitute mustard for mayonnaise. See Chapter 13 for additional tips on how to stay within your budget when you're dining out.

FISH AND SHELLFISH

Current figures show that we're eating more fish. As with poultry, much of the increased interest in fish is driven by its nutritional reputation: low in calories, low in saturated fat, rich in protein. In addition, the role of fish oil in the prevention of heart attacks has been widely reported. Says Dr. William Connor of the Oregon Health Sciences University, "Fish oil contains a component called Omega-3 that is instrumental in reducing the risk of heart attack by lowering cholesterol and keeping the blood from clotting." An article in the *New England Journal of Medicine* counseled that eating "as little as two fish dishes a week, about 7½ ounces of fish total, may cut the risk of dying from heart attack in half."

This positive link to cardiac health seems to hold true for all types of fish, from oily salmon to leaner cod, from ocean fish to freshwater varieties, and applies to shellfish as well. According to Dr. William Castelli of the Framingham

Study, shellfish are no longer condemned for high-cholesterol content. "The Omega-3's contained in shellfish tend to offset their higher cholesterol content," he says. As a result, shrimp, lobster, crab, scallops, mussels, clams, oysters and squid can now be included in a healthy diet. There is no more reason to avoid shellfish than to give up red meat.

Another factor in the popularity of fish is the availability of better quality. No longer does "fish" mean sole, salmon, flounder and a few local varieties. Today we can choose from a wide variety of seafood: monkfish, mako shark, halibut, scallops, lobster, crab, shrimp, orange roughy, bass, oysters, red snapper and catfish, to name but a few. Also, thanks to better handling and transportation methods, fresh and fresh-frozen fish is available throughout the country. And finally, people are finding new and interesting ways to prepare fish and shellfish. Stir-fried scallops, calamari salad, seafood fettucine, salmon grilled in fennel—these are meals that can compete well with red meat and poultry in appearance, taste and satisfaction.

Leaner Fish

Fish tends to have fewer calories than red meat. Most of the calories in fish, except for the oiliest varieties, come from protein. By comparison, most of the calories in red meat come from fat. As the amount of fat (in the form of oil) varies from species to species of fish, so does the amount of calories. A good example of a lean fish is Dover sole, which contains one gram of fat and 91 calories in a 3½-ounce serving. A good example of an oily fish is Chinook salmon, with 10.5 grams of fat and 178 calories in a 3½-ounce serving.

If eaten in moderation, as all animal foods should be, even the oiliest of fish will not upset your personal fat budget. In the following table, types of seafood have been grouped according to fat content. This can serve as a guide for making leaner choices.

Type of Fish (3.5 oz.)	Total Calories	Grams of Fat	% of Calories from Fat
Under 1.0 grams of fat			
Abalone	105	.7	6%
Cod	81	.7	9
Crab, Alaskan king	84	.7	8
Haddock	88	.7	8
Lobster, northern	91	.7	7
Pike, northern	88	.7	8
Pollock	91	.7	7
Scallops	88	.7	8
1–3 grams of fat			
Clams, cherrystones or littlenecks	147	1.9	12%
Crab, blue	88	1.1	11
Crayfish	88	1.1	11
Flounder	91	1.0	19
Grouper	91	1.0	19
Halibut, Atlantic/Pacific	140	2.1	13
Monkfish	73	1.5	18
Mussels	84	2.3	25
Ocean perch	95	1.5	9
Oysters, eastern	66	2.3	31
Oysters, Pacific	80	2.3	26
Pike, walleye	91	1.1	11
Shrimp	105	1.5	12
Snapper, red	98	1.1	10
Sole, Dover	91	1.0	19
Squid	91	1.5	15
3–6 grams of fat			
Bass, freshwater	112	3.5	28%
Bluefish	122	4.2	31
Catfish, Channel	115	4.2	33
Croaker, Atlantic	105	3.1	26
Lox (smoked salmon)	115	4.2	33
Salmon, Coho	144	5.8	36
Shark	130	4.2	29
Sturgeon	105	3.9	33
Swordfish	119	3.9	29
Trout, rainbow	115	3.5	27
Tuna	143	4.6	29
Whitefish	133	5.8	39

Type of Fish (3.5 oz.)	Total Calories	Grams of Fat	% of Calories from Fat
6–10 grams of fat			
Mackerel, Spanish	137	6.2	40%
Pompano, Florida	165	9.3	50
Roughy, orange	126	7.0	50
Salmon, Atlantic	140	6.2	40
Salmon, sockeye	168	8.5	45
Over 10 grams of fat			
Herring, smoked kippered	210	12.8	55%
Mackerel, Atlantic	203	13.6	60
Sablefish	192	15.1	70
Salmon, Chinook	178	10.5	53
Sardines, Pacific	178	12.0	60
Shad	196	13.6	62

Source: USDA.

Cooking Methods

Frying can turn low-fat fish into a high-fat food. For example, two ounces of uncooked striped bass has just 29 calories per ounce. But see what happens when the bass is breaded and fried: breading (bread crumbs, milk and eggs) adds about 6.5 calories to each ounce, and frying in butter adds another 12 calories per ounce. The result? Your striped bass has gained 16.5 calories per ounce—an increase of 57%, mostly from added fat. If you do fry, avoid butter, margarine, oil and lard. Instead of deep-frying, use a nonstick pan with a little cooking spray.

Fattier fish, such as salmon and trout, lend themselves to grilling, baking or broiling. Leaner fish, such as cod and halibut, do better with moist cooking methods such as poaching or microwaving. Use lemon juice, lime juice or wine for liquid. Also, try cooking fish in papillotes (paper packets), parchment or foil to seal in flavor and juices. Avoid using butter or margarine for basting or in poaching liquid. If added fat is needed, brush the fish very lightly with olive, canola or safflower oil.

Budget-Busting Condiments

Say you've picked out a nice piece of swordfish and grilled it with no added fat. So far, so good. Now that you're sitting down to enjoy it, don't undo your good start by using fatty condiments—butter, butter sauce, mayonnaise, tartar sauce. A pat of butter or margarine on your fish will add 4 grams of fat. A tablespoon of mayonnaise or tartar sauce will add 10 or 11 grams of fat to your budget. It does little good to make a leaner choice—broiled halibut over spareribs, for example—and then serve it in a butter sauce. You could end up with a meal that has more fat and calories than the spareribs. Better condiment choices include fresh lemon and lime, horseradish, tomato salsa, low-sodium soy sauce, flavored vinegars, vinaigrettes and oil-free dressings.

Watch Out For...

Tuna packed in oil. In this case, the oil is typically not fish oil but vegetable oil, so there is no additional cardiac benefit from the extra oil. However, it does add a lot of calories to the tuna. A 3½-ounce serving of oil-packed tuna contains 300 calories and 20 grams of fat. A better choice is water-packed tuna. The same serving contains 131 calories and about one-half gram of fat.

Tuna salad. Used too liberally, mayonnaise can turn a low-fat fish into a high-fat salad. Better choices include diet mayonnaise, a blend of non-fat yogurt and mayonnaise, and fat-free salad dressings. Whatever dressing you choose, if it contains fat, the rule is: Go lightly.

"Light" tuna. This term has no nutritional significance. It does not mean that there are fewer calories, just that the color of the tuna is lighter. The term "white" means that the tuna is albacore.

Frozen meals. There is no better example of good food gone bad through added fat than frozen meals. Most present fish that has been breaded, deep-fried and/or drowned in a fatty sauce. Even those labeled "lite" are not low in fat, just lower than the regular line. Van de Kamp's Light Fillets may have "⅓ less fat" than their regular counterparts, but they still average about 45% of calories from fat—about the same as a trimmed four-ounce pork chop. The following are examples of frozen meals that are higher in fat:

Frozen Meal (1 pkg.)	Total Calories	Grams of Fat	% of Calories from Fat
Gorton's Salmon in Dill Sauce	410	33	72%
Fishline Cod au Gratin	430	33	69
Gorton's Crunch Fish Fillets (2)	350	26	67
Gorton's Fillets Almondine	340	24	64
Mrs. Paul's Batter Dipped Fish	430	28	59
Van de Kamp's Breaded Fish	260	15	52
Booth Shrimp in Garlic Butter	440	25	51
Mrs. Paul's Crunchy Fish Sticks (4)	200	10	45
Mrs. Paul's Fried Clams	240	13	49

Source: Individual food companies.

Fortunately, some (but not many) smarter choices exist, including:

Frozen Meal (1 pkg.)	Total Calories	Grams of Fat	% of Calories from Fat
Healthy Choices Sole au Gratin	280	5	16%
Armour Classics Lite Baby Bay Shrimp	250	6	21
Mrs. Paul's Light Haddock Fillets	220	5	20
Mrs. Paul's Light Cod	220	7	29
Oven Poppers Flounder Florentine	275	7	23

Source: Individual food companies.

So, if you like your fish in the form of frozen meals, choose very carefully. Some contain virtually the same amount of fat as fresh fish. Others have added fat to the point where they are much worse than their red meat counterparts.

Restaurants. The same rules for cooking fish at home apply in restaurants. Order fish baked, poached, broiled, grilled or steamed—but not fried. Ask that it not be cooked in butter or added fat. "Dry-grilled" is a useful term when ordering. And skip the tartar sauce and drawn butter in favor of fresh lemons, vinaigrette and low-sodium soy sauce. Be very wary of fast food: two pieces of fish at Arthur Treacher's have 355 calories and 21 grams of fat; a breaded Shrimp Platter at Long John Silver has 962 calories and 57 grams of fat. Happily, some restaurants now offer broiled fish. But if the only fish available is deep-fried, order a plain hamburger instead—or look for another restaurant. See Chapter 13 for additional tips.

DAIRY PRODUCTS

Dairy foods are one of the most important components of a nutritious diet. They are a delicious way to get vitamins and minerals, and are a prime source of calcium. As with other foods, the calories in dairy products come from carbohydrate, protein and fat. Of these three nutrients, fat is responsible for the greatest difference between one dairy food and another. This is a key concept. By making smart choices, you can receive the full nutritional benefit of dairy foods without overloading on fat. When you choose fortified non-fat milk over whole milk, for example, you're still getting protein, carbohydrate and calcium.

Milk: Skim Is Best

Milk, a staple in the U.S. diet, comes with a wide range of fat, from whole milk (the fattest) to skim (the lowest in fat).

Type of Milk (1 cup)	Total Calories	Grams of Fat	% of Calories from Fat
Whole milk	150	8.5	51%
Chocolate milk, whole	208	8.5	37
2% milk	125	5.3	38
Chocolate milk, 2%	179	5.0	25
1% milk	104	2.5	22
Buttermilk, skim	88	.4	2
Skim milk	81	.4	2

Source: USDA.

The above comparison clearly illustrates the impact of dietary fat on calories. The richer in fat the type of milk, the more calories it contains. Chocolate milk is considered high in fat and calories. But it's the milk—not the chocolate syrup—that makes the difference. You could add a tablespoon of Hershey's Chocolate Syrup (45 calories) to a cup of 1% milk (104 calories) to make a cup of chocolate milk (149 calories), and it would still have fewer calories than a cup of whole milk (150 calories).

The smartest choice is fortified skim, or non-fat, milk. Three cups a day, which meets the RDA for calcium, only "costs" your fat budget 1.2 grams. For virtually everyone, this represents a small piece of the daily fat budget. The same amount of whole milk, however, contains 25.5 grams of fat. This would "cost" someone on a 60-gram budget almost half of that budget—too much to spend for just three cups of milk. The difference in calories is also important. Drinking three glasses of whole milk a day, instead of the same amount of non-fat milk, produces enough extra calories in the course of a year to create 22 pounds of extra body fat.

Some people find skim milk difficult to drink because of a "watery" taste, but this is less a problem of taste than of timing. If you are now drinking whole milk or 2% milk, don't switch immediately to skim. Chances are good that you will not like it. A better way is to make a gradual change, which will allow your taste buds a chance to adapt. Give yourself about two months to take a series of small steps away from whole milk to 2% milk, then from 2% to 1% milk, and finally from 1% to skim milk. (If you can't get 1% milk, use a mixture of one part skim to three parts 2% milk. As time goes on, use more skim and less 2% milk, until finally you arrive at 100% skim milk.) By making this adjustment in small increments over time, you greatly increase the chance for permanent change to take place.

Another way to get used to skim milk is to put it in milk shakes. Donvier makes a great at-home milk-shake machine that uses skim milk to create a non-fat drink with the richer taste of whole milk.

Butter: 100% Fat

What more can be said? When you use butter as a spread, as a sauce or in cooking, you are adding fat and concentrated calories. A single pat is 36 calories and 4 grams of fat; a tablespoon has 100 calories and 11 grams of fat. At 22.5 grams of fat per ounce, butter is fatter than spareribs! In addition, 63% of the fat in butter is saturated, making it worse than palm oil or lard for cardiac health. Butter is an insidious product. A dab here, a pat there—it doesn't seem like much. But it doesn't take much to wreck your fat budget. The best advice concerning butter is simple. Avoid it.

At first glance, margarine made from a polyunsaturated fat such as corn oil or safflower oil looks like a better choice than butter, but this may not be so. Soft, tub-type margarine does contain far less saturated fat than butter, so it's preferable from a cardiac standpoint. But stick margarine, hardened by a process known as hydrogenation, contains trans fatty acids. New research shows that these acids work like saturated fat in raising blood cholesterol. Diet margarine is lighter (it contains more water than regular margarine) and ounce for ounce can save you half the calories of butter or regular margarine. Like whipped butter, however, it's still a source of concentrated calories and should be eaten judiciously.

Cardiac health aside, the true issue here is fat—and margarine, like butter, is 100% fat. Melt a pat on your baked potato, and you'll still use 4 grams of fat from your budget. Like butter, margarine should be avoided or severely limited.

Cream: Don't Even Think About It!

Whipped cream, table cream and half-and-half are rich enough to break your budget and saturated enough to break your heart. To get an idea of how much fat is involved, look at the following comparison:

- A tablespoon of skim milk has no fat (under 6 calories).
- A tablespoon of 1% milk has .1 gram of fat (just over 6 calories).
- A tablespoon of whole milk has .5 gram of fat (about 10 calories).
- A tablespoon of half-and-half has 1.7 grams of fat (about 20 calories).
- A tablespoon of light table cream has 2.9 grams of fat (about 32 calories).
- A tablespoon of medium cream has 3.8 grams of fat (about 36 calories).
- A tablespoon of heavy whipping cream has 5.6 grams of fat (about 51 calories).

Whipped cream is so dense in fat that the topping on a sundae can represent about 20% to 40% of an average fat budget. A tablespoon of cream or half-and-half in your coffee, three cups a day, adds up to 5.1 to 8.7 extra grams of fat. You'd be better off to use 2%, 1% or skim milk. Beware of non-dairy creamers and non-dairy whipped toppings. Most are just as fatty as cream, and worse if they contain coconut oil or palm oil and additives. Some products use unsaturated vegetable oils, such as Mocha Mix made with soybean oil. These are less of a risk to cardiac health, but have the same fat and calories as half-and-half.

In recipes that call for cream, milk or evaporated milk, good substitutions are non-fat or low-fat yogurt, low-fat buttermilk and skim evaporated milk. Buttermilk is low in calories and works well in pancake and waffle recipes. Skim evaporated milk can be used in recipes for soufflés and puddings.

Cheese: From Very High to Very Low

Cheese is a concentrated source of nutrients, including protein, riboflavin and calcium. Unfortunately, most cheese is also very rich in fat. While equal amounts of cheese and cooked lean red meat supply about the same amount of protein, some cheeses supply twice the fat and calories. Most whole-milk cheeses derive 65% to 80% of their calories from fat. One ounce of Cheddar cheese, for example, contains about 10 grams of fat. Even "part-skim" mozzarella is rich in fat—one ounce has about 5 grams of fat. Indeed, a typical 1½-ounce serving, about two slices of American cheese, contains as many grams of fat as 3½ pats of butter. Something should be clearly understood: cheese is an excellent food and should be part of a healthful diet. But if you choose high-fat varieties, and you eat too much too often, cheese can be a problem food. The key is to make smart choices.

A number of varieties of low-fat cheese are now available, but keep in mind that these products are "lower in fat" than their original versions. Many still carry a fair dose of saturated fat. Part-skim, after all, is still a long way from all-skim. But food manufacturers have managed to remove more than a third of the fat and about a quarter of the calories in some varieties without ruining the texture or taste. The trick is figuring out which cheeses are truly light. For instance, many people assume that the harder cheeses (Cheddar, Gouda, Swiss) contain less fat than softer cheeses (Brie, Camembert). This is not necessarily true.

One ounce of Cheddar is 110 calories, while the same amount of Brie is 95 calories. Swiss and Gouda both are more calorically dense than Camembert.

The most effective guideline for determining acceptable cheeses is offered by the American Heart Association. Be aware that the measurement is for one ounce of cheese, a pitifully small amount for a real cheese lover. Smart choices involve serving size as well as fat content.

Less than 1 gram per ounce
Use without restriction. Generally made from skim milk.

Baker's cheese	Low-fat (2%) cottage cheese
Dry-curd cottage cheese	Rinsed cottage cheese
Gamelost's Norwegian pot cheese	

1-2 grams per ounce
May be eaten in addition to meat, or used as an additional protein or calcium source at other times. Made chiefly from skim milk.

Borden's Lite-Line Diet Cheese	Purity's May Bud Skim Milk Cheese
Breakstone's Skim Milk Farmer's Cheese	Purity's Wisconsin Skim Milk Cheese
Chef's Delight Cheddar Cheese	Tasty Brand's Imitation Processed Cheese
Fisher's Countdown Diet Cheese	
Kraft Calorie Wise Cheese Spread	Weight Watchers Diet Cheese
Part-skim ricotta	Weight Watchers Lo-Fat Cheese Slices

3-5 grams per ounce
May be eaten in addition to meat, unless calorie intake is a factor. The saturated fat and cholesterol content of one ounce of these cheeses is similar to that of one ounce of cooked lean meat.

Borden's Skim American	Le Maigrelait Cheese
Borden's Slimline Diet Cheese	Lucerne's Semi-Soft Skim Milk Cheese
Goldbach's Slim from Switzerland	
Green River's Low-Fat Cheddar	Olympia's Diet Cheese
Green River's Skim Milk Cheese	Part-skim mozzarella cheese
Kraft Philadelphia Imitation Cream Cheese	Slim Tilsit Cheese
	Swiss Knight's Fondue Cheese
	Whole-milk farmer's cheese
Kraft Pizza Mozzarella Cheese	Whole-milk ricotta cheese

6-8 grams per ounce
Use in place of (not in addition to) meat. These cheeses are high in total fat, although those filled with corn, cottonseed, safflower or sunflower seed oils are low in saturated fat. Watch out for hydrogenated oils, rich in cholesterol-raising trans fatty acids. Avoid skim milk cheeses made with palm or coconut oils.

Bandon's Part-skim Cheddar
   Cheese
Bel Paese
Blue Cheese
Bonaards Colby Cheese
Borden's Lite Line Neufchatel
Borden's Swiss Cheese
Brie
Camembert
Danbo, regular
Edam cheese
Feta cheese
Fisher's Corn Oil Cheezola
Fontina
Kraft Grated Romano Cheese
Hickory Farm's Longhorn Lyte
   Cheese
Jarlsberg Cheese
Kraft American Cheese
Kraft Brick Cheese
Kraft Calorie Wise Neufchatel

Kraft Cheese Whiz
Kraft Grated Romano Cheese
Kraft Monterey Jack Cheese
Kraft Parmesan Cheese
Kraft Pasteurized process
   Monterey Jack Cheese
Kraft Pasteurized Process Brick
   Cheese
Kraft Swiss Cheese
Kraft Velveeta Cheese
Laughing Cow's Babybell
   Cheese
Laughing Cow's Bonbel Cheese
Leyden Cheese
Nabisco Snack Mate Cheese
Port du Salut
Purity's Farmer's Cheese
Purity's May Bella
Ski Queen's Gjetost Cheese
Tilsit cheese
Ye Olde Tavern's Cheddar Cheese

9-11 grams per ounce
Save for special occasions. These are made from whole milk with added butterfat, and there is more than a tablespoon of fat in each ounce. Be sure to slice thin or grate to make them go farther.

Bandon's Regular Cheddar
   Cheese
Borden's American Cheese
Borden's Camembert
Borden's Colby Cheese
Borden's Country Store Cheese
Borden's Longhorn Cheese
Borden's Monterey Jack Cheese
Borden's Muenster
Gruyère

Kraft Cheddar Cheese
Kraft Cracker Barrel Cheddar
   Cheese
Kraft Gouda
Kraft Philadelphia Cream
   Cheese
Lorraine's Swiss Cheese
Natural Brick Cheese
Roquefort
Tillamook Cheddar Cheese

Try to limit your cheese selections to lower-fat versions. Remember, in a ham and cheese sandwich, it's the cheese and not the ham that's responsible for most of the fat and calories.

When the occasion calls for a small slice of Brie, Havarti or other full-fat cheese, by all means enjoy it. But budget for it. Understand what it means in terms of your personal fat budget, and don't feel guilty. Flexibility is an important part of fat budgeting. You get to spend your budget any way you want. If 3 ounces of Brie is worth 24 grams of fat to you, go ahead and eat it. But be certain to restrict fat in other foods that day.

Yogurt:
Good and Bad

People in Asia and the Middle East have been eating yogurt for centuries, but Americans have acquired a taste for it only in recent years. In 1960, consumers bought just 44 million pounds of yogurt; by the late 1980s, that figure had skyrocketed to more than a billion pounds.

Yogurt is one of the most healthful foods around. Eight ounces supplies about 20% to 25% of the RDA for protein and 300 to 400 milligrams of calcium—about as much as a glass of milk. It's also a good source of riboflavin, phosphorus and potassium.

Yogurt is not necessarily a "diet food." The number of calories and amount of fat it contains depend on what type of milk it is made from (whole, part skim, or skim) and what, if anything, is added (cream, non-fat milk solids, sucrose, corn syrup, honey, fructose or other sweeteners). A wide range is available. A cup of yogurt can have 90 calories and zero fat, or it can supply 400 calories and 11 grams of fat. It can have no sugar (plain) or up to seven teaspoons (fruit flavors).

The chief thing to watch for here is fat, but that's easy to do. Look for "non-fat" and "low-fat" types of yogurt, which contain substantially less fat than whole-milk yogurt. Some smart choices are included in the list that follows.

NON-FAT
(less than 1 gram of fat per serving)
Alta Dena Non-Fat
Colombo Plain, Fruit (all flavors), Vanilla
Dannon Plain (Nonfat)
Honey Hill Plain
Mountain High Non-Fat
Weight Watchers Nonfat Plain, Nonfat Flavored, Nonfat à la Francais
Yoplait 150 Nonfat (all flavors)

LOW-FAT
(less than 20% of calories from fat)
Breyers Strawberry
Brown Cow Farm Lowfat Blueberry, Strawberry, Vanilla, Plain
Dannon Lowfat Fresh Fruit Flavors (all), Coffee, Lemon, Vanilla
Light n' Lively Lowfat Red Raspberry, Strawberry
Yoplait Original Fruit, Breakfast Style Berries, Strawberry-Banana

As a rule, non-fat yogurts have substantially fewer calories per ounce. In low-fat yogurts, extract flavorings such as vanilla and coffee tend to be lower in calories than the preserves used in the fruit-flavored yogurts within the same brand. This is one reason their calories are comparable to whole-milk yogurt even though their fat content is much less. You may want to buy non-fat or low-fat plain or vanilla yogurt and stir in your own blueberries, bananas or strawberries. Fresh fruit provides enhanced flavor as well as extra vitamins and fiber.

Plain, non-fat yogurt is also a good substitute for sour cream, mayonnaise and commercial dressings. Mix it with mayonnaise as a spread for tuna or chicken salad. Use it as a substitute for sour cream on a baked potato. Create a low-fat vegetable dip with it. Or use it in cakes and spreads in place of cream cheese.

Frozen Desserts: Choose Carefully

Americans love ice cream, and we eat about 18 pounds of it per person each year. Unfortunately, the premium brands that make up more and more of our selection are bursting with fat and calories. One cup of Häagen-Dazs Vanilla Swiss Almond, for example, is 600 calories and contains a whopping 44 grams of fat! The same is true of Ben & Jerry's, Frusen Glädjé, and Klondike. Premium brands are simply too rich to be eaten except on the most infrequent occasions.

Regular ice cream and ice milk are lighter by comparison. Then again, what wouldn't be lighter than premium ice cream? Don't be fooled into thinking these are fat bargains. One cup of Breyers Strawberry contains 6 grams of fat, while the same amount of Breyers Grand Light Vanilla has 4 grams of fat. Even these lighter versions may be too rich on a regular basis for your fat budget. Also, watch out for Tofutti and other non-dairy desserts. These are made from vegetable oils and do not contain saturated fat, but they are not low in fat. A cup of Tofutti has 26 grams of fat and 460 calories. Simple Pleasures, an ice cream made with the fat substitute Simplesse, obviously won't harm your budget; however, it's devoid of fiber, vitamins and minerals, so enjoy it occasionally.

Frozen yogurt can be a delicious alternative to ice cream. However, as with regular yogurt, fat content can vary. Yoplait Soft Frozen Yogurt (all fruit flavors, 3 fluid ounces) contains 90 calories and 3 grams of fat. Dannon Frozen Yogurt on-a-Stick (1.75 fluid ounces) contains 50 calories and just one gram of fat, while Dole Fruit 'N Yogurt Bars (2.25 fluid ounces) contain 70 calories and are virtually fat-free. Frozen yogurt sold at "stands" also varies in fat content. Dannon Vanilla Soft Frozen (4 fluid ounces) contains 100 calories and 2 grams of fat; the same amount of Colombo Lite Nonfat Frozen Yogurt, 95 calories and no fat. Check with the vendor for the amount of fat in the product, so you don't trade high-fat, high-calorie ice cream for high-fat, high-calorie frozen yogurt.

TABLE FATS AND OILS

Like so many other aspects of the American lifestyle, consumption of fats and oils is a mixture of health and indulgence. On one hand, most of us understand that saturated fats promote high cholesterol and heart disease, and this is reflected in a decline in the amount of butter and lard eaten in the United States. On the other hand, there has been a sharp increase over the last 20 years in the consumption of polyunsaturated and monounsaturated vegetable oils—seen to be more heart-healthful than saturated fats—chiefly as salad oils, cooking oils and margarine. Americans today eat about 55 pounds per year of these fats, mostly from fried foods, fatty baked goods, spreads, and commercial salad dressings.

The upshot is that we're now eating oils that may be better for our hearts (although hydrogenated oils contain trans fatty acids, which raise blood cholesterol levels), but we're not eating less fat. Once more, we've simply traded one type of fat for another.

Not All Fats Are Equal

To be sure, there are differences in healthful properties among fats, and these differences should be considered in the food selection process. All fats and oils are a mixture of three types of fat: saturated, poly- and monounsaturated. Each type has an effect on cholesterol levels. The proportion of saturated, poly- and monounsaturated fat found in any product ultimately determines its impact on cholesterol. In general, the greater the concentration of saturated fat, the more the propensity to raise cholesterol in the blood. The greater the concentration of poly- or monounsaturated fat, the more the propensity to reduce cholesterol.

Because of their impact on cardiac risk, saturated fats are

categorized as the most harmful in excess. The American Heart Association recommends that no more than 10% of total calories come from saturated fats, which are primarily derived from animal sources. Good examples are the visible fat on meat, lard, butter, whole milk, cheese, cream, egg yolks, and chicken fat.

Unsaturated vegetable oils are more beneficial to cardiac health because they tend to reduce blood cholesterol levels. Polyunsaturated oils include corn, cottonseed, safflower, sesame and sunflower oils. Monounsaturated oils include olive, canola and peanut oils. The American Heart Association recommends that 10% of daily calories come from polyunsaturated oils, and 10% from monounsaturated oils. According to Dr. Margo Denke, lipids researcher at the University of Texas Southwestern Medical Center, both mono- and polyunsaturated oils appear to be effective in keeping blood cholesterol levels down when they're substituted for saturated fats. Monounsaturated oils, particularly canola and olive oil, seem to have the most beneficial effect on blood cholesterol. See the facing page for a composition comparison of vegetable oils.

Vegetable oils in general provide less cardiac risk, but there are exceptions. A few vegetable sources of saturated fat do exist, namely, palm oil, palm kernel oil and coconut oil. These tropical oils, even more saturated than lard, are found chiefly in processed foods such as non-dairy creamers, imitation whipped cream toppings, frozen meals, salad dressings, cake mixes, pie crusts, soups, cheese-flavored snacks, chips and crackers. It's important to read food labels for evidence of tropical oils. A telltale phrase is "made with one or more of the following oils." A number of oils may be listed, but you can't tell from the description which oil is actually used. It could be a tropical oil. Another clue is the term "all-vegetable oil," which doesn't reveal the specific oil used. Coconut oil, for example, fits the "all-vegetable oil" criterion. If the label isn't specific about the type of oil used, assume the worst.

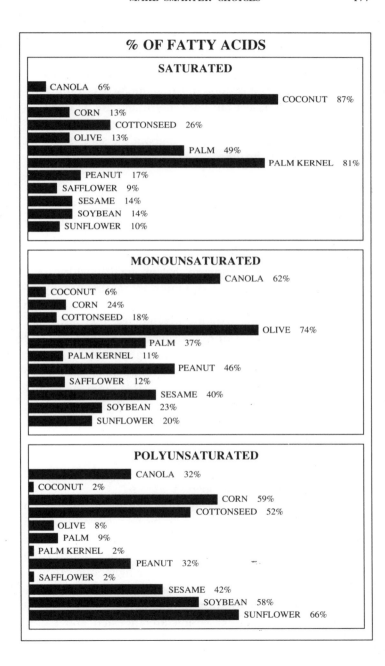

% OF FATTY ACIDS

SATURATED

- CANOLA 6%
- COCONUT 87%
- CORN 13%
- COTTONSEED 26%
- OLIVE 13%
- PALM 49%
- PALM KERNEL 81%
- PEANUT 17%
- SAFFLOWER 9%
- SESAME 14%
- SOYBEAN 14%
- SUNFLOWER 10%

MONOUNSATURATED

- CANOLA 62%
- COCONUT 6%
- CORN 24%
- COTTONSEED 18%
- OLIVE 74%
- PALM 37%
- PALM KERNEL 11%
- PEANUT 46%
- SAFFLOWER 12%
- SESAME 40%
- SOYBEAN 23%
- SUNFLOWER 20%

POLYUNSATURATED

- CANOLA 32%
- COCONUT 2%
- CORN 59%
- COTTONSEED 52%
- OLIVE 8%
- PALM 9%
- PALM KERNEL 2%
- PEANUT 32%
- SAFFLOWER 2%
- SESAME 42%
- SOYBEAN 58%
- SUNFLOWER 66%

A second exception involves hydrogenation, or the chemical process of hardening vegetable oils to produce products such as stick margarine and shortening. Unfortunately, this process results in an increase of trans fatty acids, which increase LDL cholesterol and are as likely as saturated fats to increase the risk of heart disease. This means that stick margarine may be about the same as butter in terms of cardiac health.

All Fats Are Rich in Calories

While definite cardiac advantages exist in some oils over others, do not lose sight of a major common characteristic of all fats and oils: they are uniformly rich in calories. A single tablespoon of oil, any oil, has about 120 calories and 13 grams of fat. A teaspoon of butter, margarine or mayonnaise has about 100 calories and 11 grams of fat, although "diet" margarine and "light" mayonnaise can have half that amount. Melt a pat of margarine on peas, and you still end up with a vegetable lathered in 4 grams of fat and 36 extra calories. From a calorie standpoint, there isn't much difference between cream in your coffee or a non-dairy creamer (even one made with a "good" oil, like soybean). The point is that all fats and oils, even healthful ones, have a concentration of calories that pose an increased risk for certian cancers and for becoming "overfat."

When fats and oils are added to foods, the caloric content of the meal jumps tremendously.

And that's not the only problem. Almost all the fat calories are quickly stored as body fat. As outlined in Chapter 6, the process of converting food to body fat burns up calories. It is estimated that about 23% of calories from protein and carbohydrates are lost in the metabolic process, a "handling charge" that allows only 77% of the calories consumed to be available for storage as body fat. It is not the same for fat-calories, which are digested and stored more efficiently. Of 100 calories of fat consumed in one tablespoon of mayonnaise, about 97 are converted to body fat. What it boils down to is that calorie for calorie, fat is more fattening than protein or carbohydrate. This means that 100 calories worth of baked potato is not the same as 100 calories worth of margarine.

The message on fats and oils, then, is twofold:

- If you budget fats and oils in your diet, be sure to choose the more healthful ones: poly- and monounsaturated oils. Olive and canola oil are two of the best. Avoid saturated fats, tropical oils and hydrogenated vegetable oils.
- Moderate the intake of *all* fats and oils. Overconsumption of "good" fats can have bad results.

Leaner Choices

As with all foods, the key is to make smart choices that will not upset your personal fat budget. This may seem difficult in this case, since "a fat is a fat is a fat" but it can certainly be done.

Often, smarter choices take the form of small changes:

- The most healthful margarines have a liquid polyunsaturated oil as their main ingredient. Soft, tub-type margarine is preferable to hydrogenated sticks. However, from a fat-calorie standpoint, all margarines are about the same—100% fat, 100 calories and about 11 grams of fat per tablespoon. In this respect, margarine is the same as butter and should be used very judiciously. It doesn't make much sense to switch from butter to margarine on both pieces of bread in a sandwich. A smarter choice would be to spread margarine on one piece and mustard on the other. You'll have cut the fat in half. The smartest choice, of course, would be to use mustard on both pieces of bread and eliminate any added fat.
- Consider using diet margarine and light mayonnaise as spreads. They contain about one-half the fat and calories as their regular counterparts.

Mayonnaise (1 Tbs.)	Calories	Grams of Fat
Kraft Real	100	11
Hellmann's Reduced Calorie	50	5
Kraft Light Reduced Calorie	50	5
Weight Watchers	40	4

Margarine (1 tbs.)	Calories	Grams of Fat
Soft Parkay (tub)	100	11
Diet Mazola (tub)	50	6
Promise Extra Light (tub)	50	6
Shedd's Spread Country Crock (tub)	70	7

- Use sprinkle-on powder as a butter substitute for potatoes, rice, vegetables and other hot foods. They won't do, however, for spreading on toast, sautéing or in recipes. Virtually fat-free, a single teaspoon is only about 8 calories.
- Have salad dressing served on the side. Dip your fork into the dressing before taking a bite of salad. The flavor will be rich and strong, but you won't take in much dressing.
- Add dressing to pasta salad just before serving. The flavor will be stronger, so you'll need less dressing, and the pasta will have less time to absorb excess oil.
- Make your own vinegar-and-oil dressing. The classic recipe for vinaigrette calls for a three-to-one ratio of oil to vinegar, which produces a dressing with about 90 calories per tablespoon. If you want a lighter dressing, simply use less oil. Use fresh seasonings to enrich the flavor of your own dressings: minced garlic instead of garlic powder or salt, fresh herbs (basil, coriander, dill, fennel, oregano, parsley) instead of dried. Don't overlook a wide variety of flavored vinegars such as balsamic, raspberry, blueberry and black currant to provide low-fat zip to dressings.
- Don't fry or sauté in margarine, cooking oil, lard, bacon fat or shortening. You're better off to use a nonstick pan

or a skillet seasoned with flavored vinegars (such as raspberry or strawberry), lemon juice, de-fatted broth, vermouth or wine. Simply by eliminating two teaspoons of oil, you'll save about 26 grams of fat and 250 calories. Or use a cooking spray that will add only 7 calories to cover the surface of a small pan. If you must use oils, choose canola or olive oil in very small amounts.

- Cook vegetables without added fat by steaming or micro-waving, or sauté them in broth or flavored vinegar. Don't add margarine to cooked vegetables; instead, enhance flavor with lemon juice, flavored vinegars, herbs and spices.
- Be careful about using tartar sauce with fish. A single tablespoon of Nally's Tartar Sauce will add more than 10 grams of fat to the meal.

Watch out for...

Mayonnaise salads. Although chicken, tuna and shrimp are basically low-fat foods, too much mayonnaise in the salad can turn it into a high-fat food. It's the same with coleslaw, potato salad and macaroni salad.

Mayonnaise seems to be a particular problem for women. According to government surveys on food preferences, women rank mayonnaise salads as one of the foods they eat most frequently. Perhaps because women are more con-cerned with weight control, these salads seem to be lighter choices than red meat. Often they're not. Two ounces of tuna salad can actually have more fat and calories than three ounces of lean red meat. The impact of added fat on the caloric density of such foods can be tremendous.

Salad dressings. Most commercial dressings, whether creamy or oily, are primarily fat, with about 90% of their calories coming from the oil they contain. Some dressings also contain eggs, cream and cheese. Many are rich in sodium. Two tablespoons of a ranch-style blue cheese or Russian dressing can add 150 calories and 16 grams of fat to your salad.

To place this in perspective, two tablespoons of salad dressing can have:

- As many calories as a Hershey bar
- As much fat as two slices of Domino's pizza
- As much sodium as a handful of taco chips

Be a smart shopper. Commercial dressings range from Kraft Oil-Free Italian, which contains no fat, to Newman's Own, with 9 grams of fat per tablespoon. Understand that some dressings are much more calorically dense than others. Or, put another way, you can have an entire eight-ounce bottle of Kraft Low-Calorie Italian Dressing for two tablespoons of Kraft Creamy Italian Dressing. Be aware that not all "dietetic" dressings are low in calories. While Mrs. Filbert's Imitation Mayonnaise has about 4 grams of fat per tablespoon, the same amount of Featherweight Low Sodium Soyamaise has about 11 grams. Examples of lower-fat choices include:

Good Seasons No Oil Italian Mix
Gourmet Garnishes Reduced Calorie
Heinz Oregon Trail Mary's Thin
Kraft Catalina Reduced Calorie
Pfeiffer Frenchette French
Pritikin No Oil
Richard Simmons Oriental or French
Wish Bone Lite Russian

A LAST WORD

In establishing a low-fat diet pattern, remember:

1. Low-fat eating is not a "doom and gloom" affair. Healthy meals can be tasty, appetizing and attractive.
2. There are no "good" or "bad" foods, but there are "smart" and "not so smart" choices for your food budget.

3. Changes in eating patterns take place slowly, over time. Rushing changes or expecting too much too soon usually results in failure.

The way to low-fat eating is to know your personal fat budget. It is a gauge against which to measure food choices so that you can make smarter decisions. Its value becomes apparent when examining how insidiously dietary fat can creep into the diet. For example, a person might not think of herself as a big user of table fats. She might fry an egg in margarine and spread a bit on her toast at breakfast. She might order the "dieter's tuna salad" at a restaurant for lunch. And she might melt a little margarine on vegetables and use a pat or two on bread at dinner, as well as have a salad with dressing. Doesn't sound like a lot, but watch how quickly small dabs of concentrated fat eat into her budget:

Meal	Added Fat	Grams of Fat
Breakfast:	Cook eggs in 1 tablespoon margarine	11
	Spread 2 pats of margarine on toast	8
Lunch:	Restaurant tuna salad with 2 tablespoons of mayonnaise	22
Dinner:	Salad with 2 tablespoons of French dressing	12
	Melt 1 pat of margarine on vegetables	4
	Spread 2 pats of margarine on bread	8
	Total	65

However, if the woman above has established a personal fat budget, it becomes easier to see the impact of her food choices on fat intake. The bottom line is that it provides her with a greater degree of control.

Red Meat
- Substitute poultry and fish for red meat.
- For leaner cuts of beef, choose "loin" and "round." For

pork, lamb and veal, look for "loin" and "leg." Select is the preferred grade.

- Always trim off all visible fat before cooking meat. Never eat fat.
- Broil, bake, grill, roast, stew and braise, but never fry. Cook meat to medium or well done to allow the fat to drip off.
- Use meat as a condiment. "Stretch" it to make it go further. Avoid large portions.
- Avoid luncheon meats, hot dogs, sausages and bacon. Better sandwich choices include roasted turkey or chicken breast, lean roast beef and lean ham.
- Choose frozen meals wisely. Be sure to read labels for fat content.

Poultry

- Make skinless white breast your premium choice. White meat is leaner than dark. Whenever possible, strip poultry skin before cooking. Never eat cooked skin. Remember, compared with the full range of food choices—fruits, vegetables, grains, etc.—no poultry is truly low in fat.

Medium in Fat	High in Fat	Very High in Fat
White meat of chicken and turkey, no skin	White meat, with skin Dark meat, no skin Duck, goose, no skin Ground turkey	Dark meat chicken and turkey, with skin Duck and goose, with skin

- Pay attention to food labels on chicken and turkey parts. "Chicken" or "turkey" means dark meat, fat and skin as well as breast meat.
- Use fat-reduced cooking methods—bake, broil, grill, roast, steam, poach and stew. Frying chicken or turkey parts adds tremendously to fat and calories.
- Avoid ground turkey, ground chicken, and turkey/chicken franks and cold cuts. They are not low in fat.

- Look for low-fat choices in frozen meals. Not all chicken and turkey meals are similar in fat content. Read labels.

Fish
- The amount of oil a fish contains dictates caloric content. Less oily fish has fewer calories. But don't be concerned about the oil itself, for it benefits cardiac health. All fish is acceptable, including shellfish.
- Strive for variety in types of fish and creativity in how you prepare them. Tuna with tomato and basil sauce, grilled shrimp and vegetables, scallops dijonnaise, and hickory-smoked salmon are good examples.
- Preferred cooking methods call for baking, poaching, grilling, steaming and broiling. Do not fry or deep-fry in butter, margarine, oil or lard.
- Watch out for fatty condiments such as butter, butter sauce, cream sauce, mayonnaise and tartar sauce. They will destroy your low-fat efforts.
- Choose water-packed tuna over oil-packed tuna to save fat and calories. Go light on the dressing for tuna salad.

Dairy Products
- Skim milk is the beverage of choice. Learn to drink it over time. Even 1% milk is preferable to whole or 2% milk. Use a milk-shake machine to make rich- and creamy-tasting homemade dairy drinks from skim milk.
- Avoid whipped cream, table cream and half-and-half. Watch out for non-dairy creamers made with saturated coconut oil.
- Avoid butter as a spread, sauce or cooking agent. The same goes for margarine, particularly that made from hydrogenated oils.
- Avoid frozen vegetables in butter sauce, cream soups, frozen dinners with cheese and cream sauces, and canned or bottled sauces and gravies.
- Select low-fat cheeses for regular consumption. Save medium- and full-fat cheeses for special occasions.

- Watch out for cheese cubes at cocktail parties. Generally, one cube contains fat and calories equal to one slice of American cheese.
- Choose non-fat and low-fat yogurt (regular or frozen) over whole-milk yogurt and ice cream.

Low in Fat	Medium in Fat	High in Fat	Very High in Fat
Non-fat milk	Buttermilk	Low-fat milk	Cream
Non-fat buttermilk	1% milk	Whole-milk yogurt	Most cheese butter
Non-fat yogurt	Low-fat yogurt	Whole milk	Sour cream
Non-fat frozen yogurt	Low-fat cottage cheese	2% milk	Ice cream
Dry-curd cottage cheese	Whey ricotta cheese	4% fat cottage cheese	Cream cheese
Sherbet	Ice milk		Half-and-half

Table Fats and Oils

- Watch out for tropical oils rich in saturated fat—coconut, palm, and palm kernal oil. Don't be fooled into thinking "all vegetable" oil is necessarily healthful.
- Hydrogenation, a process which hardens vegetable oils for products such as stick margarine and shortening, increases cholesterol-raising trans fatty acids. When you use margarine, choose soft, tub-type.
- Be aware of the calorie/fat difference between "diet" and regular products.
- Make your own salad dressing for the best flavor, then serve it on the side. Don't let excess dressing be your fat downfall.
- Watch out for added fat from mayonnaise in salads such as tuna, potato and chicken, and in condiments such as tartar sauce.
- Do not fry in oil, margarine, butter or lard. Use non-fat wetting agents such as de-fatted broth, wine, flavored-vinegar or cooking sprays in a nonstick pan.

CHAPTER 11

THE CARBOHYDRATE ADVANTAGE

Carbohydrates should be the primary source of calories in the diet. Indeed, the advice of the Surgeon General, the American Heart Association and others to cut down on fat is also a call to eat more foods rich in starch and fiber, two forms of complex carbohydrates. Specifically, it is recommended that the intake of carbohydrates be increased to more than 55% of total calories. The Committee on Diet and Health of the National Research Council advises, "Every day eat five or more servings (½ cup equals one serving) of vegetables and fruits, especially green and yellow vegetables and citrus fruits. Also, increase intake of starches and other complex carbohydrates by eating six or more daily servings of a combination of breads, cereals, and legumes."

Studies in various parts of the world indicate that people who habitually consume a diet high in plant foods have low risks of cardiovascular diseases, probably because such a diet is usually low in cholesterol-raising animal fat. In addition, there is evidence that a high-fiber diet, particularly one rich in green and yellow vegetables and citrus fruits, produces a decreased susceptibility to colon cancer. And finally, there is a wide body of evidence showing that an increased intake of starchy and fiber-rich foods, combined with a decrease in fat intake, is linked to the maintainance of appropriate body weight.

In short, carbohydrates are great foods. This would not be news to our ancestors, who based their diet on complex carbohydrates such as potatoes, rice, corn and beans along with fruits and vegetables. Carbohydrates are an excellent source of vitamins and minerals, and are typically far less fattening than fat-rich foods. In addition, foods rich in fiber enhance health. As recently as the turn of the century, about 60% of calories in the U.S. diet came from carbohydrates. In recent years, there has been a radical shift away from plant-based foods and toward fat-rich animal foods such as meat, fish, poultry, eggs and dairy products. With that shift has come an increased incidence of heart disease, cancer and obesity.

Many health professionals and agencies are today attempting through public education to reverse this trend. To a certain extent, the message to eat more carbohydrates has been accepted and is reflected in a rise in the consumption of fresh fruits and fresh vegetables over the last 10 years. True progress is being made in cereal and flour products. We are eating about 17% more wheat flour and rice than a decade ago, but it is still less than half the amount of bread, cereal, pasta and rice eaten by Americans in 1910. However, while there has been an increase in the consumption of potatoes, most has come in the form of fatty potato chips and French fries.

Carbohydrates Aid Weight Control

One of the first things a person typically does when trying to lose weight is to swear off starchy foods—bread, potatoes, rice and pasta. Many popular low-carbohydrate diets restricted these foods in favor of high-protein animal foods combined with low-calorie fruit and vegetables. On many such diets, you could eat steak and green beans, cottage cheese and fruit, lamb chops and salad, and chicken and peas. This was due to a misconception that starchy foods are rich in calories and should be avoided. Nothing could be farther from the truth. Today, nutritionists counsel just the opposite: if you want to lose weight, eat more starchy foods.

Starchy foods—minus butter, sour cream and other fatty toppings—actually promote weight loss and long-term weight control. The reason is simple: starch is not rich in calories. Like protein, it contains 4 calories per gram, while fat contains 9 calories per gram. This difference is readily evident in a comparison of caloric density in high-fat and high-starch foods. Four ounces of lamb chops contains 405 calories, or about 100 per ounce. But four ounces of cooked white rice has only 123 calories, or 30 per ounce; the same amount of kidney beans have 133 calories, or 33 per ounce. And a baked potato, with just 110 calories, has 22 per ounce. So, it is not the starchy potato that produces excess calories. It's the fat added when the potato is fried, or turned into chips, or topped with butter, margarine, sour cream and cheese. It isn't the rice that adds pounds; it's the butter sauce. It isn't the bread; it's the butter. And it isn't the pasta; it's the sausage, meatballs and cream sauce. This is not to say that there's no room for a lean lamb chop in the diet, for there is. But the above information suggests that if you're concerned with weight control, you should cut down on animal foods and eat more starchy foods.

Despite the facts, old habits die hard. More than 35% of those responding to a Good Housekeeping Institute survey a few years ago said they consider starch to be fattening. A 1983 Nielsen survey found that 30% of the respondents avoided cereals and grains for the same reason. A number of studies should help to put this misconception to rest. At Michigan State University, two groups of overweight students were fed 12 slices of bread a day for eight weeks and were instructed to eat whatever else they wanted. The group that ate ordinary white bread averaged a weight loss of 14 pounds. The group that ate high-fiber bread lost an average of 19 pounds. The same was true for a similar study at Hunter College involving subjects who ate eight slices of bread a day for 10 weeks. They lost about nine pounds on average.

In addition to being low in calories, many high-carbohydrate foods are rich in fiber. Found in unrefined grains (corn, oats, rye, wheat), dried peas and beans, fruits and vegetables, fiber is plant material that cannot be digested. Fiber-rich foods typically take a longer time to eat than fat-rich foods. Apples and carrots, for example, require a lot of chewing, which provides sufficient time (about 20 minutes) for satiety to be attained. High-fiber foods also fill the stomach with bulk, are slowly digested and "stick to the ribs," providing a psychological benefit as well—you feel that you've eaten something. In the above studies, the subjects reported that the bread kept them "full," so there was less room to overeat higher-calorie foods. Moreover, carbohydrates seem to be better than fats at informing the body that it has been fed and, when appropriate, that it has had enough. The reason is that, unlike fat, carbohydrates trigger the release of insulin, the hormone that best informs the body that food has been consumed. And finally, complex carbohydrates absorb water in the digestive system, thereby creating a feeling of satisfaction that helps to control overeating.

Starchy foods also use up more calories in the digestive process than does dietary fat, thus making fewer carbohydrate calories available for storage as body fat. Says Dr. Jean-Pierre Flatt of the University of Massachusetts Medical School, "The average person would have to eat a full 4,000 calories a day for many days before the carbohydrates in such a high-calorie regimen would be converted to fat. In reality, you get fat not from overeating carbohydrates but from the fat you eat." This does not mean, of course, that you can eat all the carbohydrates you wish and still not gain weight; if you're going to overeat, however, you're better off doing it with starch than with fat.

Carbohydrates Benefit Health

According to the Surgeon General, a diet rich in fiber and complex carbohydrates offers the best opportunity for health and longevity. In other words, we should eat more whole grains, fruits, vegetables and legumes—and less meat, convenience foods, whole milk products, snacks and other fatty foods.

There is much evidence that a high-fiber, high-carbohydrate diet reduces the risk of certain diseases. Studies show that soluble fiber in particular—found in oatmeal and oat bran, legumes, carrots, apples and barley—is effective in reducing blood cholesterol levels. According to the National Cancer Society, high-fiber, high-carbohydrate foods may reduce the risk of colon and other cancers. By pushing food through the gut faster, fiber reduces the amount of time the colon wall is exposed to potential carcinogens. Also, by displacing fats on the diet, fiber may help to prevent breast, prostate and other cancers.

Americans consume about 11 grams of fiber each day. This is short of the recommended 20 to 30 (but no more than 35) grams of fiber a day. Fortunately, many carbohydrate foods are low-calorie sources of fiber.

Food	Grams of Fiber
Fruits	
Blackberries (½ cup)	4.0
Apple* (1 medium)	3.5
Pear* (1 medium)	3.1
Banana (1 medium)	3.0
Strawberries (1 cup)	3.0
Blueberries (½ cup)	3.0
Orange (1)	2.6
Prunes (2)	2.0
Peach* (1)	1.9
Vegetables (⅔ cup)	
Corn	6.2
Brussels sprouts	3.5

Food	Grams of Fiber
Carrots	3.1
Potatoes, cooked	3.1
Broccoli	2.9
Spinach	2.8
Zucchini	2.4
Cereals (1 oz)	
All Bran w/ Extra Fiber	14
Fiber One +	13
100% Bran	10
Bran Buds	10
Wheat, shredded (2 biscuits)	6.1
Grape-Nuts	5.0
Oats, rolled (½ cup)	4.5
Breads	
Bran muffin (1)	4.0
Whole-wheat bread (2 slices)	3.2
Pumpernickel bread (2 slices)	3.2
Rye bread (2 slices)	2.8
Cracked-wheat bread (2 slices)	2.4
Grains	
Rice, brown (⅔ cup)	3.0
Barley, dry (⅔ cup)	2.1
Rice, white (⅔ cup)	1.1
Legumes	
Lentils, cooked (½ cup)	9.0
Kidney beans, cooked (½ cup)	9.7
Pinto beans, cooked (½ cup)	8.9
Lima beans, cooked (½ cup)	7.4

*With skin.

Source: USDA.

FRUITS AND VEGETABLES

Low in fat and calories, rich in carbohydrate, vitamins, minerals and fiber, fruits and vegetables are nutritional bargains in their own right. In addition, beta-carotene is found in carrots, sweet potatoes, winter squash, apricots, peaches, cantaloupe and most dark green leafy vegetables such as spinach. (In general, the darker the fruit or vegetable, the more beta-carotine.) The consensus of health groups is that five servings of fruits and vegetables should be eaten daily. Vitamin C is found in citrus fruits, strawberries, cantaloupe and other melons, broccoli, cabbage, tomatoes, green peppers and most dark, leafy vegetables.

Fruits and vegetables also have a high water content, providing bulk and a feeling of satisfaction that helps in the prevention of overeating and controlling the fat budget. They are good sources of natural sugars, so a bowl of strawberries can satisfy a craving for sweetness. And, of course, they are low in calories. One medium apple, a banana, 1¾ cups of cantaloupe, 30 fresh cherries, 1 medium orange, 2½ medium peaches and 2 cups of strawberries each contain about the same amount of calories as 15 jelly beans. Vegetables are even lower. A half-cup of most watery vegetables such as tomatoes, green beans, broccoli and asparagus contains under 25 calories. There are even fewer in lettuce, celery, radishes and raw greens.

| | Available Fresh in: | | | |
Fruit	Winter	Spring	Summer	Fall
Apples	X	X	X	X
Apricots		X	X	
Bananas	X	X	X	X
Blueberries			X	
Cantaloupe			X	
Cherries			X	
Figs			X	X
Grapefruit	X	X	X	X
Grapes	X	X	X	X
Honeydew melon			X	X
Kiwi		X	X	X
Kumquats	X			
Lemons	X	X	X	X
Limes	X	X	X	X
Mangoes		X	X	
Nectarines			X	

Fruit	Winter	Spring	Summer	Fall
Oranges	X	X	X	X
Peaches			X	X
Pears	X			X
Pineapples	X	X	X	X
Plums	X	X	X	X
Raspberries			X	
Strawberries		X		
Tangerines				X
Watermelon			X	

Table header: Available Fresh in:

Fresh fruits provide better nutrition than canned fruits because the canning process causes vital nutrients to be lost. If canned fruit is used as a substitute for out-of-season fresh varieties, look for those labeled "unsweetened," "packed in its own juices" or "packed in fruit juice." They will not have added sugar. Frozen fruit generally does not have added sugar. Dried fruit has more calories per ounce than fresh fruit.

Like fruit, fresh vegetables contain the most nutrients. In general, the deeper the color, the more nutritious. For example, dark green spinach packs more nutritional punch than light green iceberg lettuce. The way vegetables are stored and cooked also affects nutritional value impact. Keeping them whole until you're ready to use them is a good way to preserve vitamins. The most nutritious way to eat vegetables is raw, as in green salads. If you do cook them, do it lightly. In general, the less vegetables are cooked, the greater their nutritional value when eaten. If possible, cook them with the skin on for better nutrition. For best results:

- Steam in a vegetable steamer in a pot with a lid. Make sure the water level is well below the vegetables.
- Cook in a pan with a tight-fitting lid, using just a small amount of water.
- Stir-fry lightly in a small amount of oil, or in a nonstick

pan with de-fatted broth, wine, water, vinegar or a cooking spray.
- Microwave in a dish or bowl covered with plastic wrap. Make sure the wrap is punctured to allow steam to escape.

Canned vegetables can substitute for out-of-season varieties, but watch out for added sodium. Frozen vegetables are more nutritious, but beware of those packaged in butter/cream/cheese sauces.

BREAD

Bread can be nutritionally rich, high in fiber and low in calories. It can also be nutritionally poor, low in fiber and high in calories. The best choices are whole-grain breads:

- 100% whole-wheat bread
- Whole-grain bread
- Multi-grain bread
- Rye bread (dark)
- Whole-wheat pita
- Corn tortilla
- Oat bread with whole wheat
- Cracked-wheat bread
- Stone-ground grain bread
- Whole-wheat bagels
- Whole-grain English muffins

It's important to read the label on commercially baked bread, or you won't know what the bread contains. The words "wheat flour" instead of "whole-wheat flour" mean that the wheat bran and germ have been removed. Buy breads labeled "whole wheat," "whole grain" and "stone ground." Also, do not rely on appearance to estimate whole-grain content. Some manufacturers use caramel coloring or raisin juice to transform nutritionally deficient white bread into brown bread, without adding any nutrients or fiber. Crunchy breads such as French and Italian are low in fat, but their "crunch" provides no additional fiber. Reading labels takes time and effort, but you'll be rewarded with a wide selection of breads, rolls, English muffins and flatbreads that will not break your fat budget. And don't miss the experience of baking your own bread, either in loaves or as flatbread. Home-baked bread is often so filling that you're satisfied with less.

In addition to its positive nutritional qualities, bread can provide a great amount of variety in the diet. This is particularly true in regard to sandwiches. It's an unfortunate truth that once fatty fillings (salami, liverwurst, cheese, bacon) are eliminated, the range of sandwich choice is diminished. Sliced turkey or chicken breast, tuna salad, turkey or chicken salad, and veggies are great sandwich selections, but how often in the week can you eat a turkey sandwich without becoming bored? Different breads introduce variety. A turkey sandwich made with dark rye bread on Monday seems different from one made with French bread on Thursday.

BREAKFAST CEREALS

The primary cereal grains found in the American diet are made from wheat, corn, oats, barley, rye and rice. They contain about 70% to 80% complex carbohydrates, about 13% to 15% protein, and very little fat. Cereals are great sources of fiber as well as vitamins and minerals.

In general, whole-grain cereals are the best nutritional buy, particularly if served with skim milk and fresh fruit or berries. Some good choices include:

- Oatmeal
- Whole-grain puffed wheat, rice and corn
- Shredded wheat

- Whole-grain wheat, oat and rice flakes
- Mixed-grain hot cereals

Some whole-grain cereals are made from refined grain (i.e., the nutritious bran and/or germ has been removed in the milling process), so make sure the kind you buy is "enriched" by the addition of nutrients.

Look for cold cereals made with whole grains, minimally processed, and no added sugar. Those with the highest fiber content include Kellogg's All Bran with Extra Fiber, General Mills Fiber One, Nabisco 100% Bran and Kellogg's Bran-Buds. Each contains 10 or more grams of fiber in a one-ounce serving. Other good choices include Shredded Wheat, Shredded Wheat 'n Bran, Nutrigrain Corn, Nutrigrain Wheat, Nutrigrain Nuggets, Wheat Chex, Oat Bran O's, Wheaties, Cheerios and Grapenuts. Watch out for cereals loaded wth sugar. Four grams of "sucrose and other sugars" (listed in the nutritional data on the cereal label) equals one teaspoon of sugar. Be aware that granola is high in sugars (honey, molasses), fats (oil, nuts, seeds, coconut) and calories. Also, "one serving" (¼ cup) contains about 130 calories. Since virtually no one eats that size "serving," it's easy to overdose on calories.

A good general buying guide is:

Per Serving
- 2 grams or more of fiber
- No added fat
- 5 grams or less sucrose

POTATOES

Potatoes provide high nutritional value at a low caloric cost. A medium-size potato with only 90 to 110 calories is bursting with vitamins, minerals, trace nutrients, and about 3.2 grams of high-quality protein. Indeed, a diet of only potatoes would provide an adult with nearly all needed nutrients. But when you add fat as a condiment or in cooking, this great food is adulterated. With baked potatoes, skip the fatty add-ons: butter, margarine, sour cream, bacon bits and cheese. Instead, use toppings of non-fat yogurt, salsa, black pepper, garlic powder, chopped dill, parsley and chives. For mashed potatoes, use de-fatted gravy. This can be done by placing ice cubes in the gravy or by refrigerating it so that congealed fat can be skimmed. For boiled or steamed potatoes, use a vinaigrette of lemon juice, black pepper and a hint of olive oil.

Frying potatoes changes the nutritional balance by adding fat. French fries, potato chips and potato sticks get about 85% to 90% of their calories from fat. The effect on caloric impact is tremendous:

Food (8 oz.)	Total Calories	Calories per Ounce
Baked potato	170	21
French fries	620	78
Potato chips	1,200	150

To put this into perspective, you'd have to walk for 25 minutes at a pace of 4 mph, or cycle for 19 minutes at 10 mph, to offset the calories in one ounce of potato chips.

Baking sliced or French-fry cut potatoes on a nonstick cooking sheet is a good alternative to French fries. For frying potatoes, toss slices lightly with olive or canola oil (one tablespoon of oil will cover four large potatoes), then cook in a nonstick pan.

PASTA

Sloughing its reputation as a cheap, fattening food with little to offer nutritionally, pasta is emerging as the most elegant health food of our time. And with good reason.

Pasta can be a nutrient-laden food with much to offer. Two ounces of enriched dry pasta (almost all varieties are enriched) makes one cup cooked and provides starch, riboflavin, niacin, thiamin, about 10% of the RDA for protein, and less than one gram of fat—all for just over 200 calories.

Available in over 600 shapes and sizes, and almost every color of the rainbow, pasta lends itself to an assortment of dishes. Linguine, rigatoni, penne, fettucine and, of course, spaghetti are great main dishes. Rotelle, fusilli, rotini and shells make terrific salads with fresh vegetables. Tortellini and pastina make hearty soups, and orzo is a tasty side dish. Many pastas today come flavored and colored with vegetables, including spinach, carrots and tomatoes. Whole-wheat pasta has considerably more fiber than regular pasta and can be higher in protein and iron as well. And fresh pasta is now sold regularly in supermarkets as well as gourmet shops.

The type of pasta you select is less important than what you put on it. Even the most healthful pasta will become a high-fat dish if drenched in Alfredo sauce (butter, cream and cheese) or served with a pound of sausage. A better choice is a simple marinara sauce, delicious yet low in fat and calories. One cup of pasta with a quarter-cup of tomato sauce and a tablespoon of grated Parmesan cheese contains about 260 calories, or about the same as a cup of low-fat yogurt sweetened with fruit preserves. Better yet, only 25% of the calories in the pasta come from fat. You can also add a small amount of olive oil with moderate servings of mussels, clams, shrimp or scallops to your red sauce to make a heartier meal. Low-calorie salad dressings or herb dressings are perfect for pasta salads.

And finally, don't overlook noodles such as saifun and soba. Found primarily in the Oriental sections of supermarkets and in Japanese and Chinese markets, these noodles are excellent in soups and as side dishes.

RICE AND OTHER GRAINS

Rice is a low-fat, nutrient-rich food, depended upon by millions as a basic food. Polished white rice is a favorite because polishing seems to make it more digestible. Unfortunately, the process strips some protein, fiber, and many important vitamins and minerals from the rice. Parboiled, or converted, white rice is a better choice because the process of parboiling does not cause such a great vitamin loss. Instant and "minute" rice cook quickly but are lowest in nutritional content. The best choice is whole-grain brown rice; not subject to processing, it retains all its nutrients.

Like pasta, rice is a food that is often adulterated by fatty add-on's. One cup of cooked brown rice, for example, has 230 calories. The same amount of white rice has 220, and instant rice about 180. The fat calories in rice will soar, however, if it's drenched in butter or gravy. You're better off topping a bowl of rice with a low-fat chicken stir-fry or vegetable dish, or serving it on the side with a few drops of sodium-reduced soy sauce. Wild rice is also excellent as a stuffing for poultry.

Other grains worth knowing about include barley (excellent in hearty soups and as a side dish), bulgur (a tasty alternative to rice) and couscous (the main ingredient in tabbouli, a delicious salad). Don't overlook corn, an excellent source of protein and carbohydrate. Try cornmeal, polenta (Italian cornmeal) and cornbread.

LEGUMES

Legumes, or vegetables borne in pods, are chock-full of protein, complex carbohydrates, fiber, B vitamins, iron, potassium, zinc and magnesium, yet are very low in fat and sodium content and free of cholesterol. In addition, recent research has turned up more nutritional good news. The type of fiber contained in legumes (soluble) may lower blood cholesterol levels.

The most common types of legumes are beans, peas and lentils. These foods have been used as rich sources of protein since they were cultivated by Greeks, Romans and Egyptians some 9,000 years before Christ. Today, legumes continue to serve as the main source of dietary protein for millions of people throughout the world. Good examples of ethnic dishes that incorporate beans are black beans and rice (Cuba), pasta e fagioli (Italy), chili and refried beans (Mexico), falafel and hummus (Middle East), and dal (India).

Despite the twin virtues of rich nutrition and taste, legumes have yet to take their proper place in our diet. One reason is that people often think beans are fattening, when in fact one-half cup of cooked beans (such as black beans, kidney beans, lentils and lima beans) has only 100 to 200 calories. Another factor is the popular misconception that beans need to be cooked for hours. When purchased dried, beans need to be soaked from 2 to 12 hours before cooking. Cooking time, however, is generally about an hour. Lentils, split peas and black-eyed peas cook even more quickly, about 30 to 45 minutes. In addition, once cooked, beans store easily—four to five days in the refrigerator and several months in the freezer. You can also buy canned or frozen beans, which may come already cooked, but watch out for extra sodium. Pouring off the packing liquid and rinsing with fresh water will reduce sodium content, although some vitamins are lost in the process.

The secret to great bean-base recipes is seasoning. Chilies, cumin, tumeric, coriander, oregano, garlic and thyme all draw out the flavor in beans. Some good ways to work beans into your fat budget include:

- Substitute pinto beans for ground beef in tacos or burritos.
- Add lentils, split peas or black beans to a hearty soup or stew to make it even heartier.

- Flavor kidney beans with chopped onion, garlic, green pepper, tomatoes and oregano, and serve over rice.
- Add navy, kidney and garbanzo beans to salads.
- Try hummus, made of cooked chickpeas and ground sesame seeds seasoned with lemon juice, garlic and olive oil, as a dip for pita bread and vegetables.

A LAST WORD

Fruits, vegetables, whole grains and legumes should be at the center of a healthful diet pattern. High-carbohydrate, high-fiber foods are nutritious, low in calories and fat, and high in satisfaction. They are an aid to weight control and contribute to reduced risk of heart disease and cancer. Remember:

- High-carbohydrate foods are very low in fat. They will not break your fat budget.
- It is recommended that the diet contain 25 to 30 grams of fiber daily. Complex carbohydrates are the premium sources.
- Eat five fruits and vegetables (two and a half cups) daily. Look for vegetables with deep color.
- The best bread is 100% whole grain.
- Watch out for added sugar in cold cereals. Check labels for "sucrose and other sugars"—4 grams equals a teaspoon of sugar.
- Potatoes and rice are not fattening, but added fat makes them so.
- Think pasta! This versatile, tasty food can be served in soups, as a salad and as a main dish. Pasta is very low in fat calories and high in complex carbohydrates. Best choices for sauce include marinara, vegetable and red sauce with fish and shellfish.
- Add beans, peas and lentils to your diet. They are a rich source of protein and fiber, yet contain no more calories than red meat and none of the cholesterol or saturated fat.

CHAPTER 12

THE CONVENIENCE FACTOR

Societal changes have created a new market, a population short on time and enamored with convenience, and food producers have designed products to fit that market. The result is an ever widening range of canned, bottled, packaged and frozen foods designed to fit the needs of people on the go. According to the consulting firm of Booz, Allen & Hamilton, prepared convenience foods now represent the fastest-growing segment of the food business. "Times are gone," they state in a report to the grocery industry, "when shopping trips were made to restock the pantry. Sales are declining for foods bought for later preparation, so-called 'inventory' foods such as flour and shortening. Consumers today care more about convenience."

PREPARED FOODS

Many canned and bottled foods are not really new. Libby's Corned Beef Hash, Nally's Chili, Campbell's Tomato Soup and Ragu Spaghetti Sauce have been around for many years. They may seem a bit dated for fast-paced, modern Americans, but they still sell. Prepared soup, for example, is a $2.4 billion-a-year industry.

Other convenience foods are old favorites that have been updated, repackaged and given a new name. Dinty Moore Beef Stew and Chef Boyardee Tic Tac Toe's, for example, no longer come in cans. They are encased within snazzy new high-tech microwavable plastic containers which, like cans, don't need to be refrigerated. Now called "shelf-stable" products, they are packaged to look like frozen foods. In less than five years, "shelf-stable" products have grown into a $200 million market. Who is buying them? According to the Center for Science in the Public Interest, it's a mixture of canned-food fans who like two-to-three-minute preparation times, parents who want something their kids can throw into the microwave after school, and people who think they're getting frozen meals that don't need to be refrigerated.

The segment of convenience foods with the most phenomenal growth is frozen meals. As America has moved from a society that cooks to one that reheats, sales of frozen meals have soared. The first reason for their popularity is, obviously, convenience. In this microwave age, frozen meals are quickly and easily heated. Even children can prepare them in minutes. Second, frozen meals have been repackaged and redesigned to shuck their TV dinner image. With upscale choices like Stouffer's Chicken à L'Orange with Almond Rice and Armour's Steak Diane, the frozen meals of today have distanced themselves from the TV dinners of the 1950s. And third, frozen meals are cashing in on America's fascination with perpetual dieting. For many people trying to lose weight, "light" or "lean" frozen meals seem to provide a means to control calories.

No two ways about it, convenience foods live up to their name. But are they healthful? And more specifically, are they low in fat?

The answers depend on the food involved.

The Importance of Labels

Confusing and misleading information often makes it very difficult to ascertain the true fat content of convenience foods. "Consumers need to be linguists, scientists and mind-readers to understand food labels," complains Dr. Louis Sullivan, secretary of Health and Human Services. "The grocery store has become a Tower of Babel." The result is that food labels, in theory designed to educate, in reality confuse the consumer. Manufacturers routinely mis-use terms like "light" and "lean," and often arbitrarily reduce "serving size" to provide an illusion of lower calories. It is important to know how to read the nutritional information on food labels, and to use it as a tool to ensure that the product will not break your fat budget. Remember, the goal is to have less than 30% of calories come from fat. As a general rule, this means a frozen meal or entrée should have no more than 3 grams of fat per 100 calories.

The importance of reading labels for information on fat content is illustrated by the vast differences in similar foods:

- One-half cup of Chef Boyardee Regular Tomato Sauce contains 60 calories and one gram of fat; the same amount of Prego Chunky with Sausage and Pepper is 170 calories and 9 grams of fat. Another way to look at this is: Buitoni Red Clam Sauce is 28 calories an ounce; the same amount of Contadina Alfredo Sauce is 322 calories!
- A serving of Impromptu's shelf-stable Lite Chicken and Vegetables is just 200 calories and one gram of fat. You might expect this of chicken, but what about fish, another healthful choice? Not if you select Top Shelf's Lemon Cod. One serving provides 400 calories and 19 grams of fat.
- Ten ounces of Campbell's Chicken Noodle Soup contains 88 calories and 3 grams of fat. At the other end of the spectrum is Campbell's Chunky Chicken Mushroom Soup with 304 calories and 24 grams of fat.

Like any other food, frozen meals can fit into your fat budget. However, reading labels for nutritional data is essential if you are to make an informed choice. Do not rely on advertising claims. Many "lean" frozen meals are called "diet" dinners because of reduced calories, mostly due to smaller portion size. But they are not necessarily low in fat. Weight Watchers Southern Fried Chicken Patty contains only 270 calories but has almost 16 grams of fat; Lean Cuisine Salisbury Steak has 270 calories and 13 grams of fat; Gorton's Light Recipe Shrimp Scampi has 350 calories and weighs in with a whopping 24 grams of fat.

Each of the following frozen dinners is advertised as "light" and "low in calories," and most are, but upon examination it becomes obvious that these claims may have little to do with fat content. Some of the meals meet the low-fat criterion (no more than 3 grams per 100 calories); others do not.

Entrèe	Calories per Serving	Grams of Fat	% of Calories from Fat
Armour Dinner Classics			
Lite Chicken Breast Marsala	270	7	23%
Lite Chicken Cacciatore	240	4	15
Lite Steak Diane	290	9	28
Budget Gourmet Slim Selects			
Chicken-au-Gratin	260	11	38%
Glazed Turkey	270	5	17
Mandarin Chicken	290	6	19
Sirloin of Beef in Herb Sauce	290	12	37
Sirloin Enchilada Ranchero	290	15	47
Healthy Choice			
Chicken and Pasta Divan	310	4	11%
Chicken Oriental	210	1	4
Shrimp Creole	230	2	9
Le Menu			
Lifestyle Chicken Cannelloni	250	5	18%
Lifestyle Veal Marsala	260	6	21

Entrèe	Calories per Serving	Grams of Fat	% of Calories from Fat
Lightstyle Chicken Chow Mein	260	4	14
Lightstyle Herb Roasted Chicken	220	6	25
Mrs. Paul's Light Seafood			
Fish au Gratin	270	9	30%
Fish Dijon	210	9	39
Stouffer's Lean Cuisine			
Chicken à L'Orange with			
Almond Rice	270	5	17%
Chicken Chow Mein with Rice	250	5	18
Filet of Fish Divan	270	9	30
Salisbury Steak (Italian Style)	270	13	43
Vegetables & Pasta Mornay			
with Ham	280	13	42
Weight Watchers			
Beef Fajitas	270	7	23%
Broccoli and Cheese Baked			
Potato	280	7	23
Cheese Enchiladas			
Ranchero	370	22	54
Chopped Beef Steak	280	17	55
Sweet 'n Sour Chicken Tenders	250	2	7

Source: *Environmental Nutrition.*

The message is clear: if you want to know what you're eating, read the nutritional label and not the advertising. A meal can be made low in calories simply by reducing portion size, but this doesn't mean the fat content has been reduced. Theoretically, if you reduced the portion size of a frozen meal of double pork chops enough, it would be "low-calorie"; however, you'd still be eating a high-fat meal.

In addition to identifying legitimately low-fat entrées, consider what you will serve with them. You can increase the fat content of the meal by accompanying a low-fat frozen entrée with high-fat foods. Make smarter choices: fresh fruit as an appetizer or dessert, a salad with low-cal dressing, and a glass of non-fat milk. These items will not add fat to the meal and can help to keep you within your fat budget.

Homemade Convenience

Packaged convenience foods, marketed as time-savers, do not necessarily take less time to prepare than meals from scratch. Indeed, there are many low-fat, healthy meals that can be prepared in 20 minutes or less. Poached or pan-fried scallops, for example, cook in under five minutes. Put them together with rice and a tossed salad, and you have a tasty and nutritious meal in quick-to-fix fashion. Pan-fried chicken breasts take less than 20 minutes to cook, and so do vegetable stir-fries. A little planning ahead can make meals come together more easily. The next time you prepare marinara sauce for pasta, make extra and freeze it. When you want a quick meal, cook the pasta while the sauce is being defrosted and heated. Put together a green salad with vinaigrette or lo-cal dressing, a loaf of Italian bread, and fruit for dessert. In 20 minutes, you have a feast.

If you like the calorie-control aspect of frozen meals, or if you appreciate their convenience but would like to improve food quality, consider making your own frozen meals. They're easy to prepare and provide a multitude of benefits:

- As the person doing the cooking, you can use fresh and low-fat foods to reduce the higher levels of fat, calories and sodium found in many commercial meals.
- You can include foods richer in whole grains and fiber, notoriously lacking in commercial meals, and avoid preservatives and additives.
- You save money by making your own. While commercial frozen dinners may be affordable for a single person or a couple, the cost of feeding an entire family on them would be prohibitive.

The preparation of frozen meals does not require much in the way of equipment. All you need are some freezer bags and/or freezer paper, wire twisters, small aluminum tins, microwave containers (if appropriate), strong tape, and a marking pencil to label your meals (foods, portion size, date frozen and, if you wish, calories). You can put together as many as 10 or more frozen meals in just a few hours. When you want to eat one, it will take no more time to reheat than it does to pop a commercial meal in the oven.

SNACKS

Americans are snacking more than ever. The combined expenditure for two favorite snacks, potato chips and candy, last year topped $2.5 billion. Sales of cakes, pastries, cookies, doughnuts and muffins are up substantially. For many people with "fat tooth" cravings, these snack foods go to the heart of the matter.

Because sugar tends to mask fat in baked goods and candy, people have little concept of the tremendous amount of fat contained in them. One Hostess Apple Danish pastry, for instance, contains 20 grams of fat. That's about one-quarter of the recommended fat content for a 2,500-calorie diet! A single jelly-filled Dunkin' Donut is even worse—22 grams of fat. It doesn't take many snacks like these to maximize your fat intake. Luckily, there are a number of healthy options. Snacking doesn't have to be a dietary disaster.

Make Vegetables and Fruit the Premium Snacks

Fresh fruits and vegetables are high in vitamins, minerals and fiber, and they contain satisfying natural sugars. Many are crunchy and will keep your jaws occupied. They're also low in fat and calories. The fact is, you can have a lot of vegetables for one 365-calorie piece of chocolate cake. Cucumbers, radishes, zucchini, celery, red and green peppers, cauliflower, mushrooms and broccoli are under 10 calories per ounce. They also contain a lot of water, and research shows that many people snack because they're thirsty rather than hungry; they just can't tell the difference between the body's signals for thirst and for hunger. By keeping the body hydrated, vegetables help to control snacking impulses. (This is also an important reason to drink five to eight glasses of water a day.)

Fresh fruits work in much the same way. Their high sugar content provides a satisfying taste without fat. Calorically, fruit is a real bargain. One hundred calories will get you any of the following:

an apple	2 peaches
5 apricots	1 pear
a banana	14 plums
half a cantaloupe	a cup of raspberries
20 cherries	2 cups of strawberries
one grapefruit	2–3 tangerines
29 grapes	10 ounces of watermelon
1–2 oranges	1/5 of a honeydew melon
a nectarine	

This compares well with 100-calorie portions of other snack foods: two-thirds ounce of Planters Roasted Peanuts, two-fifths ounce of Ruffles Regular Potato Chips, a third of a Sara Lee Oat Bran Muffin, one and one-fifth Nabisco Almost-Home Oatmeal Raisin Cookie, or one-third of a piece of Pepperidge Farm Boston Cream Cake.

Popcorn: Fast, Fun and Low in Fat

Popcorn is about as American as apple pie, and it's a whole lot better for you. Prepared in a low-fat manner and not drenched in butter or margarine, popcorn offers a satisfying, low-calorie snack. Air-popped, one cup contains just 27 calories. For a richer taste, use one tablespoon of oil to pop one-half cup of kernels in a covered wok. The oil will provide more flavor yet add only 11 calories per cup to the popcorn. Many acceptable brands of microwave popcorn exist, but you must read labels to identify them. A number of brands have too much added fat, and often coconut oil is used.

Other Low-Fat Choices

A number of other low-fat snacks are available:

Crunchy & Chewy: Pretzels, rice cakes, polenta chips, toasted corn tortillas, Armenian crackerbread, cereals, breadsticks, anisette toast, bagels, ginger snaps, fig bars, plain meringue cookies, animal crackers.

Sweet & Smooth: Fruit sorbet, fruit-flavored gelatin, popsicle, fruit pie filling, non-fat yogurt, non-fat frozen yogurt, skim milk, honey/jelly/jam, angel food cake, cocoa (non-fat milk with non-fat chocolate syrup or powder), dried fruits, fruit juice, ice milk, sherbet, tapioca, hard candy.

Don't Eat It All

What if fruit, popcorn or other low-fat choices just won't satisfy you? You've been dreaming about a chocolate éclair all afternoon, and by golly, you're going to have one. Then by all means have it! Don't deny yourself to the point where you feel deprived, overdose on a forbidden dessert, wreck your fat budget, and then junk your attempt to establish low-fat eating habits. It's better to recognize that "fat tooth" cravings do exist and to satisfy them in a reasonable way. Having a couple of peanut butter cookies or sharing a piece of apple pie with a friend will not break your fat budget if it's done from time to time. But be honest with yourself. "A couple" of cookies isn't license to finish off the entire box. "From time to time" doesn't mean every day or even every other day. It means infrequently. If you do opt for a fatty snack food, plan your other foods accordingly. Don't decide on a slice of cake after a heavy dinner. If you want the cake, eat a lighter dinner to compensate.

Make Smart Choices

A healthful diet allows for occasional treats. Following are a few examples of trade-offs that will help you cut down on fat and calories when you splurge.

| | | Savings | |
		Calories	Grams of Fat
Instead of:	Choose:		
Nabisco Almost-Home Oatmeal Raisin Cookie	Entenmann's Fat-Free Oatmeal Raisin Cookie	31	6
Sara Lee Carrot Cake	Sara Lee Lights Carrot Cake	133	9
Pepperidge Farm Chocolate Supreme Cake	Weight Watchers Chocolate Cake	140	11
Sara Lee French Cheesecake	Sara Lee Lights French Cheesecake	144	15
Hostess Chocolate Cupcake	Hostess Lights Chocolate Cakes	80	4
Pringle's Cheez-ums Chips (1 oz.)	Snyder's Old-Fashioned Pretzels (1 oz.)	70	13
Dunkin' Donuts Blueberry Muffin	Keebler Blueberry Elfin Loaves	93	7

Source: Individual food companies.

A LAST WORD

Food industry experts estimate that convenience foods now make up more than half of what we eat today. Like it or not, the concept of three squares home-cooked by Mom has virtually disappeared from the scene. Convenience eating can be a disaster for your fat budget, but it doesn't have to be. Remember:

- Know your personal fat budget.
- Convenience foods, particularly frozen and "shelf-stable" meals, are a part of our modern lifestyle. Read their labels for fat content and make smart choices. Don't be taken in by "light" or "low-fat" claims. Balance out your packaged entrée with other low-fat foods to produce a healthful meal.
- Don't trade nutrition for convenience. Look to make homemade foods more convenient. There are many meals that can be made in less than 20 minutes. Or, consider making your own frozen dinners. A little time invested up front will save you much time later on—without sacrificing good nutrition.
- Look for healthy alternatives to fatty snacks: vegetables, fresh fruit, popcorn and low-fat munchies. If you do choose candy or a doughnut, be realistic. The "fat tooth" cannot be controlled when fatty snacks make up much of the diet.

CHAPTER 13

THE RESTAURANT CHALLENGE

I f you cook and eat at home, budgeting the fat in your diet can be simple. At home, you have better control over what you eat, how much you eat, and how it's prepared. But many people today neither cook nor eat at home regularly. This is particularly true of those in the 24-to-42 age group, which one health report categorizes as the "Young and Reckless." This group is generally cognizant of health-related values but makes little effort to practice them. Often, there just isn't time. Their fast-paced lifestyle—which often includes two-income families, long commute times, and even longer hours at work—is designed primarily to juggle an active career and social life. It typically leaves very little time for planning, cooking or even eating meals. This is not the only age group facing such a situation. According to a *USA Today* poll, 54% of adults of all ages say the greatest obstacle to cooking is "lack of time." The most pressed: married couples with kids, of whom 62% cite time pressures.

A good part of the problem is that while women have been free to pursue careers, men have not stepped forward to more fully share domestic responsibilities—particularly those in the kitchen. Indeed, research shows that men and women cook for different reasons. To him, cooking is haute cuisine. To her, it's a family need. He calls it pleasure; she calls it pressure. When asked why they play chef, men say they find it "creative and relaxing" and that they "like to prepare meals for others." Women are driven by practical motives: they cook because they care about good nutrition and balanced meals, and because "everyone has to eat." Most women still feel a sense of responsibility for domestic duties, while men feel chores are optional. Men cook because they want to; women, because they have to.

The upshot, according to a 15-year study on trends in American eating behavior, is that "the American woman has stopped cooking, at least as we've known it in the past. Cooking from scratch has been abandoned. No one has the time. 'Let someone else do the cooking' has become the new battle cry. There is a premium today on foods of convenience, for meals that can be put together quickly and easily, and consumed by different family members at different times. If the current trends continue, the family meal as we have known it could be extinct by the year 2000."

The result has been an increased reliance on restaurant food, including fast food and take-out. Consider this:

- On average, Americans are eating out about three and a half times a week, often spending close to 40% of their food budgets on restaurants.
- There are now over 75,000 fast-food restaurants in the United States.
- The market for take-out has surpassed $60 billion a year.

There is much to criticize about this aspect of the modern diet, but the fact is that convenience eating is now an accepted part of American life. Calling for a roll-back of the clock to the time of Ozzie and Harriet won't work. The answer, then, is not to ignore the world we live in, but to make smarter choices in the face of a lifestyle and culture that promotes fatty eating habits. In essence, the challenge is to eat healthfully in the real world.

FAST-FOOD RESTAURANTS

Fast food, with its tremendous influence on contemporary eating habits, is a good place to start. The availability of fast, filling, inexpensive food is seen as a positive thing by many people. Indeed, most of the adult population of the 1990s has never lived without fast food, so its inclusion in the diet seems natural. No segment of the restaurant industry has benefited more from recent societal changes than fast food. In 1973 there were 21,000 hamburger and 3,500 pizza franchises in operation in the United States. Today those numbers have risen to 35,000 hamburger and 20,000 pizza franchises. It is estimated that more than one-fifth of the American population eats at a fast-food restaurant every day.

It may be tasty and inexpensive, but fast food is not necessarily nutritious. Most contains an inordinate amount of fat, as well as too much sodium, sugar and calories. According to the *New England Journal of Medicine*, a typical fast-food meal gets from 45% to 55% of calories from fat. A Wendy's Triple Cheeseburger, as an example, has 1,040 calories and 68 grams of fat. The amount of fat in this burger is equal to that found in two-thirds of a stick of butter. A Burger King Whopper with Cheese (45 grams of fat) and a McDonald's Big Mac (35 grams of fat) are not much better. A typical meal of a quarter-pound cheeseburger, fries and a shake can have more than 1,000 calories and 50 grams of fat. In other words, this meal eats up more than half the daily fat budget for a moderately active 166-pound man or an active 125-pound woman. With fast food being so fat and eaten so often, it's easy to understand why more than 30% of calories on the U.S. diet come from fat.

While fish and chicken seem like logical lower-fat alternatives, they can be booby-trapped with vast amounts of hidden fat by fast-food cooks. At McDonald's, the Chicken McNuggets and Filet-O-Fish sandwich provide more fat calories than a Quarter-Pounder. The chicken nuggets are "processed"—a combination of ground chicken, chicken skin, salt and additives. Burger King's chicken sandwich with special sauce contains 40 grams of fat, as much as can be found in a heaping cup of hot-fudge topping. Says Connie Roberts, R.N., a dietitian at Brigham and Women's Hospital in Boston, "People are aware of the benefits of chicken and fish. But most are surprised to find that total fat in a single hamburger may be 13 grams, while just six chicken nuggets may have 20 grams. And a fish sandwich, by the time it's coated and has a slice of cheese, is up to 25 grams of fat."

Fast foods are calorically dense because they're rich in fat, and fat has over twice the calories per ounce as carbohydrate and protein. The following examines a variety of fast food in calories per ounce:

Food Item	Total Calories	Calories per Ounce
Kentucky Fried Chicken's Extra Crispy Wing (1.86 oz.)	201	108.1
Dairy Queen's Onion Rings (3 oz.)	280	93.3
Burger King's French Fries, large (4⅛ oz.)	360	87.3
Arby's Turkey De Luxe Sandwich (6 oz.)	510	85.0
McDonald's Big Mac (6.5 oz.)	541	83.3
Arthur Treacher's Fish Sandwich (5.5 oz.)	440	80.0
Taco Bell's Beef Burrito (6.5 oz.)	466	71.8
Wendy's Double Cheeseburger (11.5 oz.)	797	69.6

Even the fast-food items most likely to appeal to nutrition-conscious customers, such as baked potatoes and salad bars, are compromised. By itself, a baked potato is an excellent nutritional food. Even topped with a pat of margarine, it's still a wise choice. But in fast-food restaurants baked potatoes are topped with fatty condiments—bacon and cheese or sour cream, chili and cheese. A Wendy's

Baked Potato with Bacon and Cheese, for instance, has 570 calories and almost 30 grams of fat.

Salad bars fare no better. To be sure, if you stick with lettuce, mushrooms, beets, broccoli, tomato, pepper and cucumber, and you use a moderate amount of dressing, you can put together a meal with under 300 calories. But if you add bacon bits (40 calories per tablespoon), croutons (41 calories per half-cup) and shredded cheese (110 calories per quarter-cup), and a dab of coleslaw, chicken salad, potato salad and macaroni salad made with mayonnaise (each over 200 calories for one-half cup), and a ladle of Thousand Island dressing—you can create a meal in the 1,000 or so calorie range, with most of the calories coming from fat.

You can bury your fat budget at the salad bar with dressing alone. Two packets of McDonald's Thousand Island dressing will make a salad with more calories than a Big Mac.

McDonald's Salad Dressing (1 pkg.)	Total Calories	Grams of Fat	% of Calories from Fat
Peppercorn	400	44	98%
1000 Island	390	38	87
Blue Cheese	350	34	88
Ranch	330	34	94
Caesar	300	31	92
French	230	21	81
Red French	160	8	43
Oriental	100	.5	4
Lite Vinaigrette	60	2	30

Source: McDonald's USA.

A smarter choice is a low-calorie dressing such as Lite Vinaigrette, served on the side. Dip your fork into it before each bite of salad. You'll be amazed at the flavor, yet fat intake will be minimal. Also, be aware that not all prepackaged salads are low in fat. McDonald's Chicken Salad Oriental contains just 3 grams of fat, but their Chef's Salad has 13 grams of fat.

More and more people are starting their day with fast-food breakfasts like McDonald's Egg McMuffin and Burger King's Croissan'wich. In general, these items rate no better than other fast foods. A Burger King Bacon, Egg and Cheese Croissan'wich has 24 grams of fat.

Despite these well-known nutritional pitfalls, of the 66 million Americans who eat at least one meal a day away from home, 33% choose fast food. If you eat fast foods, it's important to make smart choices if you want to stay within your fat budget. This means identifying high-fat items and replacing them with those lower in fat. For example, stay away from the "crispy" or "extra-crispy" coatings, since they generally contain extra fat and salt, and look instead for skinless chicken and fish items that are broiled or charcoal-grilled. In some locations, you can walk into a Kentucky Fried Chicken, Arby's or McDonald's restaurant and order roasted chicken or a grilled, skinless chicken sandwich. Kentucky Fried Chicken's Monterey Broil—marinated, broiled chicken parts—has just 166 calories and 9.9 grams of fat. Long John Silver is serving a baked fish dinner with vegetables. Arthur Treacher's has a five ounce broiled fish sandwich that has only 245 calories and 14 grams of fat. These smart choices may not as yet be universal, but they are a start.

Watch out for fatty "special sauces." Much of the fat in fast food comes from add-on's: mayonnaise, tartar sauce and cheese. The difference between red seafood sauce and creamy tartar sauce on seafood is more than 120 calories and 11 grams of fat. A hamburger with mayonnaise contains 100 extra calories and 11 extra grams of fat.

If you're in the mood for meat, roast beef sandwiches and fajitas (chicken or beef) are almost always leaner than burgers. In some McDonald's locations, a Lean Deluxe quarter-pounder—310 calories and 10.1 grams of fat—is available. As a general rule, however, if you do order a hamburger, order it single and plain. Hold the mayonnaise and "special sauce." Skip the cheese and bacon. Instead, load up on onion, tomato and lettuce.

Pizza can be a good nutritional selection. If you maximize the tomato sauce and vegetable toppings (mushrooms, onions and green peppers are good choices), and moderate the cheese, you get a balance of protein, vitamins and carbohydrates. Two slices of Domino's cheese pizza, for example, contain only 340 calories and 6 grams of fat—certainly not a budget-busting amount.

Mexican fast-food restaurants are another popular alternative with nutritious fare. Bean burritos (not deep-fat fried), tacos and tostadas are made with beans, lettuce, tomato and small amounts of beef or chicken. And most chili contains far less fat than fried chicken or fish.

Smart selections do exist. It is possible to meet or come close to meeting the guidelines for eating fat. According to *HeartCorps* magazine, some of the best choices include:

Food Item	Total Calories	Grams of Fat	% of Calories from Fat
Arby's: Jr. Roast Beef Sandwich	218	9	33%
Burger King Plain Hamburger	275	12	39
Carl's Jr California Roast Beef Sandwich	300	7	21
Domino's Cheese Pizza (12″, 2 slices)	340	6	16
Jack in the Box Chicken Fajita Pita	292	8	25
Long John Silver Broiled Halibut Steak	140	4	26
McDonald's Plain Hamburger	263	11	39
Roy Rogers Roast Beef Sandwich	317	10	28
Wendy's Chicken Sandwich w/Multi-Grain Bread	320	8	28

In the final analysis, fast food does not have to be "fat food." While a steady diet of cheeseburgers, fried chicken and fish, fries and shakes would bankrupt your budget, making smart food choices can keep it balanced.

TRADITIONAL RESTAURANTS

Most sit-down restaurants pose less of a problem. They offer a wider range of food selections than most fast-food restaurants, such as fruit, vegetables; whole-grain breads, broiled chicken and fish. In addition, many are using more healthful cooking methods. Red Lobster, which 10 years ago offered only fried seafood entrées, is now broiling, steaming and baking a large portion of their menu items. Steak & Ale, a chain known for its meat-and-potatoes fare, now offers seafood. Indeed, a number of restaurants even include "heart-healthy" items that conform to American Heart Association guidelines for meals lower in fat and calories. And finally, sit-down restaurants are typically more willing to prepare foods to your specifications: no buttersauce, dressing on the side, skinless chicken, and so forth.

As with fast food, managing your fat budget in a restaurant is a product of sensible food selections.

Plan to stay on your budget.

Don't think of restaurant eating as something distinct from your at-home efforts to control fat. Instead, see it as an extension of those efforts. Understand how eating out fits in with your overall dietary plan. Above all, concentrate on what you can have rather than on what you cannot have. Remember, fatty food doesn't have to happen to you. You can be in control.

Pick a restaurant that serves food you can eat.

If you don't, your options may be limited. A restaurant that specializes in oversize portions of prime rib, for example, spells trouble for your fat budget. Almost all restaurants do have some smart choices. Seafood restaurants generally offer a range of low-fat foods: broiled swordfish, baked salmon, steamed clams. The key is to have seafood cooked and served without butter. In a steak house, order a small piece of London broil, filet mignon or round steak, and ask that no butter be added in broiling. Ask for the fat to be trimmed before cooking. And order a baked potato or rice instead of French fries.

Ethnic restaurants offer a number of options. In Italian restaurants, order pasta with meatless marinara, vegetables or red shellfish sauce. Veal piccata, chicken cacciatore, pizza with cheese and vegetable topping, and scampi sautéed in white wine also rate high for low fat and calorie content. Avoid sausage, cream sauces, garlic bread, pizza with pepperoni and sausage, and too much Parmesan cheese. Whatever the choice for a main dish, it's best to end an Italian meal the way they do in Italy—with fresh fruit or fruit-based ice.

Chinese restaurants feature rice, noodles and vegetables. Choose stir-fried or steamed dishes with chicken, fish and vegetables. Avoid deep-fried and fried items such as pork fried rice, spareribs, egg rolls and pressed duck.

Japanese restaurants offer a vareity of low-fat foods: fish, chicken, seafood, rice, noodles and clear soup. Sauces such as teriyaki and miso are oil-free. Avoid tempura and other deep-fried items, and fried dumplings. Smarter choices include sukiyaki, sushi, sashimi, Japanese vegetables, chicken and fish teriyaki, rice and noodles, and yosenabe, a combination of seafood and vegetables.

Mexican food is naturally high in complex carbohydrates. Unfortunately, in the United States we have learned to add fat to Mexican dishes in the form of sour cream, guacamole, grated cheese and lard. Deep-fried taco chips are high in fat. Avoid beef and bean burritos with cheese, refried beans, nachos, beef enchiladas, chimichangas, and sour cream tacos. Better choices include taco salad with lean beef or chicken, chicken or bean burrito, grilled chicken or fish, chicken fajitas, steamed corn tortillas, and rice. Beans that are not refried in lard are fine. Salsa has sodium but usually no oil.

Look for French restaurants that specialize in the foods of southern France (Provençale), which use wine and olive oil rather than the butter, cream, pork lard, goose fat and eggs featured in northern French cooking. Avoid quiche, duck or goose pâté, fondue, Béarnaise and Hollandaise sauces, croissants, and rich pastry. Smarter choices are poached or broiled fish, salad Niçoise, coq au vin, bouillabaise and fresh fruit.

If a restaurant is new to you, call ahead of time to learn about its menu. That will keep you from being surprised.

Don't plan to overeat.

If you skip meals all day long because you're going out for dinner, you'll arrive at the restaurant famished and will overeat. Eat low-fat meals at breakfast and lunch to compensate for increased fat at dinner, but be sure to eat. You might want to have a glass of skim milk, a piece of fruit, or some non-fat yogurt an hour or two before dinner to take the edge off your hunger. If you're very hungry at the restaurant, order a first course right away: a broth-based soup, steamed or raw seafood, or fresh melon. Stay away from bowls of chips, nuts or fried noodles, or you'll risk using up your fat budget before the entrée arrives. Watch out for alcohol—it doesn't contain fat, but it may make you ravenous and lower your resistance to fatty foods. And finally, don't feel compelled to eat everything just because you paid for it. Enjoy what you eat, but resist the urge to lick your plate clean.

Ask about the menu.

Ask how foods are prepared. Are they broiled? Grilled? Fried? Are fats added—oil, butter, cream, or sour cream? The way to keep salmon from being served in a butter sauce, or chicken Florentine served with skin, or vegetables served under melted cheese, is to tell the server what you want . . . and what you don't want. You, the customer, should have the final say over what you eat. Waiters often appreciate your interest and are willing to ask the cook to make small changes in preparation methods for you.

Make low-fat choices.

Choose fish, shellfish, chicken and veal over steaks and chops. Choose items that are poached, steamed, broiled and roasted. Avoid the creamed, pan-fried and sautéed items, as well as those described as "buttery," "cheesy" or "crispy." Ask that visible fat and/or skin be removed before cooking.

Have sauces and dressings served on the side.

You can taste the chef's special sauce if you wish, but without compromising the meal. Hollandaise has both butter and egg yolks, as does Béarnaise. Mayonnaise has oil and egg yolks. Tartar sauces and remoulade are flavored mayonnaises. Brown sauces such as Bordelaise or Bourguignonne are stock-based and may be lower in fat if they've been skimmed and no butter has been added. Tomato sauces are likely to be less oily. Dishes with Russian names (Stroganoff, Orloff) usually contain butter and sour cream.

Salad dressings, which can add 150 or so calories in two tablespoons, should be kept on the side for good control. Choose vinaigrette over creamy or cheesy dressings. Also, be aware that many restaurants add cheese, bacon bits or butter-fried croutons to salads. Ask your waiter to leave these items off your salad.

Take just a bite of rich desserts.

Fresh fruit is the dessert of choice, but sometimes it just won't do. When your "fat tooth" craving is working overtime, you could eat all the peaches in the world and still have a taste for a piece of creamy cheesecake. So, order the cheesecake—but share it. One piece split among four people gives everyone a taste without doing irreparable damage to your fat budget.

A LAST WORD

Eating out does not mean you have to sacrifice nutrition. Regardless of whether you're at a family favorite down the street or at a four-star restaurant across town, you have an opportunity to make smart choices based on your personal fat budget. Luckily, more low-fat food is showing up on the menu. That's not to say that 12-ounce steaks, asparagus with Hollandaise sauce, or chocolate cake will soon disappear, but it's nice to know that they're not the only foods offered.

To make smart choices in a restaurant, remember:

- Know your personal fat budget.
- Fast foods are fat- and calorie-intensive. Watch out for deep-fried chicken, fish and fries. Don't let salad bars, cheese or "special sauces" increase your fat intake. Best choices include plain hamburgers, vegetable/cheese pizza, tacos and, where available, roasted chicken and broiled fish.
- Choose restaurants that serve food you can eat. Look for tasty, low-fat choices in Italian, Oriental, French, Mexican and seafood restaurants.
- Make smart restaurant decisions. Have all dressings and sauces served on the side. Ask for items to be broiled, grilled, baked or poached but not fried. Stay away from fatty condiments like sour cream. Share desserts—one bite of a rich chocolate cake can provide a great deal of satisfaction.

CHAPTER 14

IN THE FINAL ANALYSIS

B usiness guru Tom Peters tells us that instead of researching and researching, we might be better off to focus on the goal, get off the mark and adapt as we get new information. I think he's right.

In 1977, when I underwent bypass surgery and began to change my diet, the general population wasn't concerned about reducing cholesterol. To be sure, heart disease was the number one killer and cholesterol was identified by medical professionals as the root of the problem, but data were not complete. Cholesterol was still being "researched." While not all the "i's" were dotted or the "t's" crossed on the research, as a heart patient I understood that enough was known about the link between diet and cholesterol to provide a strong rationale for eating prudently. Yet it wasn't until seven years later, when the National Institutes of Health released their study on cholesterol, that dietary changes designed to lower cholesterol began to get national attention.

The point is that we do not always have the luxury of 100%-completed data before making judgments on a prudent way to live. There is still much to be learned about the impact of dietary fat on the risk of disease, the science of food selection, and the mechanics of "fat tooth" cravings. But sufficient information does exist to create a medically approved goal: to restrict dietary fat to less than 30% of total daily calories. If we were to focus on this goal and accomplish it, the impact on our health and appearance would be tremendous.

So, here's what we do know:

1. That the U.S. diet derives about 37% of calories from fat, which is far above the recommended goal. According to the Surgeon General and other health authorities, the overabundance of fat provided by our national diet bears much responsibility for an epidemic of diet-induced diseases and conditions, especially cardiovascular disease, certain cancers, obesity and high blood pressure.

2. That dietary habits have not changed dramatically over the last two decades. USDA studies show a reduction in some obvious sources of fat, particularly artery-clogging saturated fat (red meat, whole milk), yet other sources have taken their place (fast food, frozen meals, cheese, snack food). The net result has been to exchange one group of fatty foods for another.

3. That the attractiveness of fatty foods is in part due to the "fat tooth," a physiological predilection for fat determined by brain chemistry. Although many of us mistakenly link the desire for ice cream, chocolate and pastries to a "sweet tooth," in actuality we may be craving fat.

4. That the pace of modern living, coupled with societal changes, has created an environment that fosters high-fat eating habits. In trading nutrition for convenience, many people simply eat what is quick, easy and available. This has caused fast food, frozen meals, take-out and snacks to become staples of the U.S. diet.

We know much about the problem, high-fat eating habits, but we also know some things about the solution. Studies have shown that regular exercise may offset "fat tooth" cravings at the brain chemistry level. In addition to improving cholesterol, burning body fat, conditioning muscles and dissipating stress, the impact of exercise on eating habits is another reason to be physically active.

We also know that management techniques can help to manage fat intake. None is more important than a personal fat budget. Once you've established your ideal weight and level of physical activity, and know the calories needed to maintain that weight and activity, it's easy to determine your budget.

SUGGESTED DAILY FAT INTAKE

Total Daily Calories	30% of Calories from Fat Expressed as:	
	Fat-Calories	Grams of Fat
1,000	300	33
1,200	360	40
1,500	450	50
1,800	540	60
2,000	600	67
2,500	750	83
3,000	900	100

Your personal fat budget is a criterion against which to measure your food choices. You can "spend" your budget any way you want. No food is "good" or "bad." Just stay within your budget, and you'll automatically be within the guidelines for good health.

And, most important, we know that small dietary changes in the form of smarter choices can produce nutritional fitness. Made gradually over time, these changes can be simple and painless. A study published in *Archives of Internal Medicine* showed that 184 women aged 45 to 69 successfully cut their fat intake in half (from 40% to 20%) and kept it there for at least two years simply by eating ordinary foods but making smarter choices:

- Choosing leaner cuts of beef, trimming fat and stretching portions.
- Choosing skinless white-meat poultry breast, fish and shellfish as primary sources of animal protein.
- Avoiding fried foods; using nonstick pans; employing fat-

reducing cooking methods, such as broiling, grilling, roasting, steaming and poaching, and de-fatting soups by skimming fat.

- Choosing non-fat or low-fat dairy products over those made with whole milk (non-fat for whole milk, non-fat yogurt for sour cream, low-fat over full-fat cheese).
- Reducing all fats and oils in cooking and at the table. This reduction includes not only fats harmful to cardiovascular health (butter, lard) but those that do not penalize (olive, canola, safflower oils). The key concept is a reduction of *all* fat.
- Centering the diet around high-carbohydrate, fiber-rich, low-fat foods: dark green and orange vegetables and fruits, whole-grain cereals and breads, pasta, brown rice, barley, potatoes and beans. Not adulterating these foods with fatty sauces or condiments.
- Making smart choices in restaurants, such as a lean roast beef sandwich over a triple cheeseburger in fatty "special sauce."
- Making smart choices with convenience foods; comparing the labels on similar "lite" frozen meals to find out which are lower in fat.
- Knowing how to read food labels to understand true fat content; knowing how to judge legitimately low-fat packaged foods: no more than 3 grams of fat per 100 calories.
- Understanding that it is not the fat content of any one food that is of greatest importance, but how all foods chosen go together to produce a meal (and a day) in which fat constitutes less than 30% of total calories.

We know enough today to understand that a diet low in fat, high in carbohydrates, nutrient-dense, calcium-rich, full of fiber, and big on fish and poultry is one that will improve health, vitality and appearance. And we also know that a diet encompassing these elements can be achieved through smart choices. Barbara Posner, R.D., Dr./P.H., director of nutrition for the Framingham Study, sums it up succinctly:

"Being smart about food choices doesn't just make a change, it makes a difference."

A BALANCED DIET

The aim of a balanced diet is to reduce elements that can be harmful in excess, such as fat, saturated fat, sugar and sodium, and to eat a variety of tasty foods so that normal weight and health are maintained. Such a diet should be established in accord with nutritional recommendations based on scientific knowledge. In 1990 a special report entitled "The Healthy American Diet," a consensus on dietary guidelines for all healthy Americans over the age of two, was presented by 10 major voluntary and governmental health agencies: the American Heart Association, American Academy of Pediatrics, American Cancer Society, American Diabetes Association, American Dietetic Association, U.S. Centers for Disease Control, National Cancer Institute, National Heart, Lung and Blood Institute, and the U.S. Departments of Agriculture and Health and Human Services. The guidelines included:

- Eat a nutritionally adequate diet consisting of a variety of foods.
- Reduce the consumption of fat to no more than 30% of daily calories. Daily intake of cholesterol should be no more than 300 milligrams.
- Achieve and maintain a reasonable body weight.
- Increase the consumption of complex carbohydrates and fiber.
- Reduce intake of sodium.
- Consume alcohol in moderation, if at all.

According to Dr. Alan Chiat, chairman of the American Heart Association's Nutrition Commission and professor of medicine at the University of Washington, these six concepts deal with nutritional needs and with reducing the risk of heart disease, cancer, stroke and diabetes.

COOKBOOK

COMMENTS FROM THE COOK

by Bernie Piscatella

It's one thing to understand the basic principles involved in low-fat eating. But it's quite another to make those principles work in real life. My first understanding of this hard fact came when Joe returned home from the hospital after open-heart surgery. The first meal we shared was lunch—a tuna sandwich. In the past, it would have contained a lot of mayonnaise as well as pickles and olives. But now I was so paranoid about eating healthfully that the tuna contained no mayonnaise, yogurt, or any fat whatsoever, and the bread—purchased at a health food store—was so full of grains and seeds that it was barely chewable. It was healthful, all right. Direct as always, Joe's comment was: "Look, Bernie, I might have survived the surgery, but I don't think I'll survive this lunch."

This was an early demonstration to us both of the importance of "quality of life" issues as part of a healthy diet. To be sure, we wanted (indeed, needed) to eat healthfully, but we also wanted to eat food that looked appetizing, tasted good and didn't take three hours to prepare. In addition, I had no desire to turn the kitchen into a chemistry lab where every morsel of food had to be weighed and analyzed.

It was then that I decided to become less rigid, to rely less on lists of "good" and "bad" foods, and to spend more time and energy modifying my own recipes to combine good taste and good health. And to do it within a reasonable time. I found that by making smarter choices I could prepare foods that the entire family enjoyed, yet ones that conformed to our low-fat needs. It certainly wasn't a "diet"; it was a new way of eating for a lifetime.

Many of my recipes are found in our two previous books, *Don't Eat Your Heart Out Cookbook* and *Choices for a Healthy Heart*. There are more than 220 new recipes in

Controlling Your Fat Tooth. I have tried to make them meet the following three criteria.

1. The recipes taste and look good, and provide variety. They range from Taco Pizza, Grilled Chicken with Salsa, and Roasted Cajun Turkey to Sea Bass with Shrimp and Seafood Primavera. There are soups, salads, side dishes and even a variety of desserts to satisfy your "fat tooth."

2. The recipes are low in fat. Each recipe uses low-fat ingredients and fat-reduced cooking methods. In addition, each provides a nutritional analysis covering fat, cholesterol and fiber. Fat is given both in grams and as a percentage of calories so that you'll know how the recipe fits into your personal fat budget.

3. The recipes are designed to work in the real world. The vast majority of the recipes are quickly and easily prepared. They offer a flexibility that conforms to modern needs. The key to making them work is planning.

Often, eating healthfully requires a change in habits and menus. It is vitally important to spend a few minutes each week making a meal plan. Take into account the menu, the drinks, the company, and preparation time. We use a weekly format as a guide: pasta on Monday, seafood on Tuesday, main-meal salads on Wednesday, and so forth.

If you plan to have Black Bean Soup as a main meal on Tuesday, for example, be sure to prepare the broth on Saturday or Sunday to allow the fat time to congeal so it can be easily skimmed off. If the beans need to be soaked overnight, remember to do that on Monday. Being organized and planning ahead will actually save time in the end and make cooking and eating healthfully more realistic.

It also helps to have back-up plans for meals that you know can be prepared quickly. If, for example, you remember while at work that you've forgotten to take the meat out of the freezer for dinner, your alternative could be Clam and Black Bean Chowder. With preplanning, most of the ingredients are easy to have on hand. Served with a green salad and a loaf of French bread, it offers a simple alternative and is much more healthful than picking up fast food, take-out or hot dogs.

When planning meals, it's important to be realistic about the needs of each family member. We do not all need the same amount of food. For example, my daughter and I are always watching calories. A main-dish salad such as Two-Salsa Pasta Salad is perfect for us. We can eat a good serving of it, particularly if we limit the dressing. Joe needs more calories, so he will eat a bigger serving. But our teenage son, who comes home from football practice in a ravenous state, will eat several bowls and then ask, "What's for dinner?" For him, I'll need to have on hand a small chicken or turkey breast that is quick to fix, perhaps a taco or taco salad that is left over from the night before, or just a sandwich. The point is that his needs are different from mine. He doesn't want to eat what I do, and I couldn't eat what he does. With flexible meal planning, each family member's needs can be met.

And finally, if you slip and overeat or eat too much fat, don't worry about it. Just get back on track right away. It's the little changes made over time that add up to healthier lifestyle habits. Remember, food is fun. If you approach fat budgeting with a "doom and gloom" attitude, your good intentions aren't likely to last.

Low-fat eating does not have to be boring or tasteless, and sticking to a low-fat diet does not have to take a test of willpower. The suggestions, recipes and information in this book will help give you the tools to manage your fat budget without sacrificing taste or enjoyment.

NUTRITIONAL CONTENT ANALYSIS

A nutritional analysis is provided for each recipe on a per-serving basis. The analysis includes: total calories;

grams of fat; percentage of calories from fat; grams of protein, carbohydrates and dietary fiber; and milligrams of cholesterol and sodium.

For the sake of consistency and clarity, certain decisions were made concerning the analyses:

- When a range is given for an ingredient, the midpoint amount is analyzed.
- When the ingredient listing gives one or more options, the first ingredient listed is the one analyzed.
- Figures are rounded off to whole numbers, so there may be slight discrepancies between an analysis for a whole meal and the sum of its parts.
- Fat grams are rounded off to whole numbers, so there may be slight discrepancies in the percentage of calories from fat.
- In many cases, salads and dressings are analyzed separately. The amount of dressing, which is an individual choice, can greatly change the calories and the fat content of a salad.
- Recipes that call for chicken or beef stock or broth are analyzed based on homemade. Commercially prepared broth is quicker but is much higher in sodium.
- Some recipes are so low in calories that even a trace of fat causes a high fat percentage. These have been identified with a notation. Do not be overconcerned with the fat content.
- In recipes calling for oil-based marinades, only ½ or ¼ of the marinade was used in the nutritional analysis if the marinade is drained off before cooking. It's important always to drain off the marinade thoroughly.

The menus and recipes are designed to ensure that meals fall within the American Heart Association's guidelines for fat, cholesterol and sodium. Sometimes a single recipe may exceed the fat guideline—no more than 30% of calories from fat—but the whole meal is in line when other foods are included for nutritional balance.

Every effort has been made to ensure the accuracy of nutritional data information; however, we cannot guarantee its suitability for specific, medically imposed diets. People with special dietary needs should consult with their physician and dietitian.

Recipes have been analyzed for nutritional content using Nutritionist III by N-Squared Computing. The primary sources of values used in Nutritionist III computerized data base are (in order from most usage to least usage):

1. *Agriculture Handbooks* #8-1 through #8-21. USDA, 1977–1989.

2. *Nutritive Value of American Foods in Common Units* (Handbook 456). USDA, 1975.

3. *Provisional Table on the Nutrient Content of Bakery Foods and Related Items.* USDA, May 1981.

4. *Nutrient Content of Beverages.* USDA, September 1982.

5. *Provisional Table on the Nutrient Content of Frozen and Canned Vegetables.* USDA, April 1979.

6. *Table of Amino Acids in Fruits and Vegetables.* USDA, May 1983.

7. *Vitamin E Content of Foods.* USDA, December 1979.

8. *Folacin in Selected Foods.* USDA, December 1979.

9. *Recommended Dietary Allowances,* Tenth Edition. National Research Council, 1989.

10. *Food Values of Portions Commonly Used,* Fourteenth Edition. Bowes & Church, 1985.

11. *The Dictionary of Sodium, Fats, and Cholesterol* by Barbara Kraus. Grosset & Dunlap, 1974.

12. *The Complete Book of Food Counts.* Dell Publishing, 1988.

13. *Margo Feiden's The Calorie Factor: The Dieter's Companion.* Simon & Schuster, 1989.

NOTES ON INGREDIENTS

All the ingredients described below are available in most supermarkets. Often, it's a case of knowing where to look: some foods, such as whole spears of small baby corn, can be found in the Oriental section with the water chestnuts and soy sauce. In the gourmet or international food sections, you may find Oriental noodles and rice, Mexican pure ground chili powder, and various spices and flavorings. Check spices and condiments, canned goods, rice, grains and frozen-food sections. If you don't find what you're looking for, ask the manager to order it.

For a delightful adventure, familiarize yourself with Oriental, Italian and other ethnic markets in your area, as well as gourmet and health food stores.

ARROWROOT

is a delicate thickener for sauces and gravies. It's neutral in flavor and does not mask or alter natural flavors. Because it reaches maximum thickening power before boiling, it produces very clear sauces and gravies. Use 2 teaspoons arrowroot in place of 1 tablespoon cornstarch. Use 1½ teaspoons arrowroot in place of 1 tablespoon flour. Combine arrowroot with 2 tablespoons cold water. Gradually add to hot sauces, soups or gravies to thicken.

ARTICHOKE HEARTS

are available packed in water or oil. Unless otherwise stated, all recipes in this book refer to those packed in water. The water must be drained before use. In recipes specifically calling for artichokes marinated in oil, look for brands packed in nonhydrogenated, unsaturated oils such as soy bean oil or safflower oil.

BABY CORN (WHOLE SPEARS)

is miniature ears of corn that are canned in water. Look for it in the Oriental section of the supermarket.

BEANS

used in these recipes are usually canned beans. Home-cooked dried beans are preferable, but canned can be used to shorten cooking time. Progresso makes a heart-healthy canned black bean, as well as a cannellini bean and kidney bean. Canned beans tend to be higher in sodium than home-cooked beans, so watch the sodium intake in the other foods consumed throughout the day. Rinsing canned beans will reduce their sodium content by one-half.

BEAN CURD or TOFU

is available in the produce section of most supermarkets. This high-protein, low-calorie, no-cholesterol product, made from the milk of puréed soybeans, is best in stir-fried dishes and in soups.

BREADS

should be whole-wheat and whole-grain whenever possible. There are several recipes in this book for homemade bread. Once you make bread a few times, it's easy—and the smell of bread baking in the kitchen makes it worth the effort. Try it on a Saturday or Sunday, when you may have more time. During the week, use shortcuts; for example, for the Cheese-and-Herb or Cajun Flatbreads, use a prepared heart-healthy pizza crust (some pizza parlors sell their crusts). Another shortcut is to use a heart-healthy frozen dough, as in the recipe for Hot Cross Buns.

BROTH or STOCK

(whether chicken, beef or fish) will have the maximum flavor and quality when it's homemade and then reduced by one-third (see stock recipes). Commercially canned stock or broth can be substituted for homemade broth or stock in most recipes and is convenient to have on hand. Be sure to refrigerate it overnight or place it in the freezer for 30 minutes. The fat will congeal and rise to the top, and can then be skimmed. Remember: using commercially prepared broth instead of homemade will increase the milligrams of sodium.

GRAINS AND RICE

ALA is a cracked-wheat bulgar available in the rice or gourmet section of most supermarkets.

COUSCOUS, a wheat grain, is a delicious alternative to rice. It's available in the rice or gourmet section of most supermarkets.

ORIENTAL-STYLE RICE is the long- or short-grain, sticky type of white rice that is served in Chinese restaurants. Look for it in Oriental markets or in the Oriental section of the supermarket.

HERBS AND SPICES

Fresh herbs and spices are much more flavorful than dried. Substitute three parts fresh for one part dried.

BASIL should be used fresh whenever possible; the flavor is markedly superior to dried. Fresh basil is now often available in produce markets year round. Preserve fresh basil by standing the stems, with roots intact, in a jar of water; loosely cover the leaves with a plastic bag. Store in refrigerator.

CHILIES are available in many supermarkets and in Spanish and Mexican markets. Although the flavor may not be quite the same, any mild fresh chilies or canned jalapeño peppers can be substituted for serrano.

Negro, ancho, poblano, pasilla and mulatto are available in many supermarkets and Spanish or Mexican markets. Although the flavor will be slightly different, any hot dried chilies may be substituted. The same is true for Anaheim chilies, which are also called New Mexico, Texas, California, Colorado, guajillo, long red or long green chilies.

Arbol, chimayo, Thai or bird chilies are also hot.

CHILI POWDER, for maximum flavor, should be made from (and labeled) pure ground chili powder. Take the time to search for a Spanish or Mexican market or a supermarket that carries pure ground chili powder. Pure ground chili powder is made by grinding dried chilies, and the flavor is far superior to that of commercial chili powder, which is most often 40% salt and 20% additives. It comes in mild, medium-hot and hot.

CRUSHED RED PEPPERS are especially good as a topping for pasta dishes. They're available in the spice section of most supermarkets.

GINGERROOT adds a distinctive, spicy flavor to many Chinese dishes. It's especially good on chicken and fish. To use, peel the tan skin and thinly slice the root. To obtain ginger juice, peel the gingerroot and grate the root with a fine grater; squeeze the pulp to extract the juice. Look for gingerroot in the produce section of most supermarkets.

LEMON JUICE is most flavorful when it's freshly squeezed. For maximum quality, do not substitute bottled juice or lemon extract in recipes calling for lemon juice.

REDUCED-SODIUM SOY SAUCE contains 46% less sodium than regular soy sauce, with little or no difference in flavor. Reduced-sodium soy sauce has 80 milligrams of sodium per ½ teaspoon. By comparison, ½ teaspoon of salt has 1,150 milligrams of sodium.

SALT content in these recipes is for those just beginning to change to a healthier eating pattern. The goal should be to reduce the amount of salt gradually, first by one-fourth and then, when taste buds are ready, by one-half.

SAFFRON, made from the dried stigmas of a type of crocus, adds both color and flavor. A small amount goes a long way. The most costly of all seasonings, it's available in the spice section or gourmet section of most supermarkets.

WASABI (JAPANESE HORSERADISH) comes in a tube or little can and is available in Oriental markets or in the Oriental section of most supermarkets.

NOODLES

BUCKWHEAT (CHUKA SOBA) NOODLES are curly noodles made with wheat flour. They're available in Oriental markets and in the Oriental section of most supermarkets.

MAIFUN BEAN NOODLES or CELLOPHANE NOODLES are dry, thin, transparent noodles. You'll find them in Oriental markets and in the Oriental section of most supermarkets.

PASTA can differ greatly in quality among brands. It's important to use the best pasta available, since the quality of the meal is only as good as the quality of the pasta. Many supermarkets and Italian markets offer high-quality imported and domestic brands. (*Al dente* is an Italian term meaning "firm to the tooth." Pasta or vegetables cooked *al dente* should be just barely tender.)

OILS

Of the monounsaturated oils, olive and canola oils are the most highly recommended.

CANOLA OIL, the lowest in saturated fat, has a light taste and is particularly good in recipes calling for butter, margarine or lard.

OLIVE OIL ranges from mild-flavored to rich-flavored. Use a lighter variety for cooking and a stronger one for salads. The finest quality, labeled "extra-virgin" or "virgin," has a more intense flavor, so the amount of oil can be reduced. Remember: light olive oil has no less fat or fewer calories than regular olive oil.

Of the polyunsaturated oils, safflower oil is the most unsaturated, followed in order by soybean, sunflower, corn, cottonseed and sesame.

SESAME OIL is made from toasted sesame seeds. It's available in Oriental markets and in the Oriental section of most supermarkets.

CHILI OIL (LA YU) is oil flavored with red hot peppers. It can be found in Oriental markets and in large supermarkets.

MARGARINE made from safflower or corn oil is a good choice. Tub-style is the best. Stick margarine, which has been hardened or hydrogenated, contains cholesterol-raising trans fatty acids. Diet margarines made with water are lower in fat and calories.

SAFFLOWER MAYONNAISE is mayonnaise made with unsaturated safflower oil. Mayonnaise is high in calories, and most of the calories are from fat, so be judicious in its use.

PARMESAN CHEESE

should be used only sparingly. Avoid the preground, packaged variety, which is very expensive and almost flavorless. Buy a small wedge of fresh Parmesan and grate as needed. Or have the delicatessen or dairyperson freshly grate the amount you need.

PRICKLY PEAR CACTUS LEAVES

(also called nopalitos) are available in many supermarkets or Spanish markets. Although they add to the texture of salads, they are not essential to the flavor.

SHALLOTS

have a delicate garlic flavor. They're available near the garlic and onions in most supermarkets.

SHIITAKE

(dried forest mushrooms) are available in Oriental markets and in the Oriental section of most supermarkets. To reconstitute the dried mushrooms, soak them in enough water to cover for about 30 minutes, or until soft. Drain. Squeeze out excess water. Remove and discard stems.

TOMATOES

ITALIAN PLUM TOMATOES, CANNED, are the best substitute for fresh or home-canned tomatoes. It's important to buy the best available. Progresso Plum Tomatoes and S&W Pear

Tomatoes are especially good, as are many of the imported brands. The better the grade, the more flavorful the sauce. For recipes in this book that call for diced plum tomatoes, buy the whole plum tomatoes and dice them yourself.

TOMATILLOS are Mexican-style green tomatoes. They are available fresh and canned in many supermarkets or Spanish markets.

TOMATO SAUCE, TOMATO PURÉE and TOMATO PASTE should be of the highest grade available. Progresso and Contadina are among the best. Freeze any leftover paste by the tablespoonful on a sheet of waxed paper. Once frozen, remove to a plastic freezer bag and store in the freezer for later use.

TORTILLAS

are available in flour and corn. Always buy flour tortillas that are made with soy bean oil, not with lard. Corn tortillas generally do not contain oil or shortening, so they're more heart-healthy and lower in calories.

VINEGARS

BALSAMIC VINEGAR has a mellow, sweet-and-sour flavor. Good on salads, cold chicken and fish, or drizzled over warm vegetables, it's found in the gourmet section of most supermarkets.

RICE VINEGAR is a mild vinegar made from fermented rice. It's available in the Oriental section of most supermarkets.

WHITE ONIONS

(sometimes called Bermuda onions or Walla Walla sweet onions) are the best onions for salads and sandwiches.

WONTON or SPRING ROLL WRAPPERS

are a quick and easy way to prepare tortellini and ravioli. (I think the quality is equal to those made with homemade pasta.) Look for them in Oriental markets and in the gourmet frozen-food sections of the supermarket.

SOUPS & STEWS

BLACK BEAN SOUP

Makes 10 cups

4 cups Chicken Broth (page 272) or canned broth*
6 cloves garlic
1 medium onion, chopped
1 cup chopped celery
1 teaspoon ground coriander
¼ teaspoon ground red pepper
¼ teaspoon salt
3 15-ounce cans black beans, drained**

In a medium stockpot, simmer chicken broth, garlic, onion, celery and seasonings 1 hour. In a blender or food processor, purée 1 can of the black beans; add to stockpot. Stir in remaining 2 cans of beans and heat through.

*Canned broth is higher in sodium.
**Rinsing will reduce sodium in canned beans by half.
VARIATION: Add 1 cup cooked elbow macaroni or shell-shaped pasta.

APPROXIMATE NUTRITIONAL CONTENT PER CUP

Total calories: 125
Fat: 1 g
Percentage of calories from fat: 7%

Carbohydrates: 20 g
Protein: 9 g
Cholesterol: Tr
Sodium: 696 mg
Dietary fiber: 4 g

PASTA-AND-BEAN SOUP

Makes 12 cups

1 28-ounce can Italian plum tomatoes, diced
1 cup Snappy Tom or Mr. & Mrs. T Bloody
   Mary Mix
1 cup Beef Stock (page 268) or canned broth*
1 tablespoon freshly squeezed lemon juice
5 cloves garlic
½ cup chopped white onion
½ teaspoon ground cumin
½ teaspoon Tabasco sauce
½ teaspoon crushed basil
2 15-ounce cans cannellini beans,** drained, or
   3 cups cooked white kidney beans
1 cup chopped green pepper
2 cups cooked elbow macaroni

In a small stockpot, combine tomatoes, Snappy Tom, beef stock, lemon juice, garlic, onion, cumin, Tabasco and basil. Heat just to boiling, then reduce heat and simmer 25 minutes. Stir in beans and green pepper, and simmer 10 minutes. Add macaroni and heat through.

*Canned broth is higher in sodium.

**Rinsing will reduce sodium in canned beans by half.

SERVING SUGGESTION: Serve with Italian Bread (page 276) and Lemon Meringue Pie (page 476).

APPROXIMATE NUTRITIONAL CONTENT PER CUP

Total calories: 98	Carbohydrates: 18 g
Fat: 1 g	Protein: 5 g
Percentage of calories from fat:	Cholesterol: Tr
9%	Sodium: 523 mg
	Dietary fiber: 1 g

CLAM AND BLACK BEAN CHOWDER

Makes 14 cups

1	teaspoon olive oil
1	cup chopped white onion
1	cup chopped celery
1	28-ounce can Italian plum tomatoes
1	6-ounce can V-8 juice
3	6 ½-ounce cans chopped clams with liquid
1 ½	pounds potatoes, cubed and steamed or microwaved until crisp-tender
½	teaspoon Worcestershire sauce
1	15-ounce can black beans, drained*
¼	teaspoon salt (optional)
¼	teaspoon black pepper

In a nonstick pan, heat olive oil; add onions and celery, and sauté 8–10 minutes or until tender. Purée tomatoes in a blender or food processor. Combine all ingredients in a medium stockpot. Simmer 20 minutes.

*Rinsing will reduce sodium in canned beans by half.

NOTE: This is a great last-minute lunch or light supper, easy to prepare and using ingredients that often are on hand.

VARIATION: Omit the beans for a delicious, quick-to-fix clam chowder.

SERVING SUGGESTION: Particularly good with Seafood Salad (page 315), Italian Pizza Bread with Garlic and Rosemary (page 280) and fresh fruit.

APPROXIMATE NUTRITIONAL CONTENT PER CUP

Total calories: 106	Carbohydrates: 19 g
Fat: 1 g	Protein: 6 g
Percentage of calories from fat:	Cholesterol: 24 mg
9%	Sodium: 304 mg
	Dietary fiber: 2 g

BEAN AND TOMATO SOUP

Makes 14 cups

2   teaspoons olive oil
1   onion, sliced
2   cloves garlic, minced
2   15-ounce cans cannellini beans
3   large ripe tomatoes, diced
1   28-ounce can Italian plum tomatoes, diced
2   cups Beef Stock (page 268) or canned broth*
1   15-ounce can black beans, drained
1   teaspoon salt or to taste
½   teaspoon black pepper
4   cups cooked cavatelli or other shell-shaped pasta

In a nonstick skillet, heat olive oil; add onion and garlic, and sauté 4–5 minutes or until onion is tender. Add 1 can cannellini beans with liquid, and diced ripe tomatoes; simmer 5 minutes. Pour into a medium stockpot. Add diced plum tomatoes and simmer.

Drain remaining can of cannellini beans and purée beans in a blender or food processor; add to stockpot. Add beef stock, black beans, salt and pepper; simmer 4–5 minutes. Add pasta and heat through.

*Canned broth is higher in sodium.

SERVING SUGGESTION: Serve for lunch or light supper with Pan Rolls (page 295) and Baked Apples (page 495).

APPROXIMATE NUTRITIONAL CONTENT PER CUP

Total calories: 147
Fat: 2 g
Percentage of calories from fat:
   11%

Carbohydrates: 26 g
Protein: 7 g
Cholesterol: Tr
Sodium: 548 mg
Dietary fiber: 2 g

LENTIL SOUP

Makes 14 cups

> 8 cups Bean Soup Stock (page 269)
> 1 6-ounce can tomato paste
> 2 medium carrots, diced
> 1 large potato, diced
> 1 large onion, chopped
> 3 cloves garlic, minced
> ¼ teaspoon powdered thyme
> 1 cup lentils
> ¾ teaspoon salt or to taste

In a medium stockpot, bring stock, tomato paste, carrots, potato, onion, garlic and thyme just to boiling. Add lentils and reduce heat. Cover and simmer 1½–2 hours or until lentils are cooked. Season with salt.

VARIATION: Add ½ cup alphabet pasta during last 15 minutes of cooking.

SERVING SUGGESTION: Especially good for lunch on a cold winter day. Serve with Winter Vegetable Salad (page 335). For a fun dessert, try Hot Cross Buns (page 288).

APPROXIMATE NUTRITIONAL CONTENT PER CUP

Total calories: 55
Fat: Tr
Percentage of calories from fat:
  10%

Carbohydrates: 10 g
Protein: 3 g
Cholesterol: 3 mg
Sodium: 591 mg
Dietary fiber: 2 g

BARLEY MUSHROOM SOUP

Makes 12 cups

1　cup pearl barley
3　cups water
8　cups Beef Broth (page 274) or canned broth*
2　teaspoons olive oil
2　cloves garlic, minced
1　onion, coarsely chopped
3　stalks celery
½　pound extra-lean ground round steak
½　pound fresh mushrooms
1　teaspoon Worcestershire sauce
⅛　teaspoon powdered thyme
⅛　teaspoon marjoram
½　teaspoon salt or to taste
¼　teaspoon black pepper

Soak barley in 3 cups water overnight. In a medium stockpot, bring beef broth to a boil; add barley with soaking liquid and cook, covered, about 45 minutes or until barley is tender. Meanwhile, heat olive oil in a nonstick skillet; add garlic and onions, and sauté 5–6 minutes. Add celery and sauté 3–4 minutes. Add ground round and sauté 5–6 minutes. Add mushrooms and sauté 4–5 minutes. When barley is tender, season with Worcestershire sauce, thyme, marjoram, salt and pepper. Stir in beef-onion mixture.

*Canned broth is higher in sodium.

NOTE: This is a hearty, great-tasting soup that can be ready in under an hour after soaking the barley overnight.

APPROXIMATE NUTRITIONAL CONTENT PER CUP

Total calories: 109
Fat: 2 g
Percentage of calories from fat: 17%

Carbohydrates: 15 g
Protein: 7 g
Cholesterol: 11 mg
Sodium: 477 mg
Dietary fiber: 3 g

TWO-MUSHROOM SOUP

Makes 4 servings

    3 cups Chicken Broth (page 272) or canned broth*
    1 6-ounce can straw mushrooms, drained
    1 8-ounce can button mushrooms, drained

In a saucepan, heat chicken broth just to boiling. Stir in mushrooms. Simmer 5 minutes. Ladle into bowls.

    *Canned broth is higher in sodium.

    SERVING SUGGESTION: An easy-to-prepare first course. Good with chicken and fish.

APPROXIMATE NUTRITIONAL CONTENT PER SERVING

Total calories: 48
Fat: 1 g
Percentage of calories from fat:
    19%

Carbohydrates: 4 g
Protein: 5 g
Cholesterol: Tr
Sodium: 486 mg
Dietary fiber: 1 g

STRAW MUSHROOM SOUP WITH GREEN ONION

Makes 4 servings

3 cups Chicken Broth (page 272) or canned broth*
1 6-ounce can straw mushrooms, drained
1 green onion, thinly sliced

In a saucepan, heat chicken broth just to boiling; stir in mushrooms. Simmer 5 minutes. Ladle into bowls. Sprinkle with green onions.

*Canned broth is higher in sodium.

NOTE: This soup has few calories and is an especially quick-to-prepare first course. Good with chicken and fish.

APPROXIMATE NUTRITIONAL CONTENT PER SERVING

Total calories: 38
Fat: 1 g
Percentage of calories from fat:
  24%

Carbohydrates: 2 g
Protein: 4 g
Cholesterol: Tr
Sodium: 486 mg
Dietary fiber: Tr

TORTELLINI-AND-VEGETABLE SOUP

Makes 15 cups

8 cups Chicken Broth (page 272) or canned broth*
1 cup peas, cooked 1–2 minutes
1 cup carrots, cut into julienne strips 1 inch long and cooked 2–3 minutes or just until crisp-tender
1 8-ounce can mushroom stems and pieces, drained
⅔ pound tortellini, cooked *al dente*
½ cup freshly grated Parmesan cheese

In a medium stockpot, bring chicken broth just to boiling. Add peas, carrots, mushrooms and pasta. Ladle into bowls. Sprinkle with Parmesan.

*Canned broth is higher in sodium.

SERVING SUGGESTION: Excellent as a main meal soup. Serve with assorted melons or Fresh Blackberry Pie (see page 478).

APPROXIMATE NUTRITIONAL CONTENT PER CUP

Total calories: 196
Fat: 5 g
Percentage of calories from fat: 22%

Carbohydrates: 20 g
Protein: 17 g
Cholesterol: 46 mg
Sodium: 748 mg
Dietary fiber: 2 g

Using fresh mushrooms in place of canned will reduce sodium by 44 mg per cup.

THE BIG CHILI

Makes 10 servings

½   cup chopped serrano chilies
⅔   cup chopped red onion
⅔   cup chopped green pepper
⅔   cup chopped celery
1   cup chopped leek, white part only
3   cloves garlic, minced
2   tablespoons dried oregano
4   cups Chicken Broth (page 272) or canned broth*
2¼   cups frozen corn, thawed
3   cups cubed uncooked turkey breast
2   tablespoons ground coriander seeds
2½   tablespoons chili powder
1   tablespoon ground cumin
½   teaspoon granulated sugar
½   teaspoon salt or to taste
¼   teaspoon black pepper
¼   cup all-purpose flour
½   cup cold water
3   15-ounce cans red kidney beans,** drained

In a large stockpot, combine chilies, onion, green pepper, celery, leek, garlic, oregano and chicken broth, and simmer 45 minutes or until vegetables are tender.

In a blender or food processor, purée 1¼ cups of the corn. Pour into a medium bowl; add remaining corn, turkey, coriander, chili powder, cumin, sugar, salt and pepper. Set aside.

Bring chicken broth just to boiling. In a jar with cover, combine flour and water; gradually add to chicken broth, stirring constantly until broth begins to thicken. Add corn, turkey and seasonings. Stir in beans. Simmer 15–20 minutes. (Your kitchen will smell terrific.)

*Canned broth is higher in sodium.

**Rinsing will reduce sodium in canned beans by half.

NOTE: Serrano chilies are available in many supermarkets and in Spanish and Mexican markets. Although the flavor won't be quite the same, any mild fresh chilies may be substituted.

VARIATION: Substitute black beans for red beans or use half black beans and half red beans.

SERVING SUGGESTION: Serve with Vegetable Crudités with Tomato and Chili Salsa (page 363), and warm tortillas.

APPROXIMATE NUTRITIONAL CONTENT PER SERVING

Total calories: 282
Fat: 2 g
Percentage of calories from fat:
   7%

Carbohydrates: 35 g
Protein: 32 g
Cholesterol: 57 mg
Sodium: 770 mg
Dietary fiber: 7 g

COUNTRY STEW

Makes 5 servings

2½ cups Chicken Broth (page 272) or canned broth*
 9 cloves garlic
 1 large white onion, cut into 1½-inch strips
 1 large green pepper, cut into 1½-inch strips
 1 large red pepper, cut into 1½-inch strips
 3 Italian plum tomatoes or 1 large ripe tomato, cut
    into 1½-inch strips
 2 teaspoons olive oil
 1 tablespoon fresh lime juice
 2 cups cooked orzo

In a medium stockpot, combine all ingredients except orzo. Simmer 30–40 minutes or until vegetables are just barely tender. Divide orzo among individual soup bowls. Ladle stew over top.

*Canned broth is higher in sodium.

SERVING SUGGESTION: Serve with Black Beans with Vegetables and Shrimp (page 331) and Cheddar Cheese Bread (page 285).

APPROXIMATE NUTRITIONAL CONTENT PER SERVING

Total calories: 142
Fat: 3 g
Percentage of calories from fat:
  20%

Carbohydrates: 23 g
Protein: 6 g
Cholesterol: Tr
Sodium: 281 mg
Dietary fiber: 2 g

SEAFOOD GAZPACHO

Makes 8 cups

    1 28-ounce can Italian plum tomatoes, diced
    1 cup Snappy Tom or Mr. & Mrs. T Bloody
         Mary Mix
    ½ cup peeled and chopped English cucumber
    ⅓ cup chopped green pepper
    ½ cup chopped white onion
    1 cup Beef Broth (page 274) or canned broth*
    1 tablespoon freshly squeezed lemon juice
    2 teaspoons olive oil
    1 tablespoon minced garlic (about 5 whole cloves)
    ½ teaspoon ground cumin
    ½ teaspoon Tabasco sauce
    ½ teaspoon salt
    ½ teaspoon crushed basil
    ½ pound cooked shrimpmeat

In a large glass bowl, combine all the ingredients except shrimp. Chill at least 2 hours. Just before serving, add shrimp.

*Canned broth is higher in sodium.

SERVING SUGGESTION: Serve with Cracked Dungeness Crab (page 364) or smoked or grilled salmon and Napoleon Caesar Salad (page 342).

APPROXIMATE NUTRITIONAL CONTENT PER CUP

Total calories: 76
Fat: 2 g
Percentage of calories from fat:
    23%

Carbohydrates: 8 g
Protein: 8 g
Cholesterol: 55 mg
Sodium: 592 mg
Dietary fiber: 1 g

SOUTHWEST JAMBALAYA

Makes 5 servings

    1 head garlic
    3 fresh Anaheim chilies or 1 large green pepper
    2 sweet yellow wax peppers
    2 large red peppers
    1 quart Chicken Stock (page 264) or canned broth*
    6 cloves garlic, sliced
    ½ fresh jalapeño pepper, seeded, stemmed and
         chopped
    ½ teaspoon black pepper
    ½ teaspoon chili powder
    ¼ teaspoon ground mace
    ⅛ teaspoon cayenne pepper
    ½ pound medium prawns, shelled and deveined
    ½ pound halibut, cut into 2-inch cubes
    2 tablespoons quick-cooking tapioca
    2 cups cooked short-grain white rice
    2 cups cooked rotelle, wagon-wheel or tube-type
         pasta

Wrap garlic head in foil and arrange chilies and yellow and
red peppers in a roasting pan. Broil 2 inches from heat 15–
30 minutes or until skins bubble and char on all sides.
Remove chilies and peppers to a paper bag; close bag and
let cool 15–20 minutes. If garlic head is still firm after
broiling, bake in a 400°F oven until it feels soft when
pressed; set aside.

When cool, pull off and discard stems, skin and seeds of
broiled chilies and peppers. Cut into strips ¼ inch wide.

In a medium stockpot, combine chicken stock, garlic
cloves and jalapeño pepper. Heat just to boiling (do not
boil); reduce heat. Add black pepper, chili powder, mace
and cayenne pepper; simmer 10 minutes. Return just to
boiling; add skinned chilies and peppers, prawns, halibut

and tapioca. Reduce heat and cook 3–4 minutes or until prawns are pink and halibut is just opaque.

Spoon ½ cup rice and ½ cup pasta into each soup bowl. Ladle jambalaya over top.

Pull apart head of roasted garlic. Squeeze garlic from skin into the jambalaya.

*Canned broth is higher in sodium.

NOTE: Anaheim chilies, also called Texas, California, New Mexico, Colorado, guijillo, long red or long green chilies, are usually available in Spanish and Mexican markets and in most supermarkets. Although the flavor will be slightly different, any other fresh hot chilies may be substituted.

VARIATION: Substitute green peppers for yellow peppers, and any medium-hot chilies for Anaheim chilies.

SERVING SUGGESTION: An excellent main meal soup. Serve with crusty French bread for dipping.

APPROXIMATE NUTRITIONAL CONTENT PER SERVING

Total calories: 335
Fat: 4 g
Percentage of calories from fat:
   10%

Carbohydrates: 43 g
Protein: 33 g
Cholesterol: 105 mg
Sodium: 426 mg
Dietary fiber: 2 g

SHRIMP, CHICKEN AND RICE GUMBO

Makes 12 cups

2 cups Beef Broth (page 274) or canned broth*
1 14-ounce can Italian plum tomatoes, diced
1 teaspoon granulated sugar
½ teaspoon powdered thyme
½ teaspoon chili powder
¼ teaspoon black pepper
½ teaspoon crushed red pepper
¼ teaspoon filé powder
2 teaspoons olive oil
4 large cloves garlic, chopped
1 small white onion, coarsely chopped
½ cup coarsely chopped celery
1 small green pepper, coarsely chopped
⅔ pound medium prawns, cooked, shelled and deveined
2 chicken breasts, skinned, boned, poached and cut into cubes
3 cups cooked white rice

In a medium stockpot, combine beef broth, plum tomatoes, sugar, thyme, chili powder, black pepper, crushed red pepper and filé powder. Simmer 10 minutes.

In a nonstick skillet, heat olive oil. Add garlic, onion and celery, and sauté 4–5 minutes or until onions become crisp-tender. Add green pepper and cook 2–3 minutes. Add to stockpot and simmer 10 minutes. Add prawns, chicken and rice.

*Canned broth is higher in sodium.

SERVING SUGGESTION: Excellent as a main course. Serve with crisp vegetables and Hummus (page 349), Cajun Flatbread (page 286) and assorted seasonal fruits.

APPROXIMATE NUTRITIONAL CONTENT PER CUP

Total calories: 142
Fat: 2 g
Percentage of calories from fat:
   13%

Carbohydrates: 13 g
Protein: 16 g
Cholesterol: 72 mg
Sodium: 269 mg
Dietary fiber: 10 g

TOMATO SHRIMP SOUP

Makes 4 servings

4   cups Chicken Broth (page 272) or canned broth*
2   medium tomatoes, coarsely chopped
1   cup English cucumber, peeled, seeded and cut
     into ¼-inch strips
½   cup firm tofu, cut into ¼-inch cubes
½   cup cooked shrimpmeat

In a small stockpot, bring chicken broth just to boiling. Add tomatoes and simmer 2 minutes. Add cucumber, tofu and shrimp, and simmer 1 minute.

   *Canned broth is higher in sodium.

SERVING SUGGESTION: Excellent for a light first course.

APPROXIMATE NUTRITIONAL CONTENT PER SERVING

Total calories: 128
Fat: 5 g
Percentage of calories from fat:
   32%

Carbohydrates: 6 g
Protein: 16 g
Cholesterol: 56 mg
Sodium: 623 mg
Dietary fiber: 1 g

NORTHWEST SEAFOOD CHOWDER

Makes 8 servings

1	10-ounce can tomato purée
1	8-ounce bottle clam juice
¾	cup dry white wine (Soave Bolla is good)
4	cups Chicken Stock (page 264) or canned broth*
2	medium carrots, diced
1	large bay leaf
½	teaspoon crushed red pepper
½	teaspoon basil
½	teaspoon ground coriander
16	clams in their shells
1	tablespoon olive oil
2	medium onions, chopped
4	cloves garlic, chopped
1	large green pepper, seeded and chopped
1	lemon, thinly sliced
½	pound medium prawns, shelled and deveined
½	pound small bay scallops
½	pound halibut, cut into 1-inch cubes
½	pound sea bass, cut into 1-inch cubes
½	pound cavatelli or other shell-shaped pasta, cooked *al dente*
¼	cup chopped fresh parsley

In a medium stockpot, combine tomato purée, clam juice, wine, chicken stock, carrots, bay leaf, red pepper, basil and coriander. Simmer, uncovered, 10 minutes. Add clams, cover and simmer 10–15 minutes.

Meanwhile, in a wok or heavy skillet, heat olive oil and sauté onions and garlic 3–4 minutes or until onions are crisp-tender; add green pepper and sauté 2–3 minutes. Add vegetables to stockpot.

When clams first begin to open, add lemon slices, prawns, scallops, halibut and sea bass. Cover and simmer until prawns turn pink, clams are fully opened and fish are cooked. Add pasta. Ladle into bowls. Garnish with parsley.

*Canned broth is higher in sodium.

VARIATION: Substitute 4 steamed and diced red potatoes for pasta.

SERVING SUGGESTION: A good main meal soup. Serve with Italian Eggplant Dip (page 350) with crudités and Italian Breadsticks (page 290).

APPROXIMATE NUTRITIONAL CONTENT PER SERVING

Total calories: 335
Fat: 5 g
Percentage of calories from fat: 14%

Carbohydrates: 34 g
Protein: 34 g
Cholesterol: 99 mg
Sodium: 652 mg
Dietary fiber: 3 g

A NOTE ON BASIC STOCKS AND BROTHS

Many recipes in this book call for de-fatted stock or broth made from chicken or beef. The best choice is homemade, which not only provides more flavor but allows better control over fat and sodium because you prepare it yourself. If you don't want to use homemade (or if you're just out of time!), substitute a good grade of commercial stock or broth. Whether homemade or commercial, you should refrigerate the broth or stock for a few hours before using it. Fat will rise to the surface and congeal, making it easy to skim off and de-fat the stock or broth.

Watch out for sodium. There can be quite a difference between the amount used in homemade and in commercial varieties. There are 782 milligrams of sodium in one cup of commercial beef stock or chicken broth. The stock and broth recipes included here, from *Don't Eat Your Heart Out Cookbook* and *Choices for a Healthy Heart,* provide you with lower-sodium options. Don't be too concerned with the high percentage of calories from fat in these recipes. The calories of the stocks and broths are so low that even a trace of fat elevates the percentage.

• One cup of our Chicken Stock, which is very flavorful because it is reduced in cooking by one-third, has just 226 milligrams of sodium—a saving of 556 milligrams of sodium.

• One cup of our Beef Stock contains just 275 milligrams of sodium, a saving of 507 milligrams over commercial.

• One cup of our Chicken or Beef Broth contains 550 milligrams of sodium. That's a saving of 226 milligrams over the same amount of commercial broth.

Depending on your desire to control sodium intake, you have a range of choice in broth or stock.

CHICKEN STOCK

Makes 4½ quarts

2 pounds meaty chicken pieces*
3 pound chicken trimmings (carcass, bones, backs)**
4 quarts cold water
3 leeks, roots and green stems removed
3 carrots, peeled
3 stalks celery with leaves
1 large yellow onion, quartered
2 cloves garlic
2 teaspoons salt
1 tablespoon white peppercorns

In a shallow baking dish, combine meaty chicken pieces; bake at 350°F. 20–25 minutes. Remove to stockpot; add chicken trimmings and water. Bring slowly to a boil, removing scum and fat as they float to the top. Add remaining ingredients and simmer 3½ hours. (Do not boil, or fat will be reabsorbed into the stock and will make it cloudy.) Cover only partially with lid so that steam can escape. Strain stock. Refrigerate overnight. Skim fat from surface and discard.

Return stock to stockpot. Simmer, uncovered, 3 hours or until stock is reduced by one-third. Test seasoning; sparingly add salt, if needed. Use stock at once, or store in freezer or up to 2 weeks in refrigerator. (You may want to freeze some stock in ice-cube trays to use for stir-frying or sautéing vegetables.)

*Remove breasts and other meaty pieces from stock as soon as they are cooked (about 45–60 minutes). Reserve for stews, soups, salads and sandwiches. Return any bones, scraps and skin to stockpot for remainder of cooking.

**Do not use the liver or giblets when making stock, since they impart a bitter taste.

VARIATION: For Turkey Stock, substitute turkey pieces for chicken.

APPROXIMATE NUTRITIONAL CONTENT PER CUP

Total calories: 27
Fat: 1 g
Percentage of calories from fat:
  30%

Carbohydrates: Tr
Protein: 4 g
Cholesterol: 2 mg
Sodium: 275 mg
Dietary fiber: 0

CHICKEN-AND-BEEF STOCK

Makes 7½ quarts

1½ pounds beef chuck, cut into 2-inch pieces*
2½ pounds chicken parts
2 pounds beef soupbones
7 quarts cold water
3 cloves garlic
3 leeks, roots and green stems removed
1 large yellow onion, quartered
3 stalks celery with leaves
3 carrots, peeled
3 ripe tomatoes, quartered
2 bay leaves
¼ cup chopped fresh parsley
1 teaspoon thyme
1 tablespoon salt
3 black peppercorns
4 white peppercorns

In a stockpot, combine beef, chicken parts, soupbones and water; bring slowly to a boil, removing scum and fat as they float to the top. Add remaining ingredients and simmer 3½ hours. (Do not boil, or fat will be reabsorbed into the broth and will make it cloudy.) Cover only partially with lid so that steam can escape. Strain broth. Refrigerate overnight. Skim fat from surface and discard.

Return broth to stockpot. Simmer, uncovered, 3 hours or until stock is reduced by one-third. Test seasoning. Sparingly add additional salt, if needed. Use at once, or store in freezer or up to 2 weeks in refrigerator. (It's a good idea to freeze some stock in ice-cube trays to use for stir-frying or sautéing vegetables.)

*Remove meaty chicken parts and beef chuck from stock as soon as they are cooked (about 45–90 minutes). Reserve for stews, soups, salads and sandwiches. Return any bones, scraps and skins to stockpot for remainder of cooking.

APPROXIMATE NUTRITIONAL CONTENT PER CUP

Total calories: 37
Fat: 1 g
Percentage of calories from fat:
   30%

Carbohydrates: Tr
Protein: 5 g
Cholesterol: 2 mg
Sodium: 275 mg
Dietary fiber: 0

BEEF STOCK

Makes 7½ quarts

4 pounds beef chuck, cut into 2-inch cubes*
4 pounds beef marrow bones
7 quarts cold water
3 cloves garlic
3 leeks, roots and green stems removed
1 large yellow onion, quartered
3 stalks celery with leaves
3 carrots, peeled
3 ripe tomatoes, quartered
2 bay leaves
¼ cup chopped fresh parsley
1 teaspoon thyme
1 tablespoon salt
3 black peppercorns
4 white peppercorns

In a stockpot, combine beef chuck, marrow bones and water; bring slowly to a boil, removing scum and fat as they float to the top. Add remaining ingredients and simmer 3½ hours. (Do not boil, or fat will be reabsorbed into the stock and will make it cloudy.) Cover only partially with lid so that steam can escape. Strain stock. Refrigerate overnight. Skim fat from surface and discard.

Return stock to stockpot. Simmer, uncovered, 3 hours or until stock is reduced by one-third. Test seasoning. Sparingly add salt, if needed. Use stock at once, or store in freezer or up to 2 weeks in refrigerator. (You may want to freeze some stock in ice-cube trays to use for stir-frying or sautéing vegetables.)

*Remove choice pieces of meat from stock as soon as they are cooked (about 1½ hours). Serve for dinner with steamed red potatoes and Stir-Fried Snow Peas (page 443).

APPROXIMATE NUTRITIONAL CONTENT PER CUP

Total calories: 37

Fat: 1 g

Percentage of calories from fat: 30%

Carbohydrates: Tr

Protein: 5 g

Cholesterol: 2 mg

Sodium: 275 mg

Dietary fiber: 0

BEAN SOUP STOCK

Makes 3 quarts

- 2 tablespoons dried parsley
- 1 tablespoon thyme
- 1 tablespoon marjoram
- 2 bay leaves
- 2 tablespoons celery seed
- 1 meaty ham hock, about 2½–3 pounds
- 3 quarts water
- 1 tablespoon salt

Measure parsley, thyme, marjoram, bay leaves and celery seed into a square of cheesecloth and tie cloth securely at the top with a string. Combine with ham hock, water and salt in a stockpot. Bring slowly to a boil, removing scum and fat as they float to the top. Cover and simmer 2½–3 hours. (Do not boil, or fat will be reabsorbed into the broth and will make it cloudy.) Refrigerate overnight. Skim and discard fat that floats to the top. Cut ham off bone, reserving only very lean meat. Dice and return to stockpot with seasoning pouch. Discard ham bones and ham fat. Use stock at once, or store in freezer or up to 2 weeks in refrigerator.

APPROXIMATE NUTRITIONAL CONTENT PER CUP

Total calories: 33

Fat: Tr

Percentage of calories from fat: 31%

Carbohydrates: Tr

Protein: 3 g

Cholesterol: 5 mg

Sodium: 550 mg

Dietary fiber: 0

VEAL STOCK

Makes 7½ quarts

1   pound veal chuck, cut into 2-inch pieces*
3   pounds veal bones
2   carrots, peeled
1   large yellow onion, quartered
3   quarts cold water
2   stalks celery with leaves
2   cloves garlic
1   bay leaf
2   teaspoons white peppercorns
½   teaspoon thyme
2   teaspoons salt
2   tablespoons tomato paste
½   cup white wine

In a shallow baking dish, combine veal chuck, veal bones, carrots and onion; bake at 350°F. 15–20 minutes. Remove to stockpot; add water. Bring to a boil, removing scum and fat as they float to the top. Add remaining ingredients and simmer 5 hours. (Do not boil, or fat will be reabsorbed into the stock and will make it cloudy.) Cover only partially with lid so that steam can escape. Strain stock. Refrigerate overnight. Skim fat from surface and discard.

Return stock to stockpot. Simmer, uncovered, 3 hours or until stock is reduced by one-third. Test seasoning. Sparingly add salt, if needed. Use stock at once, or store in freezer or up to 2 weeks in refrigerator. (You may want to freeze some stock in ice-cube trays to use for stir-frying or sautéing vegetables.)

*Remove choice pieces of meat from stock as soon as they are cooked (about 1–1½ hours). Serve for dinner with fresh asparagus and a hearty pasta, such as penne, with marinara sauce.

APPROXIMATE NUTRITIONAL CONTENT PER CUP

Total calories: 27
Fat: Tr
Percentage of calories from fat:
  30%

Carbohydrates: Tr
Protein: 3 g
Cholesterol: 3 mg
Sodium: 258 mg
Dietary fiber: g

CHICKEN BROTH

Makes approximately 3 quarts

    1 large chicken
    3 quarts cold water
    2 stalks celery with leaves
    2 carrots, peeled
    1 large onion, quartered
    2 cloves garlic
    ¼ teaspoon basil
    4 peppercorns
    1 tablespoon or less salt
    ⅛ teaspoon black pepper

Place chicken and water in a stockpot. Cover and simmer 2½ hours or until chicken is tender and pulls away from bone. Strain. Remove meat from bones. (Use meat for soup or sandwiches, or freeze for later use.) Refrigerate broth overnight. Skim fat from surface and discard.

Heat broth to boiling; add vegetables and seasonings. Simmer, uncovered, 2 hours; strain. Reserve vegetables for soup or later use. Reheat broth, or store in freezer or up to 2 weeks in refrigerator. (It's a good idea to freeze some broth in ice-cube trays to use for stir-frying or sautéing vegetables.)

NOTE: For maximum economy, buy a whole chicken when making a recipe that calls for cooked chicken breasts. Skin and bone breasts. Discard skin. Freeze the bones along with the giblets, necks, wings and backs in a plastic freezer bag. When 5–6 pounds accumulate, or when you have a chicken carcass after a meal of roast chicken, remove bones from freezer bag to a stockpot and add water to cover by 2 inches. Add vegetables and seasonings as in above recipe. Bring to a boil. Cover, reduce heat and simmer 5–6 hours. Strain. Discard bones and vegetables, since they will be greasy. Refrigerate broth overnight. Skim and discard fat.

VARIATION: For a richer broth, add another chicken or additional chicken parts, or simmer de-fatted broth, uncovered, 2–3 hours or until reduced by one-third.

APPROXIMATE NUTRITIONAL CONTENT PER CUP

Total calories: 37
Fat: 1 g
Percentage of calories from fat:
   30%

Carbohydrates: Tr
Protein: 5 g
Cholesterol: 2 mg
Sodium: 550 mg
Dietary fiber: 0

BEEF BROTH

Makes approximately 2 quarts

6 pounds beef bones or 2–3 pounds beef shank
  or short ribs
9 cups water
3 stalks celery with leaves, diced
2 carrots, diced
1 onion, chopped
1 tomato, quartered
2 bay leaves
2 cloves garlic
¼ teaspoon thyme
¼ teaspoon marjoram
8 black peppercorns
2 teaspoons salt

Place meat, bones and water in a stockpot. Simmer, uncovered, 3 hours (do not boil). Strain. Remove any meat or marrow from bones. Add marrow to broth; reserve meat for soup. Chill broth overnight; skim fat from the surface and discard. Bring broth to boiling; add remaining ingredients and simmer, uncovered, 2 hours. Strain. Reserve vegetables for soup or later use. Reheat broth, or store in freezer or up to 2 weeks in refrigerator. (You may want to freeze some broth in ice-cube trays for use for stir-frying or sautéing vegetables).

VARIATION: For a hearty soup, do not strain broth. Add 2–3 cups cooked pasta.

APPROXIMATE NUTRITIONAL CONTENT PER CUP

Total calories: 37
Fat: 1 g
Percentage of calories from fat:
  30%

Carbohydrates: Tr
Protein: 5 g
Cholesterol: 2 mg
Sodium: 550 mg
Dietary fiber: 0

TURKEY BROTH

Makes approximately 2½ quarts

1 turkey carcass with meaty bones
water to cover (about 3 quarts)
2 cloves garlic
¼ teaspoon basil
4 peppercorns
1 tablespoon or less salt
⅛ teaspoon black pepper
4 stalks celery with leaves
4 carrots, peeled
1 large onion, quartered

Place turkey carcass in a stockpot; add water to cover. Add seasonings; bring to a boil. Add vegetables. Cover, reduce heat and simmer 6–8 hours. Strain; discard bones and vegetables since they will be very greasy. Remove meat from bones and reserve for later use. Refrigerate broth overnight. Skim fat from surface and discard. Reheat broth, or store in freezer or up to 2 weeks in refrigerator. (You may want to freeze some broth in ice-cube trays to use for stir-frying or sautéing vegetables.)

APPROXIMATE NUTRITIONAL CONTENT PER CUP

Total calories: 37
Fat: 1 g
Percentage of calories from fat:
   30%

Carbohydrates: Tr
Protein: 5 g
Cholesterol: 2 mg
Sodium: 660 mg
Dietary fiber: 0

BREADS & SANDWICHES

ITALIAN BREAD

Makes two 18-inch loaves

> 2 cups warm water (110°–115°F.)
> ½ teaspoon granulated sugar
> 2 packages active dry yeast
> 5 cups unbleached flour
> 1 teaspoon salt
>   tub-style safflower margarine
>   cornmeal
> 1 egg white, slightly beaten
> 1 tablespoon cold water

In a small bowl, combine water and sugar; sprinkle yeast over top. Let stand 10 minutes. In a large mixing bowl, combine 2 cups of the flour, salt and dissolved yeast. Mix with a wooden spoon about 30 seconds to combine ingredients. Gradually add 2 more cups of the flour.

Knead by hand or by machine, gradually adding remaining 1 cup flour, until dough is smooth and elastic. Put dough in a bowl greased with safflower margarine, turning once to coat top. Cover and let rise in a warm place until double in size, about 1½ hours.

Punch dough down. Turn out onto lightly floured surface and divide in half. Cover and let rest 10 minutes. Roll each half into 15 x 10-inch rectangles. Roll up from long sides and seal well. Taper ends. Using a very sharp knife, make 3 or 4 diagonal cuts about ¼ inch deep across loaves. Place seam side down on bread pans greased with safflower margarine and lightly sprinkled with cornmeal. Cover and let rise until nearly double, about 1 hour. To check if the dough has risen sufficiently, poke your finger in about 2 inches. If hole remains and does not close up when you remove your finger, the dough has risen enough.

Bake in a 375°F. oven 20 minutes. Push loaves out of pans and onto oven racks. Bake 10 minutes longer. Combine egg white and cold water, and brush loaves. Bake on oven racks 1–15 minutes longer or until loaves sound hollow when tapped. Cool on wire racks.

APPROXIMATE NUTRITIONAL CONTENT PER ½-INCH SLICE

Total calories: 33	Carbohydrates: 6 g
Fat: Tr	Protein: 1 g
Percentage of calories from fat: 2%	Cholesterol: 0
	Sodium: 31 mg
	Dietary fiber: Tr

COUNTRY ITALIAN BREAD

Makes two 18-inch loaves (20 slices per loaf)

2	cups warm water (110°–115°F.)
¼	teaspoon granulated sugar
1½	teaspoons active dry yeast
5	cups unbleached flour
1	tablespoon salt
2	tablespoons olive oil
	tub-style safflower margarine

In a bowl, combine water and sugar; sprinkle yeast over top. Let stand 10 minutes. In a mixing bowl, combine flour, salt and olive oil. Add dissolved yeast and mix with a wooden spoon to form a soft dough.

Knead by hand or by machine until smooth and elastic. Put dough in a bowl greased with safflower margarine, turning once to coat top. Cover and let rise in a warm place until double in size, about 1½ hours.

Punch dough down. Cover and return to warm place. Let rise until double in size, about 1 hour. Punch down again. Divide dough in half. Roll each half into a loaf shape. Place in bread pans greased with safflower margarine. Return to warm place and let rise until nearly double in size, about 1 hour.

Bake in a 450°F. oven 15–20 minutes. (Bake on a pizza stone if available.) Remove loaves from pans. Reduce heat to 350°F. and continue baking about 30 minutes or until loaves sound hollow when tapped.

APPROXIMATE NUTRITIONAL CONTENT PER SLICE

Total calories: 63	Carbohydrates: 12 g
Fat: 1 g	Protein: 1 g
Percentage of calories from fat:	Cholesterol: 0
12%	Sodium: 160 mg
	Dietary fiber: Tr

EASY PIZZA CRUST

Makes 1 pizza crust (10 slices per crust)

    1 heaping teaspoon active dry yeast
    2 tablespoons warm water (110°–115°F.)
    ½ teaspoon salt
    1 tablespoon olive oil, plus 1 teaspoon
 1 ½ teaspoons honey
    6 tablespoons cool water
 1 ½ cups all-purpose flour
       dash tub-style safflower margarine

Dissolve yeast in the warm water. Let stand 10 minutes.

In a small bowl, combine salt, 1 tablespoon olive oil, honey and cool water; add dissolved yeast. In a mixing bowl or food processor, combine the honey-yeast mixture and flour. Knead by hand or by machine until dough is smooth and elastic. If dough is too sticky, add up to ½ cup additional flour.

Place dough in a bowl that has been greased with safflower margarine, turning once to coat top. Cover and let rest for 30 minutes.

Using a rolling pin, flatten dough into a circle about 12 inches in diameter. Slide onto a nonstick pizza pan. Brush dough with 1 teaspoon olive oil.

Bake in a 500°F. oven that has been preheated for 30 minutes with a pizza stone inside. (Pizza stone is optional.) Bake 8 minutes or until golden brown.

APPROXIMATE NUTRITIONAL CONTENT PER SLICE

Total calories: 88
Fat: 2 g
Percentage of calories from fat:
   24%

Carbohydrates: 14 g
Protein: 2 g
Cholesterol: 0
Sodium: 112 mg
Dietary fiber: 1 g

ITALIAN PIZZA BREAD WITH GARLIC AND ROSEMARY

Makes 10 slices

¾ teaspoon active dry yeast
1 cup warm water (110°–115°F.)
2½ cups unbleached flour
¾ teaspoon salt
   tub-style safflower margarine
5 cloves garlic, thinly sliced
⅓ cup fresh sprigs rosemary
2 teaspoons olive oil
¼ teaspoon black pepper

Dissolve yeast in the cup of warm water. In a bowl, combine flour and ½ teaspoon of the salt; add dissolved yeast. Knead by hand or by machine until smooth. Place dough in a bowl greased with safflower margarine, turning once to coat top. Cover and let rise in a warm place 1½ hours or until double in size.

Punch dough down. Put it back in bowl and let rise again until double in size, about 1 hour.

Punch down. Roll dough out to ½-inch thickness. Transfer to nonstick pizza pan. Make indentations at frequent intervals over the surface of dough. Insert a slice of garlic and a sprig of rosemary into each indentation. Drizzle olive oil over dough's surface and spread oil with hands to coat evenly. Sprinkle with remaining ¼ teaspoon salt and pepper.

Bake in a 400°F. oven 20–25 minutes or until crust is cooked and golden brown. (Bake on a pizza stone if available.) Remove garlic and rosemary. Slice into wedges. Serve at once.

SHORTCUT SUGGESTION: In place of homemade dough, use a heart-healthy, uncooked crust purchased from a local pizza parlor. Be sure it's made with olive oil or an unsaturated, nonhydrogenated oil such as safflower, soybean or corn oil. Do not use a crust made with hydrogenated shortening, lard, palm oil or coconut oil. Consider purchasing several crusts at one time to keep in the freezer.

APPROXIMATE NUTRITIONAL CONTENT PER SLICE

Total calories: 128
Fat: 1 g
Percentage of calories from fat:
   10 %

Carbohydrates: 24 g
Protein: 3 g
Cholesterol: 0
Sodium: 163 mg
Dietary fiber: 1 g

BREAKFAST PIZZA

Makes 1 pizza (10 slices per pizza)

> 1 Easy Pizza Crust (page 279)
> 1 teaspoon olive oil
> ⅔ cup finely chopped white onion
> ½ teaspoon cumin
> ½ teaspoon fresh thyme
> ⅔ cup shredded part-skim mozzarella cheese
> 3 eggs
> ½ cup commercial tomato salsa

Salsa Cruda
> 4 large ripe tomatoes, diced
> 2 cups finely chopped white onion
> 2 jalapeño peppers, chopped
> ½ cup fresh lime juice
> 3 tablespoons olive oil
> ½ teaspoon black pepper
> 1 teaspoon salt

Prepare pizza crust and bake 8 minutes according to instructions.

Meanwhile, in a medium bowl, prepare Salsa Cruda by combining tomatoes, onion, jalapeño peppers, lime juice, olive oil, black pepper and salt; set aside.

In a nonstick skillet, heat the olive oil. Add onion and sauté 4–5 minutes or until onion is tender. Sprinkle with cumin and thyme.

When crust is lightly browned, sprinkle with half the mozzarella cheese, then some of the diced tomatoes and onions from the Salsa Cruda. Break one egg over each third of the pizza. Prick yolk with a fork to break. Sprinkle remaining cheese over top. Bake in 500°F. oven about 20 minutes or until eggs are cooked. (Use a pizza stone if available.)

Top each slice of pizza with Salsa Cruda, then with the commercial tomato salsa.

NOTE: Serve this pizza with fresh fruits or other low-fat accompaniments to reduce percentage of calories from fat in the total meal.

SHORTCUT SUGGESTION: In place of homemade dough, purchase a heart-healthy, uncooked crust from a local pizza parlor. Be sure it's made with olive oil or an unsaturated, nonhydrogenated oil such as safflower, soybean or corn oil. Do not use a crust made with hydrogenated shortening, lard, palm oil or coconut oil.

APPROXIMATE NUTRITIONAL CONTENT PER SLICE

Total calories: 217

Fat: 11 g

Percentage of calories from fat: 44%

Carbohydrates: 22 g

Protein: 9 g

Cholesterol: 72 mg

Sodium: 418 mg

Dietary fiber: 2 g

CHEESE POPOVERS

Makes 8 popovers

> 2 eggs, room-temperature
> 1 egg white, room-temperature
> 1 ¼ cups non-fat milk
> 1 ¼ cups unbleached white flour
> ¼ teaspoon salt
>   tub-style safflower margarine
> ½ cup shredded part-skim Cheddar cheese

In a mixing bowl, beat eggs and egg white with a rotary beater until lemon-colored and frothy. Add milk and beat 1 minute. Add flour and salt, and beat 1–2 minutes or until batter is smooth and foamy on top.

Generously grease popover pans, individual custard cups or standard muffin pans with safflower margarine. Fill each cup ⅓ full with batter. Sprinkle with 1 tablespoon cheese. Top with ⅓ cup more batter. (If using standard muffin pans, grease and fill alternating cups to prevent sides of popovers from touching.)

Bake at 450°F. 15 minutes (do not open oven). Reduce heat to 350°F. and bake 20–25 minutes or until high, hollow and golden brown. Remove from oven. Insert a sharp knife into each popover to allow steam to escape. Remove from pans. Serve hot.

NOTE: The eggs and milk must be room-temperature or the popovers will not rise. Well-greased cups and pans (including tops) will prevent popovers from sticking.

APPROXIMATE NUTRITIONAL CONTENT PER POPOVER

Total calories: 143
Fat: 4 g
Percentage of calories from fat:
  25%

Carbohydrates: 17 g
Protein: 9 g
Cholesterol: 62 mg
Sodium: 178 mg
Dietary fiber: Tr

CHEDDAR CHEESE BREAD

Makes 1 loaf (20 slices per loaf)

    1 package active dry yeast
 1 ¼ cups warm (110°–115°F.) water
    1 tablespoon granulated sugar
 1 ½ teaspoons salt
    2 tablespoons olive oil or canola oil
    2 cups all-purpose flour
    1 cup whole-wheat flour
   ¾ cup diced, low-fat Cheddar cheese
 1 ½ teaspoons ground cumin
 1 ½ teaspoons cornmeal

Dissolve yeast in water and set aside. In a mixing bowl, combine sugar, salt, olive oil and flours; add dissolved yeast. Knead dough by hand or by machine until soft, about 3–5 minutes. Knead in cheese and cumin. Shape into a round loaf; flatten slightly and dust with cornmeal. Bake on a nonstick baking sheet at 375°F. 30–35 minutes or until bread sounds hollow when tapped.

SHORTCUT SUGGESTION: In place of homemade dough, use a heart-healthy frozen bread dough. Read the label to be sure it is made with olive oil or an unsaturated, nonhydrogenated oil such as safflower, soybean or corn oil. Do not use a brand made with hydrogenated shortening, lard, palm oil or coconut oil.

SERVING SUGGESTION: Good with soups and stews.

APPROXIMATE NUTRITIONAL CONTENT PER SLICE

Total calories: 93	Carbohydrates: 15 g
Fat: 2 g	Protein: 3 g
Percentage of calories from fat:	Cholesterol: 2 mg
22%	Sodium: 181 mg
	Dietary fiber: 1 g

CAJUN FLATBREAD

Makes 14 slices

¾   teaspoon active dry yeast
1   cup warm water (110°–115°F.)
2½ cups unbleached flour
½   teaspoon salt
    tub-style safflower margarine
2   teaspoons olive oil
    black pepper
    white pepper
    cayenne pepper
    paprika

Dissolve yeast in the cup of warm water. In a bowl, combine flour and salt; add dissolved yeast. Knead by hand or by machine until smooth. Place dough in a bowl greased with safflower margarine, turning once to coat top. Cover and let rise in a warm place 1½ hours or until double in size.

Punch dough down. Put back in bowl and let rise again until double in size, about 1 hour. Punch down again. Roll dough out to ½-inch thickness. Transfer to nonstick pizza pan. Drizzle olive oil over pizza. Sprinkle lightly with seasonings (about ⅛ teaspoon of each). Spread oil and seasonings with hands to coat evenly.

Bake in a 400°F. oven 20–25 minutes or until crust is cooked. (Bake on a pizza stone if available.) Slice into wedges.

SHORTCUT SUGGESTION: In place of homemade dough, use a heart-healthy, uncooked crust purchased from a local pizza parlor. Be sure it's made with olive oil or an unsaturated, nonhydrogenated oil such as safflower, soybean or corn oil. Do not use a crust made with hydrogenated shortening, lard, palm oil or coconut oil. Consider purchasing several crusts at one time to keep in the freezer.

SERVING SUGGESTION: Especially good with soups and Creole dishes.

APPROXIMATE NUTRITIONAL CONTENT PER SLICE

Total calories: 88
Fat: 1 g
Percentage of calories from fat:
   10%

Carbohydrates: 17 g
Protein: 2 g
Cholesterol: 0
Sodium: 87 mg
Dietary fiber: Tr

CHEESE-AND-HERB FLATBREAD

Makes 14 slices

  ¾ teaspoon active dry yeast
  1 cup warm water (110°–115°F.)
2½ cups unbleached flour
  ½ teaspoon salt
     tub-style safflower margarine
  2 teaspoons olive oil
  3 tablespoons freshly grated Parmesan cheese
  1 teaspoon oregano
  1 teaspooon basil
  ¼ teaspoon black pepper

Dissolve yeast in the cup of warm water. In a bowl, combine flour and salt; add dissolved yeast. Knead by hand or by machine until smooth. (If dough is sticky, gradually add up to ½ cup additional flour.) Place in a bowl greased with safflower margarine. Turn dough once to coat top. Cover and let rise in a warm place 1½ hours or until double in size.

Punch dough down. Put back in bowl and let rise again until double in size, about 1 hour. Punch down again. Roll dough out to ½-inch thickness. Transfer to nonstick pizza pan. Drizzle olive oil over dough's surface and spread oil with hands to coat evenly. Sprinkle with Parmesan, oregano, basil and pepper.

(continued on next page)

(continued from previous page)

Bake in a 400°F. oven 20–25 minutes or until crust is cooked. (Bake on a pizza stone if available.) Slice into wedges.

SHORTCUT SUGGESTION: In place of homemade dough, use a heart-healthy, uncooked crust purchased from a local pizza parlor. Be sure it's made with olive oil or an unsaturated, nonhydrogenated oil such as safflower, soybean or corn oil. Do not use a crust made with hydrogenated shortening, lard, palm oil or coconut oil. Consider purchasing several crusts at one time to keep in the freezer.

APPROXIMATE NUTRITIONAL CONTENT PER SLICE

Total calories: 94
Fat: 1 g
Percentage of calories from fat:
   10%

Carbohydrates: 17 g
Protein: 3 g
Cholesterol: 1 mg
Sodium: 105 mg
Dietary fiber: Tr

HOT CROSS BUNS

Makes 18 buns

5	cups unbleached flour
2	¼-ounce packages active dry yeast
⅓	cup granulated sugar
¼	teaspoon ground nutmeg
½	teaspoon salt
1½	teaspoons cinnamon
¾	cup non-fat milk
¼	cup olive oil or canola oil
½	cup water
3	eggs
1¾	cups raisins
1	egg white, lightly beaten
1	tablespoon cold water
	Vanilla Glaze (page 485)

In a large mixing bowl, combine 1½ cups of the flour, undissolved yeast, sugar, nutmeg, salt and cinnamon. Set aside.

In a 1-quart saucepan, heat milk, olive oil and water to 125°F.; gradually add to dry ingredients. Beat 2 minutes at medium speed of electric mixer. Add eggs and ¾ cup of the flour; beat 2 minutes at high speed. Using dough hook or wooden spoon, gradually add remaining flour to make a soft dough. Knead by hand on a lightly floured surface or by machine until dough is smooth and elastic. Cover and let rest 20 minutes.

Punch dough down. Knead in raisins. Divide dough into 18 equal pieces. Roll into smooth balls. Arrange rolls in 2 nonstick 8 x 8 inch-square baking pans. Cover and let rise in a warm place 30–60 minutes or until nearly double in size.

Bake in a 375°F. oven 10 minutes. Meanwhile, combine egg white and cold water; brush over rolls. Bake 10 minutes longer or until done. When done, rolls will pull away easily from edges of pan. Remove rolls from pans. Cool on wire racks. Drizzle glaze in a cross shape over tops.

VARIATION: Substitute Orange Glaze (page 486) for Vanilla Glaze or drizzle half the buns with Orange and half with Vanilla.

APPROXIMATE NUTRITIONAL CONTENT PER BUN

Total calories: 262
Fat: 4 g
Percentage of calories from fat: 14%

Carbohydrates: 51 g
Protein: 6 g
Cholesterol: 35 mg
Sodium: 92 mg
Dietary fiber: 2 g

ITALIAN BREADSTICKS

Makes 20 breadsticks

    ¼ teaspoon granulated sugar
    1½ cups warm water (110°–115°F.)
    1½ teaspoons active dry yeast
    3¾ cups unbleached flour
     2 teaspoons salt
     2 tablespoons olive oil
        tub-style safflower margarine

In a small bowl, combine sugar and water; sprinkle yeast over top. Let stand 10 minutes.

In a mixing bowl, combine flour, salt and olive oil. Add dissolved yeast and mix with a wooden spoon to form a soft dough.

Knead by hand or by machine until dough is smooth and elastic. Put dough in a bowl greased with safflower margarine, turning once to coat top. Cover and let rise in a warm place until double in size, about 1½ hours. Punch dough down and divide into 4 parts. Roll each part into a 5 x 8-inch rectangle. Cut each rectangle crosswise into 5 pieces. Roll each piece between palms to a ¾ x 4-inch rope. (Be sure to keep standing dough covered while working.) Arrange on nonstick baking pans, cover and let rest 10 minutes.

Bake in a 400°F. oven 20–25 minutes or until lightly browned. Remove to napkin-lined basket and serve at once.

SHORTCUT SUGGESTION: In place of homemade dough, use a heart-healthy frozen bread dough. Read the label to be sure it is made with olive oil or an unsaturated, nonhydrogenated oil such as safflower, soybean or corn oil. Do not use a brand made with hydrogenated shortening, lard, palm oil or coconut oil.

SERVING SUGGESTION: Good with soups and stews and for after-school snacks.

APPROXIMATE NUTRITIONAL CONTENT PER BREADSTICK

Total calories: 98	Carbohydrates: 18 g
Fat: 2 g	Protein: 2 g
Percentage of calories from fat: 15%	Cholesterol: 0
	Sodium: 215 mg
	Dietary fiber: Tr

ROASTED GARLIC BREAD

Makes 1 loaf (12 slices per loaf)

- 1 head garlic, cloves separated but not peeled
- 1 tablespoon olive oil
- ½ teaspoon salt
- ¼ teaspoon black pepper
- 1 12-inch French baguette

Arrange garlic in a 8 x 8 x 2-inch ovenproof baking dish. Add olive oil, salt and pepper. Bake at 350°F. 30–40 minutes or until garlic is soft. Release garlic from peels right into the baking dish. Stir cooked garlic into the oil, salt and pepper.

Slice the baguette in half lengthwise. Rub each half with the garlic-oil. Place under the broiler 2–3 minutes or until lightly toasted. Delicious!

VARIATION: Serve the bread warm, not toasted. Place the garlic-oil mixture in the center of the table and let each person dip bread into the warm oil.

APPROXIMATE NUTRITIONAL CONTENT PER SLICE

Total calories: 111	Carbohydrates: 18 g
Fat: 2 g	Protein: 3 g
Percentage of calories from fat: 20%	Cholesterol: 0
	Sodium: 232 mg
	Dietary fiber: 1 g

HONEY OAT BREAD

Makes 2 loaves (10 slices per loaf)

⅓	cup honey
2	cups warm water (110°–115°F.)
3	packages active dry yeast
1½	cups rolled oats
¼	cup olive oil or canola oil
1	egg
1	tablespoon salt
2	cups whole-wheat flour
3¼	cups all-purpose flour
	tub-style safflower margarine

Combine honey with water; add yeast. Let stand 5 minutes.

In a mixing bowl, combine oats, olive oil, egg, salt, whole-wheat flour and all but 1 cup of the all-purpose flour. Mix with wooden spoon to form a soft dough.

Knead the dough by hand or by machine, gradually adding remaining 1 cup all-purpose flour, until smooth and elastic. Place dough in a 2½-quart bowl greased with safflower margarine, turning once to coat top. Cover and let rise in a warm place until double in size, about 1½ hours. Dough is ready if indentation remains when touched.

Punch dough down; divide into halves. Let rest 5 minutes. Flatten each half with hands or rolling pin into an 18 x 9-inch rectangle. Roll into a cylinder. Place seam side down in loaf pans greased with margarine. Cover and let rise until double in size, about 1 hour.

Bake in a 350°F. oven 20–30 minutes. When dough is set, remove from pans to oven rack and cook 10–15 minutes longer or until bread sounds hollow when tapped. Cool on wire racks.

Total calories: 92

Fat: 2 g

Percentage of calories from fat: 18%

Carbohydrates: 16 g

Protein: 2 g

Cholesterol: 5 mg

Sodium: 162 mg

Dietary fiber: 1 g

APPLE OAT BRAN MUFFINS

Makes 18 muffins

    3 cups oat bran
 2 ½ cups whole-wheat flour
    ½ teaspoon salt
    2 teaspoons baking soda
    2 eggs
    ¼ cup molasses
    ¼ cup olive oil or canola oil
    2 cups apple juice concentrate
    2 cups skim milk
 2 ½ cups chopped Granny Smith apples (about 2
          large apples)
 1 ½ cups raisins

In a small bowl, combine oat bran, whole-wheat flour, salt and baking soda; set aside. In a large mixing bowl, beat eggs; stir in molasses. Mix in olive oil, apple juice concentrate and skim milk. Gradually add flour mixture using a wire whisk. Mix ingredients just until moistened. Stir in chopped apples and raisins. Pour into paper-lined muffin pans. Bake at 350°F. 20–25 minutes or until toothpick inserted into center comes out dry.

APPROXIMATE NUTRITIONAL CONTENT PER MUFFIN

Total calories: 201

Fat: 4 g

Percentage of calories from fat: 18%

Carbohydrates: 39 g

Protein: 5 g

Cholesterol: 23 mg

Sodium: 161 mg

Dietary fiber: 4 g

APPLESAUCE OATMEAL MUFFINS

Makes 12 muffins

2½ cups applesauce
2 eggs
¾ cup brown sugar
¼ cup olive oil or canola oil
1½ cups rolled oats
1 cup whole-wheat flour
1 cup all-purpose flour
1 teaspoon baking soda
1 teaspoon baking powder
1½ teaspoons salt
2 teaspoons cinnamon
1½ cups raisins

In a large bowl, combine applesauce, eggs, brown sugar and olive oil; set aside. In a medium bowl, combine oats, flours, baking soda, baking powder, salt and cinnamon. Add to applesauce mixture. Stir with wire whisk just until dry ingredients are moistened. Stir in raisins. Pour into paper-lined muffin pans. Bake at 350°F. 15–20 minutes or until toothpick inserted into center comes out dry.

APPROXIMATE NUTRITIONAL CONTENT PER MUFFIN

Total calories: 309
Fat: 6 g
Percentage of calories from fat:
    18%

Carbohydrates: 60 g
Protein: 6 g
Cholesterol: 35 mg
Sodium: 399 mg
Dietary fiber: 4 g

PAN ROLLS

Makes 20 rolls

1½ teaspoons active dry yeast
2   cups warm water (110°–115°F.)
5   cups unbleached flour
1   teaspoon salt
    tub-style safflower margarine

Sprinkle yeast over the warm water. Let stand 5 minutes.

In a bowl, combine flour with salt; add dissolved yeast. Mix with a wooden spoon to form a soft dough.

Knead dough by hand or by machine until smooth and elastic. Place in a bowl greased with safflower margarine, turning once to coat top. Cover and let rise in a warm place 1½ hours or until double in size.

Punch dough down. Form into a ball. Divide dough in half; then each half into 10 equal pieces. Shape 10 pieces into balls and place close together in a nonstick 9-inch round pan. Repeat with second 10 pieces. Cover and return to a warm place. Let rise until double in size, about 1 hour.

Bake at 400°F. 20 minutes. Reduce heat to 350°F. and bake 10–15 minutes longer.

SHORTCUT SUGGESTION: In place of homemade dough, use a heart-healthy frozen bread dough. Read the label to be sure it is made with olive oil or an unsaturated, nonhydrogenated oil such as safflower, soybean or corn oil. Do not use a brand made with hydrogenated shortening, lard, palm oil or coconut oil.

APPROXIMATE NUTRITIONAL CONTENT PER ROLL

Total calories: 105	Carbohydrates: 22 g
Fat: Tr	Protein: 3 g
Percentage of calories from fat:	Cholesterol: 0
3%	Sodium: 108 mg
	Dietary fiber: 1 g

SESAME WAFFLES

Makes 5 large (6" x 11") waffles

1 cup unbleached flour
1 cup whole-wheat flour
1 cup instant non-fat milk
2 tablespoons sugar
1 tablespoon baking powder
1 teaspoon salt
2 eggs, slightly beaten
2 tablespoons olive oil or canola oil
2 cups water
¾ cup sesame seeds
1 teaspoon vanilla extract

In a large mixing bowl, combine flours, instant non-fat milk, sugar, baking powder and salt. In a small mixing bowl, combine eggs, olive oil and water.

Make a well in the flour mixture; add egg mixture and blend. Fold in sesame seeds and vanilla extract. Pour ⅔ cup of mix into a waffle iron and bake 3 minutes.

NOTE: Instead of the traditional butter and syrup, try topping waffles with a mixture of puréed and whole fresh strawberries, raspberries or blueberries, powdered sugar and a dollop of non-fat yogurt.

APPROXIMATE NUTRITIONAL CONTENT PER ½ WAFFLE

Total calories: 159
Fat: 4 g
Percentage of calories from fat:
    23%

Carbohydrates: 24 g
Protein: 6 g
Cholesterol: 44 mg
Sodium: 363 mg
Dietary fiber: 2 g

SHRIMP BAGUETTE SANDWICHES

Makes 6 servings

1	12-inch French baguette
1	tablespoon safflower mayonnaise
6	tomato slices
12	English cucumber slices
1	cup shredded lettuce
½	cup alfalfa sprouts
½	pound cooked shrimpmeat

Cut a baguette in half lengthwise. Spread mayonnaise over each half. Layer bottom half with remaining ingredients. Top with remaining baguette half. Cut diagonally into 6 servings.

SERVING SUGGESTION: Serve with Asparagus, Tomato and Pasta Salad (page 323) or Marinated Peppers and Onion (page 327) and Lemon Chiffon Pie (page 247).

APPROXIMATE NUTRITIONAL CONTENT PER SERVING

Total calories: 257
Fat: 5 g
Percentage of calories from fat: 18%

Carbohydrates: 37 g
Protein: 15 g
Cholesterol: 75 mg
Sodium: 486 mg
Dietary fiber: 2 g

ORIENTAL CHICKEN SANDWICHES

Makes 12 silver dollar–size sandwiches

- 1 tablespoon Chinese Five Spice*
- 1 teaspoon salt
- 1 teaspoon granulated sugar
- ½ teaspoon black pepper
- 1 pound skinned and boned chicken breasts
- 2 teaspoons olive oil
- 1 head Bibb lettuce
- 4 green onions, thinly sliced
  - fresh cilantro (optional)
  - Black Bean Dip (page 348)
  - Oriental hot mustard
- 12 silver dollar–size baked or steamed Chinese buns
  or soft dinner rolls, split in half

Hot Chili/Soy Sauce:
- ⅓ cup reduced-sodium soy sauce
- 1 teaspoon hot chili oil (LaYu)*

Combine Chinese Five Spice, salt, sugar and pepper. Sprinkle over chicken to coat. Cover and chill overnight.

Thoroughly rinse chicken under cold running water to release salt and seasonings. Drain; pat dry with paper towels. Place chicken in an 8 x 8-inch ovenproof baking dish. Drizzle with olive oil. Bake at 350°F. 20–30 minutes or until done. Slice crosswise into pieces ¼ inch thick.

Line a platter with lettuce and arrange chicken on it. Garnish with green onions and cilantro. Surround with bowls of Black Bean Dip, Oriental hot mustard and Hot Chili/Soy Sauce. Serve rolls in napkin-lined basket. Each person may then assemble his or her own sandwich.

NOTE: This recipe takes minutes to prepare the day ahead and less than 30 minutes to prepare before serving.

*Chinese Five Spice and hot chili oil (LaYu) are available in many supermarkets and Oriental groceries.

SERVING SUGGESTION: Serve with Asparagus, Tomato and Pasta Salad (page 323) and sliced oranges with fresh pineapple and papaya.

APPROXIMATE NUTRITIONAL CONTENT PER SANDWICH

Total calories: 159
Fat: 4 g
Percentage of calories from fat:
    23%

Carbohydrates: 15 g
Protein: 14 g
Cholesterol: 32 mg
Sodium: 350 mg
Dietary fiber: 1 g

Add 23 calories per tablespoon of Black Bean Dip. Add 14 calories per tablespoon of Hot Chili/Soy Sauce. Add 18 calories per tablespoon of Oriental hot mustard.

CAJUN TURKEY SANDWICHES

Makes 4 sandwiches

½ pound Roasted Cajun Turkey Breast (page 410)
4 French rolls
1 tablespoon safflower mayonnaise
1 teaspoon Dijon mustard
2 cups shredded leaf lettuce
¾ small onion, thinly sliced
1 tomato, thinly sliced

Cut the turkey into thin slices. Spread rolls with mayonnaise and mustard. Fill with turkey, lettuce, onion and tomato.

SERVING SUGGESTION: Serve with Wild and White Rice Salad (page 333).

APPROXIMATE NUTRITIONAL CONTENT PER SANDWICH

Total calories: 267
Fat: 5 g
Percentage of calories from fat:
    18%

Carbohydrates: 34 g
Protein: 21 g
Cholesterol: 44 mg
Sodium: 400 mg
Dietary fiber: 1 g

GRILLED TURKEY SANDWICHES

Makes 6 sandwiches

2	tablespoons fresh lemon juice
1	tablespoon olive oil
¼	teaspoon black pepper
1	pound very thin turkey breast fillets
6	very fresh sesame hamburger buns
1	large ripe tomato, sliced
6	thin slices white onion
1	small head Bibb lettuce
	Dijon mustard or Lemon Mayonnaise, below (optional)

Lemon Mayonnaise

¼	cup safflower mayonnaise
1½	teaspoons fresh lemon juice
1	teaspoon grated lemon peel

In a bowl, combine 2 tablespoons lemon juice, olive oil and pepper; pour over turkey. Marinate 15–20 minutes at room temperature, turning occasionally to coat.

Grill turkey over hot coals 8–10 minutes on each side or until meat is white in center. Just before removing from grill, arrange buns over top of turkey for about 1 minute to warm. Slice turkey crosswise into pieces ¼ inch thick.

To assemble, pile turkey, tomato, onion and lettuce on bottom half of bun. Spread top half with Dijon mustard and/ or Lemon Mayonnaise, if desired.

SERVING SUGGESTION: Serve with Marinated Potato Salad (page 326), Vegetable and Black Bean Antipasto (page 330), and fresh fruit. For heartier fare, include Fresh Lemonade (page 463) and homemade raisin oatmeal cookies.

APPROXIMATE NUTRITIONAL CONTENT PER SANDWICH WITHOUT DIJON MUSTARD OR LEMON MAYONNAISE

Total calories: 249

Fat: 5 g

Percentage of calories from fat:
   18%

Carbohydrates: 23 g

Protein: 27 g

Cholesterol: 63 mg

Sodium: 283 mg

Dietary fiber: Tr

Add 18 calories per tablespoon of Dijon mustard. Add 99 calories per tablespoon of Lemon Mayonnaise.

TURKEY MEAT LOAF SANDWICH

Makes 1 sandwich

- 2 slices crusty French bread or whole-wheat bread
- 1 teaspoon Dijon mustard
- 2 slices Turkey Meat Loaf (page 408)
- 2 teaspoons spicy tomato sauce (see Turkey Meat Loaf)
- 2 slices tomato
- 2 slices white onion
- 2 lettuce leaves

Spread bread with mustard. Top 1 slice with meat loaf. Spread meat loaf with spicy tomato sauce. Top with tomato and onion, then lettuce and other slice of bread.

SERVING SUGGESTION: Serve with Two-Salsa Pasta Salad (page 320) and fresh fruit.

APPROXIMATE NUTRITIONAL CONTENT PER SANDWICH

Total calories: 357

Fat: 5 g

Percentage of calories from fat:
   13%

Carbohydrates: 54 g

Protein: 24 g

Cholesterol: 62 mg

Sodium: 425 mg

Dietary fiber: 5 g

SALADS

CRAB-AND-SHRIMP SUSHI SALAD

Makes 5 servings

Spinach

    5 cups fresh spinach leaves torn into bite-size
       pieces

Rice

  1½ cups uncooked short-grain rice
  1¾ cups water, plus 2 tablespoons
   ⅓ cup seasoned rice vinegar

In a 3-quart saucepan, rinse rice with water until water runs clear; drain. Add water to rice and bring to a boil. Reduce heat, cover and simmer 20–25 minutes or until water is absorbed. Remove from heat; stir in vinegar. Let stand at room temperature until ready to serve.

Carrots

   2 large carrots, peeled
  ⅓ cup rice vinegar
  ½ teaspoon hot chili oil (LaYu)

Cut carrots into matchstick pieces 3 inches long. In a 2-quart saucepan, bring vinegar to a boil. Add carrots and cook, stirring often, just until crisp-tender, about 60 seconds. Drain. Drizzle with hot chili oil. Set aside.

Snow Peas
> ¼ pound snow peas
> ½ teaspoon sesame oil

In a covered pan over boiling water, steam snow peas 1–2 minutes or just until crisp-tender. Drizzle with sesame oil. Set aside.

Cucumber
> 1 English cucumber, peeled
> 3 tablespoons rice vinegar

Cut cucumber into matchstick pieces 3 inches long. Toss with vinegar. Set aside.

Mushrooms
> 1 7-ounce package dried forest mushrooms (Shiitake)
> 2 cups warm water
> ¼ teaspoon granulated sugar
> 2 teaspoons sake
> 2 tablespoons reduced-sodium soy sauce

Soak mushrooms in 2 cups warm water 20 minutes or until soft. Cut off and discard hard stems. Pour mushrooms with their soaking liquid into a 2-quart saucepan; add sugar, sake and soy sauce. Bring to a boil. Cook, stirring often, until most of liquid is absorbed. Remove from pan and cut into matchstick pieces. Set aside.

(continued on next page)

(continued from preceding page)
Seafood

⅓   pound cooked shrimpmeat
⅓   pound cooked crabmeat

Dressing

⅓   cup rice vinegar
3   tablespoons granulated sugar
¼   teaspoon salt
½   teaspoon hot chili oil (LaYu)
2   teaspoons sesame oil

Combine dressing ingredients in a jar with cover.

To Assemble: Line 5 individual salad bowls with spinach leaves. Top spinach with rice. Arrange carrots, snow peas, cucumbers and mushrooms around rice. Top with seafood. Accompany with dressing.

SERVING SUGGESTION: Serve with a watermelon basket of seasonal fruits or a heartier dessert such as Berry Cobbler (see page 479).

APPROXIMATE NUTRITIONAL CONTENT PER SERVING WITH DRESSING

Total calories: 372	Carbohydrates: 65 g
Fat: 5 g	Protein: 19 g
Percentage of calories from fat: 11%	Cholesterol: 74 mg
	Sodium: 1,035 mg
	Dietary fiber: 5 g

Sushi Salad is high in sodium. Serve it with low-sodium accompaniments such as those suggested. Choosing low-sodium foods for other meals will keep the total sodium for the day under control.

CHICKEN-AND-RICE SALAD

Makes 6 servings

1 ¼	cups water
1	cup uncooked short-grain white rice
⅛	teaspoon saffron powder
2 ½	tablespoons olive oil
1 ½	tablespoons tarragon-flavored white wine vinegar
½	teaspoon salt
1	cup cooked and cubed chicken
½	medium green pepper, cubed
½	medium red pepper, cubed
1	small ripe tomato, cubed
1	6-ounce jar marinated artichoke hearts, drained and cubed
4	large green onions (some with tops), chopped
1	2-ounce jar sliced pimientos, drained

In a medium saucepan, bring water and rice to a boil; stir in saffron. Cover, reduce heat, and simmer 20–30 minutes or until rice is tender and water is absorbed. Combine olive oil, vinegar and salt; pour over rice. Toss until well coated. Cool to room temperature. Add chicken, peppers, tomato and artichoke hearts. Refrigerate 3–4 hours or until thoroughly chilled. Garnish with green onion and pimientos.

SERVING SUGGESTION: For dessert, serve seasonal fruits or Red Raspberry Cobbler (see page 479).

APPROXIMATE NUTRITIONAL CONTENT PER SERVING

Total calories: 320
Fat: 14 g
Percentage of calories from fat: 38%

Carbohydrates: 24 g
Protein: 26 g
Cholesterol: 64 mg
Sodium: 242 mg
Dietary fiber: 1 g

Water-packed rather than marinated artichoke hearts will reduce the calories per serving to 302 and the percentage of calories from fat to 26%.

HOT CHICKEN SALAD

Makes 6 servings

Noodles

    3 cups Chicken Stock (page 264) or canned broth*
    3 cups water
    1 tablespoon reduced-sodium soy sauce
    1 8-ounce package buckwheat (Soba) noodles

In a medium stockpot, bring chicken stock and water to a boil; add soy sauce and noodles. Boil 4–5 minutes or until noodles are tender. Drain.

Chicken

    ¾ pound chicken breast, skinned and boned
    1 cup Chicken Stock (page 264) or canned broth*
    1 tablespoon peeled, coarsely chopped, fresh gingerroot
    3 green onions, coarsely chopped

In a medium saucepan or Dutch oven, combine all chicken ingredients, and heat to boiling. Reduce heat, cover and simmer 20 minutes or until done. Cool in stock 10 minutes. Drain. Cool slightly. Tear chicken into julienne strips.

Vegetables

    5 cups leaf lettuce torn into bite-size pieces
    1 English cucumber, peeled, cut into thirds and julienned

Dressing

    ¼ cup reduced-sodium soy sauce
    1 tablespoon rice vinegar
    2 tablespoons hot chili oil (LaYu)

  2 tablespoons sesame oil
  1 tablespoon water
2½ teaspoons granulated sugar
  3 tablespoons finely chopped green onion
  ½ tablespoon minced garlic (about 5 cloves)
  3 tablespoons finely chopped green onion, white
    part only (about 6–8 onions)
  1 tablespoon ginger juice**

Combine all dressing ingredients in a jar with cover.

To Assemble: Line 6 salad bowls with lettuce. Top lettuce with noodles, chicken and cucumber. Drizzle with dressing.

*Canned broth is higher in sodium.

**To make ginger juice, grate a chunk of fresh ginger, then squeeze the pulp to yield desired amount of juice.

SERVING SUGGESTION: Excellent as a main meal salad. Serve with Italian Bread (page 276) and Lemon Custard (page 458).

APPROXIMATE NUTRITIONAL CONTENT PER SERVING WITHOUT DRESSING

Total calories: 254	Carbohydrates: 31 g
Fat: 4 g	Protein: 23 g
Percentage of calories from fat:	Cholesterol: 41 mg
13%	Sodium: 327 mg
	Dietary fiber: 2 g

APPROXIMATE NUTRITIONAL CONTENT PER TABLESPOON OF DRESSING

Total calories: 33	Carbohydrates: 1 g
Fat: 3 g	Protein: Tr
Percentage of calories from fat:	Cholesterol: 0
83%	Sodium: 134 mg
	Dietary fiber: Tr

Most of the sodium is in the dressing. Remember to use a moderate amount.

IMPERIAL CHICKEN SALAD

Makes 8 servings

 2 chicken breasts, skinned and boned
 3 cloves garlic
 2 tablespoons reduced-sodium soy sauce
 1 tablespoon olive oil, plus 2 teaspoons
 1 tablespoon dry sherry
 ¼ teaspoon powdered ginger
 ¼ teaspoon cinnamon
 3 cups Chicken Stock (page 264) or canned broth*
 3 cups water
 1 8-ounce package buckwheat (Soba) noodles
 20 wonton skins, cut into julienne strips
 1½ cups snow peas, steamed 2–3 minutes or just
       until crisp-tender
 1 small zucchini, peeled and cut into julienne strips
 1 cup bean sprouts
 4 cups shredded iceberg lettuce
 ⅓ cup chopped green onions
 ⅓ cup slivered almonds
 2 tablespoons toasted sesame seeds
   salt and black pepper to taste

Dressing
 ¼ cup fresh lemon juice
 ¼ cup sesame oil
 ¼ cup olive oil
 1 tablespoon reduced-sodium soy sauce
 ½ teaspoon hot chili oil (LaYu)
 ½ teaspoon powdered Oriental hot mustard
 ¼ teaspoon celery salt

In a large saucepan, place chicken breasts, garlic, soy sauce, 1 tablespoon olive oil, sherry, ginger, cinnamon and 2 cups of the chicken stock. Heat to boiling. Cover, reduce heat and simmer 20 minutes or until chicken is done. Cool in stock 10 minutes. Drain. Cool slightly. Tear chicken into julienne strips. Set aside.

In a medium saucepan, bring remaining cup of chicken stock and water to a boil. Add noodles and cook 4–5 minutes or until noodles are tender. Drain. Rinse quickly with cold water. Set aside.

In a nonstick skillet, heat 2 teaspoons olive oil and add wonton strips. Cook over high heat 2–3 minutes, stirring constantly. Set aside.

In a large salad bowl, toss chicken, noodles and vegetables. Sprinkle with almonds, sesame seeds and wontons.

Combine ingredients for dressing in a jar with cover. Drizzle salad with desired amount of dressing. Season to taste with salt and pepper.

*Canned broth is higher in sodium.

VARIATION: Imperial Chicken is also good cold. To serve cold, chill ingredients separately. Just before serving, combine ingredients and toss with dressing.

SERVING SUGGESTION: Fabulous as a main meal salad. Serve fresh fruit or Pudding Cake (page 480) for dessert.

APPROXIMATE NUTRITIONAL CONTENT PER SERVING WITHOUT DRESSING

Total calories: 308	Carbohydrates: 33 g
Fat: 9 g	Protein: 23 g
Percentage of calories from fat: 26%	Cholesterol: 37 mg
	Sodium: 482 mg
	Dietary fiber: 3 g

APPROXIMATE NUTRITIONAL CONTENT PER TABLESPOON OF DRESSING

Total calories: 110	Carbohydrates: Tr
Fat: 12 g	Protein: Tr
Percentage of calories from fat: 99%	Cholesterol: 0
	Sodium: 125 mg
	Dietary fiber: 0

Most of the fat is in the dressing, so use a moderate amount. Keep a balance for the day by selecting low-fat foods for other meals.

BEEF, NOODLE AND MUSHROOM SALAD

Makes 6 servings

⅓ cup rice vinegar
½ bunch white radishes, cut into julienne strips
4 cups Beef Stock (page 268) or canned broth*
1 8-ounce package buckwheat (Soba) noodles
½ teaspoon olive oil
8 cloves garlic, slivered
¾ pounds lean beef sirloin, cut into stir-fry strips
1 7-ounce package dried forest mushrooms
      (Shiitake), reconstituted in water to soften and
      then cut into julienne strips
⅓ pound bean sprouts
½ English cucumber, peeled, seeded and cut into
      julienne strips
6 green onions, sliced on the diagonal into thirds

Sauce

¼ cup reduced-sodium soy sauce
2 tablespoons oyster sauce
2 tablespoons rice vinegar
1 tablespoon olive oil
¼ teaspoon crushed red pepper

Pour vinegar over radishes and marinate 30 minutes at room temperature. Rinse and pat dry.

Meanwhile, in a medium saucepan, bring beef stock to a boil; add noodles and cook 5–6 minutes or until noodles are tender.

In a small saucepan, combine all the sauce ingredients and simmer 5 minutes.

In a nonstick skillet, heat ½ teaspoon olive oil, add garlic and stir-fry 1–2 minutes; add beef and julienned mushrooms, and stir-fry 2–3 minutes.

To serve, mound bean sprouts on one side of a copper skillet or large platter. Arrange noodles on the other side. Spoon beef and mushrooms over top. Garnish with radishes, cucumber and green onions. Pass the sauce.

*Canned broth is higher in sodium.

SERVING SUGGESTION: Excellent as a main meal salad. Serve with Frozen Yogurt Parfait with Fruit Sauces (page 467).

APPROXIMATE NUTRITIONAL CONTENT PER SERVING WITHOUT SAUCE

Total calories: 300	Carbohydrates: 35 g
Fat: 7 g	Protein: 23 g
Percentage of calories from fat:	Cholesterol: 45 mg
22%	Sodium: 221 mg
	Dietary fiber: 2 g

APPROXIMATE NUTRITIONAL CONTENT PER TABLESPOON OF SAUCE

Total calories: 20	Carbohydrates: Tr
Fat: 1 g	Protein: Tr
Percentage of calories from fat:	Cholesterol: Tr
77%	Sodium: 333 mg
	Dietary fiber: 0

Most of the fat and sodium are in the sauce. Remember to use a moderate amount.

ORIENTAL SHRIMP SALAD

Makes 5 servings

4   cups Chicken Stock (page 264) or canned broth*
1   8-ounce package buckwheat (Soba) noodles
3   cups fresh spinach leaves
3   cups Bibb lettuce
⅔   pound medium prawns, cooked, shelled and
       deveined
½   pound snow peas, steamed 2 to 3 minutes or
       until crisp-tender
½   pound fresh asparagus, steamed 3–4 minutes or
       until barely tender
3   carrots, sliced diagonally into 4 or 5 pieces and
       steamed 3–4 minutes or until crisp-tender
½   English cucumber, peeled and thinly sliced
1   small bunch radishes, trimmed and thinly sliced
½   cup canned water chestnuts, drained
     Wasabi Vinaigrette (page 358)

In a medium saucepan, bring chicken stock to a boil. Add noodles and boil 5–7 minutes or until noodles are tender. Drain.

Arrange spinach and lettuce leaves over chilled salad plates. Mound noodles to one side of each plate. Arrange prawns next to noodles. Surround with snow peas, asparagus, carrots and cucumber. Garnish with radishes and water chestnuts. Serve hot or cold with Wasabi Vinaigrette.

*Canned broth is higher in sodium.

SERVING SUGGESTION: Great as a main meal salad. Serve with warm tortillas and Fresh Pineapple with Papaya Purée (page 491).

APPROXIMATE NUTRITIONAL CONTENT PER SERVING WITHOUT DRESSING

Total calories: 319

Fat: 3 g

Percentage of calories from fat: 9%

Carbohydrates: 47 g

Protein: 26 g

Cholesterol: 118 mg

Sodium: 413 mg

Dietary fiber: 5 g

SHRIMP-AND-SPINACH SALAD

Makes 6 servings

- ½ cup cooked shrimpmeat
- 1 English cucumber, very thinly sliced
- ¼ cup rice vinegar
- 1 teaspoon reduced-sodium soy sauce
- 1 tablespoon granulated sugar
- ½ teaspoon salt
- 10 fresh spinach leaves, stems removed, steamed and chilled

In a salad bowl, combine the shrimp and cucumber. In a jar with cover, combine vinegar, soy sauce, sugar and salt, and pour over shrimp and cucumber. Chill 1 hour.

Just before serving, mix in spinach. Spoon into small bowls or custard cups. Serve with chopsticks.

SERVING SUGGESTION: A good light appetizer or first course to complement an Oriental meal.

APPROXIMATE NUTRITIONAL CONTENT PER SERVING WITH DRESSING

Total calories: 38

Fat: Tr

Percentage of calories from fat: 7%

Carbohydrates: 4 g

Protein: 5 g

Cholesterol: 37 mg

Sodium: 270 mg

Dietary fiber: Tr

CALAMARI SALAD

Makes 8 cups salad; dressing makes ⅔ cup

1 pound squid tubes
½ teaspoon olive oil
1 large tomato, diced
1¾ cups coarsely chopped red onion
⅔ cup chopped green onions
1 cup coarsely chopped celery

Dressing
3 tablespoons olive oil
3 tablespoons fresh lemon juice
3 tablespoons fresh lime juice
¾ teaspoon salt
1 teaspoon black pepper
1 teaspoon Tabasco sauce

Clean squid tubes and cut into ½-inch rings. Toss with ½ teaspoon olive oil. In a nonstick skillet, sauté squid 3–4 minutes or until color changes and squid are cooked. Plunge into ice water. Drain and pat dry.

In a shallow bowl, combine squid, tomatoes, red and green onions and celery; set aside.

In a jar with cover, combine all the dressing ingredients. Pour desired amount of dressing over squid and vegetables. Chill 2–3 hours, tossing 2–3 times.

SERVING SUGGESTION: Serve with Hickory-Smoked Salmon (page 368), steamed rice and seasonal fruit.

APPROXIMATE NUTRITIONAL CONTENT PER CUP OF SALAD WITHOUT DRESSING

Total calories: 72	Carbohydrates: 6 g
Fat: 1 g	Protein: 9 g
Percentage of calories from fat:	Cholesterol: 132 mg
15%	Sodium: 40 mg
	Dietary fiber: 1 g

APPROXIMATE NUTRITIONAL CONTENT PER TABLESPOON OF DRESSING

Total calories: 36
Fat: 4 g
Percentage of calories from fat:
  90%

Carbohydrates: 1 g
Protein: Tr
Cholesterol: 0
Sodium: 153 mg
Dietary fiber: Tr

SEAFOOD SALAD

Makes 6 servings; dressing makes ¾ cup

Dressing

- ⅔ cup safflower mayonnaise
- 5 cloves garlic, finely minced
- 2 tablespoons lemon juice, plus 1 teaspoon
- 1 teaspon white pepper
- ¼ teaspoon Tabasco sauce
- ¾ teaspoon salt
- 2 teaspoons fresh dill
- 2 tablespoons grated white onion

Salad

- 12 cups shredded lettuce
- ¼ cup finely chopped green onion
- 1 cup chopped celery
- ½ pound cooked crabmeat
- ¾ pound cooked shrimpmeat
- 2 medium tomatoes, cut into wedges

In a jar with cover, combine dressing ingredients. Chill at least 1 hour.

Toss lettuce, onion and celery with ¼ cup of the dressing. Add crab and shrimp. Toss. Garnish with tomato wedges. Divide salad among chilled salad plates. Pass the remaining dressing.

(continued on next page)

(continued from preceding page)

SERVING SUGGESTION: Excellent as a main meal salad. Serve with Apple Oat Bran Muffins (page 293), French bread or warm tortillas.

APPROXIMATE NUTRITIONAL CONTENT PER SERVING WITHOUT DRESSING

Total calories: 114
Fat: 1 g
Percentage of calories from fat:
   10%

Carbohydrates: 5 g
Protein: 20 g
Cholesterol: 113 mg
Sodium: 269 mg
Dietary fiber: 2 g

Add 92 calories per additional tablespoon of dressing.

APPROXIMATE NUTRITIONAL CONTENT PER TABLESPOON OF DRESSING

Total calories: 92
Fat: 10 g
Percentage of calories from fat:
   93%

Carbohydrates: 1 g
Protein: Tr
Cholesterol: 7 g
Sodium: 204 mg
Dietary fiber: 0

SEAFOOD PRIMAVERA

Makes 6 servings; dressing makes 2 cups

Dressing

   1 whole egg
   1 egg yolk
   1 tablespoon Dijon mustard
   2 tablespoons freshly squeezed lemon juice
   2 tablespoons red wine vinegar
  ½ teaspoon salt
  ½ cup fresh basil
   1 cup olive oil

Salad

½ pound snow peas
1 pound ziti or elbow macaroni, cooked *al dente*
6 green onions, thinly sliced
2 green peppers, diced
3 stalks celery, diced
½ pound cooked shrimpmeat
½ pound cooked crabmeat
2 medium tomatoes, diced
1 cup fresh basil

In a blender, combine all dressing ingredients except olive oil. Process 2 minutes. With machine running, gradually add olive oil 1 tablespoon at a time. Chill.

In a steamer over boiling water, steam snow peas 2–3 minutes or until crisp-tender.

In a large salad bowl, toss pasta, snow peas, onion, peppers and celery. Sprinkle with shrimp, crab and tomatoes. Garnish with the 1 cup basil. Chill. Serve with dressing on the side.

SERVING SUGGESTION: Excellent as a main meal salad.

APPROXIMATE NUTRITIONAL CONTENT PER SERVING WITHOUT DRESSING

Total calories: 283	Carbohydrates: 43 g
Fat: 1 g	Protein: 23 g
Percentage of calories from fat:	Cholesterol: 94 mg
4%	Sodium: 524 mg
	Dietary fiber: 5 g

APPROXIMATE NUTRITIONAL CONTENT PER TABLESPOON OF DRESSING

Total calories: 65	Carbohydrates: Tr
Fat: 7 g	Protein: Tr
Percentage of calories from fat:	Cholesterol: 13 g
96%	Sodium: 50 mg
	Dietary fiber: 0

CHICKEN, SHRIMP AND PASTA SALAD

Makes 5½ quarts (approximately 8 servings as a main course)

¼ head cauliflower, florets only
2 carrots, peeled and thinly sliced on the diagonal
½ pound snow peas
1 leek, thinly sliced
1 head Bibb lettuce
1 pound cavatelli or other shell-shaped pasta,
      cooked *al dente*
1 chicken breast, skinned, boned, poached and cut
      into strips ½-inch wide
8 medium prawns, cooked, shelled and deveined
1 7-ounce can water-packed artichoke hearts,
      drained
   Aïoli Vinaigrette (page 353)

Separately blanch cauliflower, carrots, snow peas and leek 1–2 minutes or just until crisp-tender.

Arrange lettuce over dinner plates. Mound pasta, chicken, prawns and vegetables over lettuce. Serve with Aïoli Vinaigrette.

SERVING SUGGESTION: Serve with Cheese Popovers (page 284) and fresh fruit. Or omit the popovers and fruit, and serve a dessert such as Blackberry Cobbler (see page 479).

APPROXIMATE NUTRITIONAL CONTENT PER CUP OF SALAD WITHOUT DRESSING

Total calories: 124	Carbohydrates: 22 g
Fat: Tr	Protein: 7 g
Percentage of calories from fat:	Cholesterol: 16 mg
6%	Sodium: 34 mg
	Dietary fiber: 2 g

FUSILLI WITH SMOKED TURKEY, BROCCOLI AND PEPPERS

Makes 8 servings

> 1 pound fusilli pasta, cooked *al dente*
> 1 pound smoked turkey, diced
> 1 bunch fresh broccoli, florets only, cooked *al dente*
> 1 6-ounce jar roasted red peppers, drained and diced
> ⅓ cup freshly grated Parmesan cheese

Dressing
> ¾ cup olive oil
> ¼ cup cider vinegar
> ¾ teaspoon salt
> ¼ teaspoon black pepper

In a large salad bowl, toss pasta, turkey, broccoli and peppers. Chill. In a jar with cover, combine dressing ingredients.

Drizzle salad with desired amount of dressing and sprinkle with Parmesan cheese.

VARIATION: Sprinkle with crushed red pepper flakes.

SERVING SUGGESTION: Excellent as a main meal salad. Serve with fresh fruit.

APPROXIMATE NUTRITIONAL CONTENT PER SERVING WITHOUT DRESSING

Total calories: 345	Carbohydrates: 49 g
Fat: 9 g	Protein: 21 g
Percentage of calories from fat: 22%	Cholesterol: 3 mg
	Sodium: 94 mg
	Dietary fiber: 4 g

(continued on next page)

(continued from preceding page)

**APPROXIMATE NUTRITIONAL CONTENT PER
TABLESPOON OF DRESSING**

Total calories: 89
Fat: 10 g
Percentage of calories from fat:
    99%

Carbohydrates: Tr
Protein: 0
Cholesterol: 0
Sodium: 100 mg
Dietary fiber: 0

TWO-SALSA PASTA SALAD

Makes 20 cups (approximately 8 servings as a main course)

- 14 fresh tomatillos, husks removed
- 3 fresh jalapeño peppers
- 3 cloves garlic
- 1 cup chopped white onion
- ¼ cup chopped fresh cilantro
- 1 tablespoon olive oil
- 1 pound fusilli or other curly pasta, cooked *al dente*
- 1 cup chopped red onion
- 1 medium ripe tomato, diced
- ½ green pepper, diced
- ½ yellow, gold or red pepper, diced
- 1 cup prepared prickly pear cactus leaves, chopped (optional)
- ½ cup chopped fresh cilantro or parsley for garnish
- 6-8 very thin red onion rings for garnish
  homemade or commercial tomato salsa

In a medium saucepan, boil tomatillos in just enough water to cover 7–10 minutes or just until barely tender. Drain. In a blender or food processor, combine tomatillos, jalapeño peppers, garlic, white onion and ¼ cup cilantro. Purée 5–10 seconds or just to chunky stage. Pour into medium stockpot. Add olive oil and cook 5 minutes, stirring constantly.

Arrange pasta in a shallow serving bowl. Toss with tomatillo sauce, red onion, diced tomato, peppers and cactus leaves, if desired. Garnish with cilantro or parsley and onion rings. Serve with salsa.

NOTE: One 12-ounce can tomatillos, drained, may be used in place of fresh. One 4-ounce can jalapeños may be substituted for fresh. Prickly pear cactus leaves (nopalitos), available in many supermarkets and Spanish markets, add texture but are not essential to flavor.

SERVING SUGGESTION: An excellent addition to any salad buffet. A wonderful side dish with tacos, taco salad or any Mexican meal.

APPROXIMATE NUTRITIONAL CONTENT PER CUP OF SALAD WITHOUT SALSA

Total calories: 119	Carbohydrates: 23 g
Fat: 1 g	Protein: 4 g
Percentage of calories from fat:	Cholesterol: 0
8%	Sodium: 15 mg
	Dietary fiber: 2 g

Add 20 calories per ¼ cup of tomato salsa. Sodium will vary depending on the brand of salsa selected.

PASTA-AND-BEAN SALAD

Makes 8 cups

2 15-ounce cans cannellini beans, drained and
   rinsed
1 15-ounce can black beans, drained and rinsed
2 large tomatoes, coarsely chopped
1 red onion, coarsely chopped
2 cups cavatelli or other shell-shaped pasta cooked
   al dente
2 tablespoons olive oil
2 tablespoons white wine vinegar
¾ teaspoon salt
¼ teaspoon black pepper
3 cloves garlic, minced
½ cup fresh basil (optional)

In a salad bowl, combine beans, tomatoes, onion and pasta.
In a covered jar, combine olive oil, vinegar, salt, pepper and
garlic; pour over pasta and beans, and toss. Chill at least 3
hours. Just before serving, garnish with basil, if desired.

SERVING SUGGESTION: Serve with Louisiana Chicken
Strips (page 394). Also good with grilled chicken. Great
with sandwiches.

**APPROXIMATE NUTRITIONAL CONTENT PER ½ CUP OF
SALAD WITH DRESSING**

Total calories: 84	Carbohydrates: 13 g
Fat: 2 g	Protein: 4 g
Percentage of calories from fat:	Cholesterol: 0
22%	Sodium: 260 mg
	Dietary fiber: 1 g

ASPARAGUS, TOMATO AND PASTA SALAD

Makes 16 cups

¼ cup olive oil
1 tablespoon freshly squeezed lemon juice
¼ teaspoon salt
¼ teaspoon black pepper
2 cloves garlic
1 pound elbow macaroni, cooked *al dente*
2 medium tomatoes, coarsely chopped
1 small cucumber, peeled, halved lengthwise, seeded and cut crosswise into ¼-inch strips
1 small red onion, chopped
1 8-ounce can mushroom stems and pieces, drained
1 bunch fresh asparagus, steamed 2–3 minutes and cut diagonally into 1½-inch pieces

In a jar with cover, combine olive oil, lemon juice, salt, pepper and garlic.

In a large salad bowl, toss pasta with dressing. Add remaining ingredients and toss again. Serve hot or cold.

SERVING SUGGESTION: A good side dish with hamburgers, chicken burgers or grilled poultry or seafood.

APPROXIMATE NUTRITIONAL CONTENT PER CUP OF SALAD WITH DRESSING

Total calories: 148	Carbohydrates: 24 g
Fat: 4 g	Protein: 5 g
Percentage of calories from fat: 24%	Cholesterol: 0
	Sodium: 36 mg
	Dietary fiber: 2 g

For a lighter version, reduce olive oil to 2 tablespoons. Toss with dressing just before serving. The calories per cup with dressing will be 133, fat will be reduced to 2 grams and the percentage of calories from fat will be 14%.

OLD-FASHIONED POTATO SALAD

Makes 10 cups; dressing makes 1 cup

1	egg
1	teaspoon red wine vinegar
2	teaspoons fresh lemon juice
1	teaspoon Dijon mustard
3	cloves garlic
½	teaspoon salt
1	cup olive oil
2¾	pounds russet potatoes, cooked
3	hard-boiled egg whites
2	whole hard-boiled eggs
2	stalks celery, finely chopped
½	cup finely chopped white onion
1	dill pickle, finely chopped
	salt black pepper to taste
15	ripe black olives, pitted and halved
	paprika
1	tomato, cut into wedges

In a blender or food processor, combine egg, vinegar, lemon juice, mustard, garlic and salt. With machine running, gradually add olive oil, 1 tablespoon at a time. Chill at least 4 hours.

Into a large salad bowl, cut cooled, cooked potatoes in 1-inch cubes and all egg whites in 1-inch chunks. Crumble yolks over potatoes. Add celery, onion and pickle. Chill.

Just before serving, toss the potato-egg mixture with desired amount of dressing. Season to taste with salt and pepper. Sprinkle with olives, then with paprika. Garnish with tomato wedges.

SERVING SUGGESTION: Good for a summer party or buffet. Serve with grilled meats, poultry or seafood. Accompany with other salads such as Three-Bean Salad (page 338), Two-Salsa Pasta Salad (page 320), Wild and White Rice Salad (page 333) and a tray of assorted seasonal fruits.

APPROXIMATE NUTRITIONAL CONTENT PER ½ CUP OF SALAD WITHOUT DRESSING

Total calories: 85

Fat: 1 g

Percentage of calories from fat: 11%

Carbohydrates: 17 g

Protein: 3 g

Cholesterol: 21 mg

Sodium: 111 mg

Dietary fiber: 2 g

APPROXIMATE NUTRITIONAL CONTENT PER TABLESPOON OF DRESSING

Total calories: 125

Fat: 14 g

Percentage of calories from fat: 98%

Carbohydrates: Tr

Protein: Tr

Cholesterol: 13 mg

Sodium: 80 mg

Dietary fiber: Tr

Most of the fat is in the dressing. Remember to use a moderate amount.

MARINATED POTATO SALAD

Makes 8 servings

¾ pound tiny new red potatoes, cooked until barely
    tender
¼ cup olive oil
¾ cup cider vinegar
¾ teaspoon salt
¼ teaspoon black pepper
3 ripe plum tomatoes, quartered
1 14-ounce can water-packed artichoke hearts,
    quartered
½ medium red onion, cut into rings
½ red pepper, cut into thin strips
½ green pepper, cut into thin strips
1 5-ounce can whole baby corn, drained

Into a salad bowl, cut potatoes in quarters. In a jar with
cover, combine olive oil, vinegar, salt and pepper; pour
over warm potatoes. Chill 2 hours. Add remaining ingredients. Toss to coat the salad with dressing. Chill 2 more
hours.

APPROXIMATE NUTRITIONAL CONTENT PER SERVING WITH DRESSING

Total calories: 167	Carbohydrates: 26 g
Fat: 7 g	Protein: 4 g
Percentage of calories from fat:	Cholesterol: 0
35%	Sodium: 321 mg
	Dietary fiber: 2 g

*For a lighter version, decrease olive oil to 1 tablespoon and vinegar to ¼
cup. Toss ingredients with dressing just before serving. The calories will
be reduced to 122, the fat to 2 grams, and the percentage of calories
from fat to 14%.*

MARINATED PEPPERS AND ONION

Makes 4 servings

1	medium green pepper
1	medium red pepper
½	medium white onion
½	medium red onion
1	large tomato
1½	tablespoons olive oil
1½	tablespoons fresh lemon juice
1½	tablespoons fresh lime juice
½	teaspoon salt
¾	teaspoon black pepper
½	teaspoon Tabasco sauce

Cut peppers in half, remove seeds and cut crosswise into ¼-inch rings. Cut onions in half, then into ¼-inch rings. Coarsely chop tomato.

In a covered jar, combine olive oil, lemon juice, lime juice, salt, pepper and Tabasco. Pour over vegetables and toss. Chill 2–3 hours.

APPROXIMATE NUTRITIONAL CONTENT PER SERVING WITH DRESSING

Total calories: 70	Carbohydrates: 6 g
Fat: 5 g	Protein: 1 g
Percentage of calories from fat:	Cholesterol: 0
63%	Sodium: 273 mg
	Dietary fiber: 1 g

Don't be too concerned with the percentage of calories from fat. Calories in the peppers and onions are so few that even a small amount of fat will elevate the percentage.

VEGETABLE ANTIPASTO SALAD

Makes 8 servings

  1 clove garlic, minced
  ¼ cup fresh lemon juice
  1 tablespoon olive oil
  ½ teaspoon salt
  ¼ teaspoon black pepper
  4 small carrots, peeled and thinly sliced on the
       diagonal
  1 small zucchini, peeled and sliced on the diagonal
       into matchstick strips
  ¼ pound broccoli florets
  6 tiny red potatoes, quartered
  ¼ pound fresh green beans
  ½ red onion, cut into rings
  6 plum tomatoes, quartered

In a covered jar, combine garlic, lemon juice, olive oil, salt
and pepper. Set aside.

In a steamer over boiling water, steam vegetables, one
type at a time, just until crisp-tender: carrots, zucchini and
broccoli about 2 minutes each; potatoes and green beans
about 6–10 minutes each. As each vegetable is cooked,
remove to a 13 x 9 x 2-inch glass casserole dish. Tuck onion
rings and tomatoes among vegetables as garnish. Chill at
least 3 hours. Just before serving, toss with dressing.

**APPROXIMATE NUTRITIONAL CONTENT PER SERVING
WITH DRESSING**

Total calories: 112	Carbohydrates: 22 g
Fat: 2 g	Protein: 3 g
Percentage of calories from fat:	Cholesterol: 0
16%	Sodium: 157 mg
	Dietary fiber: 4 g

MEDITERRANEAN ANTIPASTO

Makes 6 servings

- ⅓ pound fresh asparagus
- ⅓ pound fresh green beans
- ¼ cup fresh lemon juice
- 2 tablespoons olive oil
- ½ teaspoon salt or to taste
- ¼ teaspoon black pepper
- 1 head red leaf lettuce
- 1 8-ounce can garbanzo beans, drained and rinsed
- 2 ounces part-skim mozzarella cheese, cut into julienne strips

In a steamer over boiling water, steam asparagus and then green beans until just crisp-tender. In a jar with cover, combine lemon juice, olive oil, salt and pepper. Pour over asparagus and green beans while vegetables are still warm.

Just before serving, drain marinade from vegetables. Arrange leaf lettuce over small serving platter. Mound asparagus, green beans, garbanzo beans and cheese over top.

APPROXIMATE NUTRITIONAL CONTENT PER SERVING

Total calories: 92
Fat: 4 g
Percentage of calories from fat: 41%

Carbohydrates: 9 g
Protein: 5 g
Cholesterol: 5 mg
Sodium: 192 mg
Dietary fiber: 2 g

VEGETABLE AND BLACK BEAN ANTIPASTO

Makes 6 servings

- 3 carrots
- 3 stalks celery
- 2 jicama
- 1 English cucumber
- 1 head red leaf lettuce
- 1 cup Black Bean Dip (page 348)

Slice carrots, celery, jicama and cucumber diagonally into sticks. Place lettuce on chilled salad plates and arrange vegetables on lettuce. Serve with a dollop of Black Bean Dip.

SERVING SUGGESTION: An excellent accompaniment to a soup meal. Also good as an appetizer.

APPROXIMATE NUTRITIONAL CONTENT PER SERVING WITHOUT BEAN DIP

Total calories: 43
Fat: Tr
Percentage of calories from fat: 6%

Carbohydrates: 10 g
Protein: 1 g
Cholesterol: 0
Sodium: 45 mg
Dietary fiber: 3 g

BLACK BEANS WITH VEGETABLES AND SHRIMP

Makes 6 servings

1 ½ cups Chili Salsa (page 361), or commercial salsa
1   cup Black Bean Dip (page 348)
⅔   pound medium prawns, cooked, shelled and
        deveined
1   English cucumber, thinly sliced
8   stalks celery, sliced diagonally into thirds
8   carrots, sliced diagonally into thirds
     fresh parsley for garnish
1   lime, cut into wedges
1   1 inch-square piece tomato for garnish

Into the center of a medium dish, spread ½ cup of the salsa. Mound bean dip over salsa. Arrange prawns, cucumber, celery and carrots around dip. Tuck in parsley and lime wedges for garnish. Top bean dip with small piece of tomato and touch of parsley. Pour remaining cup of salsa into bowl and pass with vegetables.

VARIATION: Add tortilla chips. Be sure they are baked, not fried, using a heart-healthy oil such as safflower or corn oil.

SERVING SUGGESTION: An excellent accompaniment to a soup meal. Also good as an appetizer.

APPROXIMATE NUTRITIONAL CONTENT PER SERVING

Total calories: 183
Fat: 2 g
Percentage of calories from fat:
   7%

Carbohydrates: 28 g
Protein: 17 g
Cholesterol: 98 mg
Sodium: 600 mg
Dietary fiber: 7 g

ENSENADA SALAD

Makes 4 servings

- ½ cucumber, peeled
- 3 cups red leaf lettuce torn into bite-size pieces
- 1½ cups Bibb lettuce
- 1½ cups fresh spinach leaves
- 2 medium tomatoes, diced
  Jalapeño Vinaigrette (page 357)

Cut cucumber in half lengthwise, then slice crosswise into ¼-inch strips. In a salad bowl, toss lettuce, spinach, cucumber and tomatoes. Drizzle with Jalapeño Vinaigrette to taste.

APPROXIMATE NUTRITIONAL CONTENT PER SERVING WITHOUT DRESSING

Total calories: 27
Fat: Tr
Percentage of calories from fat:
   10%

Carbohydrates: 5 g
Protein: 2 g
Cholesterol: 0
Sodium: 40 mg
Dietary fiber: 2 g

WILD AND WHITE RICE SALAD

Makes 12 cups

1⅓ cups uncooked wild rice
1 cup beef consommé
1 cup uncooked short-grain white rice*
1 red onion, coarsely chopped
1 8-ounce can mushroom stems and pieces, drained
½ green pepper, coarsely chopped
½ red pepper, coarsely chopped
 salt and black pepper to taste

Dressing
¾ cup olive oil
¼ cup cider vinegar
¾ teaspoon salt
¼ teaspoon black pepper

Steam wild rice according to package directions, substituting 1 cup beef consommé for 1 of the cups of water. Allow 45–60 minutes' cooking time.

In a separate pan, steam white rice according to package directions. Allow 20–30 minutes' cooking time.

In a large salad bowl, combine cooked wild and white rice. Add onion, mushrooms, and green and red peppers.

In a jar with cover, combine dressing ingredients. Pour ½ cup of dressing over salad and toss. (Reserve remaining dressing for later use.) Season to taste with salt and pepper.

*Brown rice in place of white rice yields 3 times as much fiber.

APPROXIMATE NUTRITIONAL CONTENT PER ½ CUP OF SALAD WITH DRESSING

Total calories: 100	Carbohydrates: 15 g
Fat: 3 g	Protein: 1 g
Percentage of calories from fat:	Cholesterol: Tr
31%	Sodium: 111 mg
	Dietary fiber: Tr

GEORGETOWN RICE SALAD

Makes 10 cups

    4½ cups Chicken Stock (page 264) or canned broth*
     3 cups uncooked long-grain rice**
    ¼ cup olive oil
     2 tablespoons rice vinegar
     1 teaspoon dry mustard
    ¾ teaspoon salt or to taste
    ½ teaspoon black pepper
     1 yellow or red pepper, diced
     1 green pepper, diced
     3 large ripe tomatoes, diced

In a medium saucepan, bring chicken stock to a boil. Add rice, cover, reduce heat and simmer 20–30 minutes or until rice is tender and moisture is absorbed. Cool. Spoon into a low salad bowl.

In a jar with cover, combine olive oil, vinegar, mustard, salt and pepper. Pour over rice and toss.

Sprinkle diced peppers and tomatoes over rice. Toss again. Chill.

*Canned broth is higher in sodium.

**Brown rice in place of white rice yields 3 times as much fiber.

SERVING SUGGESTION: Especially good with chicken and fish or as a side dish with sandwiches.

APPROXIMATE NUTRITIONAL CONTENT PER ½ CUP OF SALAD WITH DRESSING

Total calories: 139	Carbohydrates: 24 g
Fat: 3 g	Protein: 3 g
Percentage of calories from fat:	Cholesterol: Tr
22%	Sodium: 144 mg
	Dietary fiber: Tr

For a lighter version, reduce olive oil to 1 tablespoon and increase rice vinegar to ¼ cup. The calories per ½ cup of salad with dressing will be 46, and fat will be reduced to 1 gram.

WINTER VEGETABLE SALAD

Makes 4 servings

> 3 cups romaine lettuce torn into bite-size pieces
> 1½ cups Bibb lettuce torn into bite-size pieces
> 1½ cups iceberg lettuce torn into bite-size pieces
> 6 mushrooms, sliced
> 2 medium tomatoes, cut into wedges
> ½ red onion, thinly sliced into rings
>   Creamy Garlic Dressing (page 352)

Layer lettuce onto chilled salad plates. Arrange mushrooms, tomatoes and onion rings over top. Drizzle with dressing.

APPROXIMATE NUTRITIONAL CONTENT PER SERVING WITHOUT DRESSING

Total calories: 30	Carbohydrates: 6 g
Fat: Tr	Protein: 2 g
Percentage of calories from fat:	Cholesterol: 0
10%	Sodium: 13 mg
	Dietary fiber: 2 g

FARMER'S MARKET SALAD

Makes 1 serving

- 2 leaves red leaf lettuce
- 2 leaves green leaf lettuce
- 1 broccoli floret, steamed or microwaved 1–2 minutes or until crisp-tender
- 1 cauliflower floret, steamed or microwaved 2–3 minutes or until crisp-tender
- 1 large carrot, grated
- 1 medium ripe tomato, diced
- 2 very thin raw turnip slices
- 3 very thin red onion rings
- ⅓ cup homemade or commercial tomato salsa

Layer lettuce leaves on a chilled dinner plate. Arrange the remaining vegetables on the lettuce. Accompany with tomato salsa.

VARIATION: Add ½ cup 1% or 2% cottage cheese, ½ cup couscous or ½ cup saffron-flavored rice. (To make saffron rice, stir in ¼ teaspoon powdered saffron to cooked rice.)

SERVING SUGGESTION: Excellent for lunch accompanied with a whole-wheat roll or a slice of hearty bread.

APPROXIMATE NUTRITIONAL CONTENT PER SERVING WITH SALSA

Total calories: 145	Carbohydrates: 32 g
Fat: 1 g	Protein: 6 g
Percentage of calories from fat: 7%	Cholesterol: 0
	Sodium: 100 mg
	Dietary fiber: 9 g

The sodium will fluctuate depending on the brand of salsa. Homemade tomato and chili salsa has 75 mg of sodium per ⅓ cup. Some commercial brands may have as much as 400 mg.

LETTUCE, ONION AND TOMATO SALAD

Makes 4 servings

    3 cups red leaf lettuce torn into bite-size pieces
    3 cups green leaf lettuce torn into bite-size pieces
    1 tomato, cut into wedges
       Light Dijon Vinaigrette (page 355)
    4 red onion rings

In a bowl, toss red and green leaf lettuce and tomato with desired amount of dressing. Arrange on chilled salad plates. Garnish with red onion rings.

VARIATION: Use Light Italian Vinaigrette (page 356) in place of Light Dijon Vinaigrette.

APPROXIMATE NUTRITIONAL CONTENT PER SERVING WITHOUT DRESSING

Total calories: 23
Fat: Tr
Percentage of calories from fat:
  11%

Carbohydrates: 5 g
Protein: 1 g
Cholesterol: 0
Sodium: 12 mg
Dietary fiber: 2 g

THREE-BEAN SALAD

Makes 6 cups

3 tablespoons olive oil

5 cloves garlic

2 tablespoons fresh lemon juice

1¼ teaspoons ground cumin

½ teaspoon oregano

2 teaspoons hot chili oil (LaYu)

½ teaspoon salt or to taste

¼ teaspoon black pepper

1 15-ounce can red kidney beans, drained and rinsed

1 15-ounce can cannellini beans, drained and rinsed

1 15-ounce can black beans, drained and rinsed

1 small white onion, coarsely chopped

In a blender or food processor, purée olive oil and garlic. Add lemon juice, cumin, oregano, hot chili oil, salt and pepper. Chill at least 3 hours.

In a salad bowl, combine beans. Chill. Just before serving, add onion and toss with dressing.

SERVING SUGGESTION: Especially good with grilled chicken and red meats.

APPROXIMATE NUTRITIONAL CONTENT PER ½ CUP OF SALAD WITH DRESSING

Total calories: 128	Carbohydrates: 16 g
Fat: 5 g	Protein: 6 g
Percentage of calories from fat:	Cholesterol: 0
32%	Sodium: 238 mg
	Dietary fiber: 3 g

For a lighter version, reduce olive oil to 1 tablespoon. The calories will be reduced to 108, the fat to 3 grams and the percentage of calories from fat to 17%.

CUCUMBER AND ONION SALAD

Makes 6 servings

- 1 English cucumber, thinly sliced
- 1 white onion, thinly sliced into rings
- ⅓ cup rice vinegar
- 1½ tablespoons granulated sugar
- ½ teaspoon salt
- ⅛ teaspoon black pepper

In a 2-quart glass bowl, toss cucumber and onions. In a jar with cover, combine vinegar, sugar, salt and pepper. Pour over cucumbers and onions. Chill 2 hours. Drain.

APPROXIMATE NUTRITIONAL CONTENT PER SERVING WITH DRESSING

Total calories: 26
Fat: Tr
Percentage of calories from fat:
  4%

Carbohydrates: 6 g
Protein: Tr
Cholesterol: 0
Sodium: 179 mg
Dietary fiber: Tr

PEPPER, ONION AND TOMATO SALAD

Makes 4 servings

> 4 cups leaf lettuce torn into bite-size pieces
> 2 ripe tomatoes, quartered
> ½ red pepper, cut into strips
> ½ green pepper, cut into strips
> Light Italian Vinaigrette (page 356)
> ¼ red onion, cut into rings

In a bowl, toss lettuce, tomatoes and peppers with desired amount of vinaigrette. Arrange on chilled salad plates. Garnish with red onion rings.

APPROXIMATE NUTRITIONAL CONTENT PER SERVING WITHOUT DRESSING

Total calories: 30
Fat: Tr
Percentage of calories from fat:
   10%

Carbohydrates: 6 g
Protein: 1 g
Cholesterol: 0
Sodium: 12 mg
Dietary fiber: 2 g

LETTUCE AND BERMUDA ONION SALAD

Makes 4 servings

   1 head red leaf lettuce, torn into bite-size pieces
  ¼ Bermuda onion, cut into rings
      Creamy Vinaigrette (page 354)

In a salad bowl, toss the lettuce and onion with desired amount of vinaigrette. Arrange on chilled salad plates.

APPROXIMATE NUTRITIONAL CONTENT PER SERVING WITHOUT DRESSING

Total calories: 8	Carbohydrates: 1 g
Fat: Tr	Protein: Tr
Percentage of calories from fat:	Cholesterol: 0
10%	Sodium: 2 mg
	Dietary fiber: Tr

NAPOLEON CAESAR SALAD

Makes 6 servings

1	egg, separated
2	cloves garlic
2½	tablespoons fresh lemon juice
¼	cup olive oil
2	tablespoons red wine vinegar
¾	teaspoon salt
¼	teaspoon Worcestershire sauce
¼	teaspoon black pepper
1	large head romaine lettuce
6	thinly shaved slices of Parmesan cheese

In a blender or food processor, combine egg yolk, garlic, lemon juice, olive oil, vinegar, salt, Worcestershire sauce and pepper. Add egg white; whirl 1 minute more. Use at once or chill up to 3 hours.

Arrange lettuce leaves on chilled salad plates. Drizzle with desired amount of dressing. Top each salad with a slice of Parmesan cheese.

VARIATION: Garnish each salad with 1 flat anchovy fillet.

APPROXIMATE NUTRITIONAL CONTENT PER SERVING WITHOUT DRESSING

Total calories: 18	Carbohydrates: 1 g
Fat: 1 g	Protein: 2 g
Percentage of calories from fat: 48%	Cholesterol: 2 mg
	Sodium: 59 mg
	Dietary fiber: Tr

APPROXIMATE NUTRITIONAL CONTENT PER TABLESPOON OF DRESSING

Total calories: 32
Fat: 3 g
Percentage of calories from fat:
  91%

Carbohydrates: Tr
Protein: Tr
Cholesterol: 0
Sodium: 106 mg
Dietary fiber: Tr

ROMAINE SALAD

Makes 4 servings

- ½ English cucumber, peeled and thinly sliced
- ½ red onion, cut into 1-inch cubes
- 2 medium tomatoes, cut into 1-inch cubes
  Light Italian Vinaigrette (page 356)
- 1 small head romaine lettuce, torn into bite-size pieces

In a salad bowl, toss cucumber, onion and tomatoes with desired amount of dressing. Chill 2 hours. Just before serving, add romaine and toss.

APPROXIMATE NUTRITIONAL CONTENT PER SERVING WITHOUT DRESSING

Total calories: 30
Fat: Tr
Percentage of calories from fat:
  9%

Carbohydrates: 6 g
Protein: 2 g
Cholesterol: 0
Sodium: 10 mg
Dietary fiber: 2 g

WARM SPINACH SALAD

Makes 6 servings

2	tablespoons reduced-sodium soy sauce
¼	cup sake
1	teaspoon sesame oil
1	teaspoon granulated sugar
1	bunch fresh spinach leaves, torn into bite-size pieces
¼	pound fresh mushrooms, sliced
1½	tablespoons toasted sesame seeds

In a small saucepan, combine soy sauce, sake, sesame oil and sugar. Simmer 5 minutes.

Put spinach and mushrooms into a salad bowl. Toss with warm dressing. Sprinkle with sesame seeds. Serve at once.

SERVING SUGGESTION: Especially good with grilled seafoods.

APPROXIMATE NUTRITIONAL CONTENT PER SERVING WITH DRESSING

Total calories: 47
Fat: 2 g
Percentage of calories from fat: 32%

Carbohydrates: 5 g
Protein: 3 g
Cholesterol: 0
Sodium: 167 mg
Dietary fiber: 3 g

SPINACH-AND-ONION SALAD

Makes 6 servings

> 3 cloves garlic
> 6 tablespoons fresh lemon juice
> ¼ cup olive oil
> ¾ teaspoon salt or to taste
> 1 bunch fresh spinach leaves, torn into bite-size
>   pieces
> ½ white onion, thinly sliced into rings

In a blender or food processor, combine garlic, lemon juice, olive oil and salt. In a salad bowl, toss spinach and onions with desired amount of dressing.

APPROXIMATE NUTRITIONAL CONTENT PER SERVING WITHOUT DRESSING

Total calories: 20	Carbohydrates: 3 g
Fat: Tr	Protein: 2 g
Percentage of calories from fat:	Cholesterol: 0
11%	Sodium: 66 mg
	Dietary fiber: 2 g

APPROXIMATE NUTRITIONAL CONTENT PER TABLESPOON OF DRESSING

Total calories: 46	Carbohydrates: 1 g
Fat: 4 g	Protein: Tr
Percentage of calories from fat:	Cholesterol: 0
91%	Sodium: 145 mg
	Dietary fiber: Tr

Most of the fat is in the dressing. Remember to use a moderate amount.

SUMMER FRUIT SALAD

Makes 2 servings

- 3 leaves red or green leaf lettuce
- ½ cup non-fat vanilla yogurt
- 3 large ripe strawberries, thinly sliced
- 3 slices fresh peach
- 1 slice fresh pineapple, cut into chunks
- 1 small wedge cantaloupe, cubed
- 1 small wedge honeydew melon, cubed
- 1 small wedge watermelon, cubed

Layer the lettuce on a chilled dinner plate. Spoon yogurt into individual custard cup or soufflé bowl; place on center or side of plate. Surround with fresh fruits.

NOTE: This is a great salad when you're watching calories. It looks like a lot of food, takes a long time to eat, and is a special treat in spring and early summer when fruits are just becoming available in the markets.

SERVING SUGGESTION: Serve with Applesauce Oatmeal Muffins (page 294).

APPROXIMATE NUTRITIONAL CONTENT PER SERVING

Total calories: 74
Fat: Tr
Percentage of calories from fat: 5%

Carbohydrates: 14 g
Protein: 4 g
Cholesterol: 1 mg
Sodium: 51 mg
Dietary fiber: 2 g

DIPS, DRESSINGS & SAUCES

A NOTE ON SALAD DRESSINGS

Salads provide an attractive, tasty way to add nutrients and fiber to your diet. They are filling and yet low in calories.

Salad dressings, however, are a different thing altogether. With few exceptions, salad dressings are rich in fat and calories, so even the most "low-cal" of dressings must be used judiciously. Too much dressing can turn a low-fat salad into a high-fat food.

Some experts recommend "oil-free" dressings, but many such dressings are not tasty enough to provide satisfaction. We offer a variety of interesting, flavorful dressings from which to choose. Some are low in fat (Chili Salsa is 7% fat); others are not (Aïoli Vinaigrette is 95% fat). In many instances, we've used garlic or Dijon mustard or other powerful ingredients so that less dressing is needed for full flavor. The point is this: whatever dressing you choose, be moderate in its use. Don't spoil a healthful salad with added fat. Remember, the more dressing you use, the more fat and calories you take in. Let your personal fat budget be your guide.

When high-fat dressings are used, be sure to surround the salad with low-fat foods. This will help keep the meal in balance.

A number of our dressings are made with olive oil, considered by many the most healthful of all oils. It may be better for your heart, but it's still rich in fat and calories and must be used sparingly. Virgin and extra-virgin olive oils are richer and have a more powerful taste than multipurpose or light olive oil; however, they provide no additional health benefit. Be aware also that "light" olive oil has no less fat and no fewer calories than regular olive oil.

BLACK BEAN DIP

Makes 1 cup

1   15-ounce can black beans, drained
1   tablespoon chili powder
½   teaspoon cumin

In a blender or food processor, purée beans. Add chili powder and cumin. Blend.

VARIATION: To make Red Bean Dip, substitute red kidney beans for black beans.

SERVING SUGGESTION: Serve with sliced carrots, celery, cucumber and jicama sticks.

APPROXIMATE NUTRITIONAL CONTENT PER TABLESPOON

Total calories: 23	Carbohydrates: 4 g
Fat: Tr	Protein: 1 g
Percentage of calories from fat:	Cholesterol: 0
7%	Sodium: 90 mg
	Dietary fiber: Tr

HUMMUS

Makes 2 ¾ cups

- ⅓ cup sesame paste (tahini)
- ¼ cup fresh lemon juice
- 1 tablespoon olive oil
- 2 tablespoons water
- 4 cloves garlic
- ½ teaspoon salt
- ½ teaspoon cumin
- ½ teaspoon black pepper
- 1 20-ounce can garbanzo beans (chick peas), drained
- 1 bunch watercress
- ½ red onion, coarsely chopped
- ½ white onion, coarsely chopped

In a mixer or food processor, process sesame paste until smooth. Add lemon juice, olive oil, water, garlic, salt, cumin, black pepper and garbanzo beans. Blend until beans are puréed and mixture is smooth.

Arrange watercress on a serving platter. Mound dip in center and garnish with red and white onion.

SERVING SUGGESTION: Serve with carrots, celery, radishes and homemade warm breadsticks or toasted pita bread, toasted English muffins or toasted bagels.

APPROXIMATE NUTRITIONAL CONTENT PER TABLESPOON

Total calories: 19	Carbohydrates: 2 g
Fat: 1 g	Protein: Tr
Percentage of calories from fat: 45%	Cholesterol: 0
	Sodium: 61 mg
	Dietary fiber: Tr

For lower fat, omit the olive oil. The dip will still taste good, since there is enough oil in the sesame paste. Without the olive oil, the calories will be reduced to 17 and the percentage of calories from fat will be 36%.

ITALIAN EGGPLANT DIP

Makes 1½ cups

    1 1½-pound eggplant
 1½ tablespoons fresh lemon juice
    3 cloves garlic
 1½ tablespoons sesame paste (tahini)
    1 tablespoon olive oil
   ½ teaspoon salt
   ¼ teaspoon black pepper
    2 tablespoons minced parsley
    2 tablespoons pine nuts
    1 bunch fresh parsley

Pierce eggplant all over with a fork. Place in a foil-lined ovenproof dish. Broil about 4 inches from heat, turning frequently, 20–30 minutes or until skin is charred and eggplant is mushy and falling apart. Remove from heat. Place eggplant in a colander. Slit one side and let drain ½ hour.

Scoop out the eggplant pulp (should yield about 1 cup). Put pulp into a blender or food processor; add lemon juice and purée. Add garlic, sesame paste, olive oil, salt and pepper. Process until smooth. Add minced parsley and pine nuts. Process 1 minute more. Chill, the longer the better. (Flavor is even better the second day.) Just before serving, line a salad plate with fresh parsley. Mound dip in center.

SERVING SUGGESTION: Serve with Cajun Flatbread still warm from the oven (page 286) and plenty of celery, carrots and crispy vegetables for dipping. Also excellent with toasted bagels or toasted English muffins.

APPROXIMATE NUTRITIONAL CONTENT PER TABLESPOON

Total calories: 21
Fat: 1 g
Percentage of calories from fat:
  51%

Carbohydrates: 2 g
Protein: Tr
Cholesterol: 0
Sodium: 45 mg
Dietary fiber: 1 g

GARLIC-AND-BASIL DIP

Makes 2½ cups

> 1 15-ounce container part-skim ricotta cheese
> 2 cups freshly grated Parmesan cheese
> 1 cup fresh basil leaves
> 2 eggs
> ½ teaspoon salt
> ¼ teaspoon black pepper
> 1 head red or green cabbage

In a blender or food processor, combine ricotta, Parmesan, basil, eggs, salt and pepper.

Hollow cabbage head so it becomes a bowl. Fill with dip.

SERVING SUGGESTION: Serve with a relish tray of lots of carrots, celery and other crunchy fresh vegetables.

APPROXIMATE NUTRITIONAL CONTENT PER TABLESPOON

Total calories: 42
Fat: 2 g
Percentage of calories from fat:
  57%

Carbohydrates: 1 g
Protein: 3 g
Cholesterol: 18 mg
Sodium: 136 mg
Dietary fiber: Tr

CREAMY GARLIC DRESSING

Makes 2¼ cups

1	16-ounce container low-fat (2%) cottage cheese
2	tablespoons safflower mayonnaise
½	teaspoon salt
¼	teaspoon black pepper
3	cloves garlic, finely minced (about 1½–2 teaspoons)
1½	tablespoons finely minced onion
2	tablespoons finely minced green onion
1	teaspoon minced fresh parsley or dried parsley flakes

In a medium bowl, combine all ingredients. Chill.

SERVING SUGGESTION: An excellent salad dressing, especially for Winter Vegetable Salad (page 335), and a great dip with carrot and celery sticks. Also good on baked potatoes.

APPROXIMATE NUTRITIONAL CONTENT PER TABLESPOON

Total calories: 18

Fat: 1 g

Percentage of calories from fat: 45%

Carbohydrates: 1 g

Protein: 2 g

Cholesterol: 2 mg

Sodium: 85 mg

Dietary fiber: Tr

For lower fat, reduce the mayonnaise to 1 tablespoon. To lower sodium, reduce the salt to ¼ teaspoon. The dip will still taste very good.

AÏOLI VINAIGRETTE

Makes ½ cup

> 1 egg white
> 5 cloves garlic
> 2 tablespoons red wine vinegar
> ¼ teaspoon salt
> ¼ teaspoon Dijon mustard
> ½ cup olive oil

In a blender or food processor, combine egg white, garlic, vinegar, salt and mustard. With machine running, add olive oil 1 tablespoon at a time.

APPROXIMATE NUTRITIONAL CONTENT PER TABLESPOON

Total calories: 124	Carbohydrates: 1 g
Fat: 13 g	Protein: Tr
Percentage of calories from fat: 95%	Cholesterol: 0
	Sodium: 79 mg
	Dietary fiber: 0

CREAMY VINAIGRETTE

Makes ½ cup

- 1 egg white
- ⅛ teaspoon Dijon mustard
- 2 tablespoons fresh lemon juice
- ⅓ teaspoon salt
- ½ cup olive oil

In a blender or food processor, combine egg white, mustard, lemon juice and salt. With machine running, add olive oil, 1 tablespoon at a time.

SERVING SUGGESTION: Good on Lettuce and Bermuda Onion Salad (page 341).

APPROXIMATE NUTRITIONAL CONTENT PER TABLESPOON

Total calories: 122
Fat: 13 g
Percentage of calories from fat: 97%

Carbohydrates: Tr
Protein: Tr
Cholesterol: 0
Sodium: 102 mg
Dietary fiber: 0

LIGHT DIJON VINAIGRETTE

Makes ¾ cup

¼ cup Dijon mustard
2 tablespoons red wine vinegar
2 tablespoons white wine vinegar
1 tablespoon olive oil
¼ teaspoon salt
½ teaspoon basil
⅛ teaspoon black pepper
1 tablespoon minced garlic (about 5 cloves)
1 tablespoon grated onion

In a tightly covered container, shake all ingredients.

APPROXIMATE NUTRITIONAL CONTENT PER TABLESPOON

Total calories: 19	Carbohydrates: 1 g
Fat: 2 g	Protein: Tr
Percentage of calories from fat: 70%	Cholesterol: 0
	Sodium: 194 mg
	Dietary fiber: 0

LIGHT ITALIAN VINAIGRETTE

Makes 1 cup

¾ cup cider vinegar
¼ cup olive oil
¾ teaspoon salt
¼ teaspoon black pepper

In a tightly covered container, shake all ingredients.

SERVING SUGGESTION: Good on Romaine Salad (page 343) and Pepper, Onion and Tomato Salad (page 340).

APPROXIMATE NUTRITIONAL CONTENT PER TABLESPOON

Total calories: 30	Carbohydrates: Tr
Fat: 3 g	Protein: Tr
Percentage of calories from fat:	Cholesterol: 0
91%	Sodium: 100 mg
	Dietary fiber: Tr

To further reduce fat and calories, do an extra-light version by reducing the vinegar to ¼ cup and the oil to 1 tablespoon. This will reduce total calories per tablespoon to 8 and the fat content to less than 1 gram.

JALAPEÑO VINAIGRETTE

Makes 1 cup

> 2 tablespoons freshly squeezed lime juice
> 2½ tablespoons sherry vinegar
> ½ teaspoon Dijon mustard
> 1 teaspoon salt
> ½ teaspoon black pepper
> ½ fresh jalapeño pepper, seeded
> ⅓ cup olive oil

In a blender or food processor, combine all ingredients except the olive oil and whirl 1–2 minutes. With machine running, add olive oil 1 tablespoon at a time. Chill.

SERVING SUGGESTION: Serve with Ensenada Salad (page 332) for an especially good accompaniment to a Mexican-style meal.

APPROXIMATE NUTRITIONAL CONTENT PER TABLESPOON

Total calories: 41	Carbohydrates: Tr
Fat: 4 g	Protein: Tr
Percentage of calories from fat: 95%	Cholesterol: 0
	Sodium: 135 mg
	Dietary fiber: Tr

WASABI VINAIGRETTE

Makes scant ½ cup

3 tablespoons rice vinegar
1 tablespoon olive oil
3 tablespoons reduced-sodium soy sauce
1 teaspoon wasabi (prepared Japanese horseradish)

In a small bowl, combine vinegar, olive oil and soy sauce. Stir in wasabi.

NOTE: Wasabi comes in a tube and is available in Oriental markets or in the Oriental section of most supermarkets.

APPROXIMATE NUTRITIONAL CONTENT PER TABLESPOON

Total calories: 21	Carbohydrates: Tr
Fat: 2 g	Protein: 0
Percentage of calories from fat: 86%	Cholesterol: Tr
	Sodium: 229 mg
	Dietary fiber: 0

HOT CHILI SAUCE

Makes 2 cups

½ cup Chicken Broth (page 272) or canned broth*
½ cup distilled white vinegar
3 dried negro chilies, stemmed and seeded
5 cloves garlic
1 medium white onion
1 medium tomato
1 teaspoon salt

In a saucepan, combine chicken broth, vinegar and chilies, and bring to a boil. Remove from heat and let chilies soak 5–10 minutes or until soft.

In a blender or food processor, combine broth-vinegar mixture, softened chilies, garlic, onion, tomato and salt. Blend until puréed.

*Canned broth is higher in sodium.

NOTE: Negro chilies, also called ancho, poblano, pasilla, and mulatto, are available in many supermarkets and Spanish or Mexican markets. Although the flavor will be slightly different, any hot dried chilies may be substituted.

SERVING SUGGESTION: Use as a barbecue sauce with pork, beef, chicken and shrimp.

APPROXIMATE NUTRITIONAL CONTENT PER ¼ CUP

Total calories: 36
Fat: Tr
Percentage of calories from fat: 4%

Carbohydrates: 7 g
Protein: Tr
Cholesterol: Tr
Sodium: 407 mg
Dietary fiber: Tr

HOT CHILI MARINADE

Makes ¾ cup

2 Anaheim chilies
1 teaspoon olive oil
6 cloves garlic
⅓ cup pineapple juice
2 tablespoons distilled white vinegar
½ teaspoon salt
⅛ teaspoon black pepper
¼ cup Hot Chili Sauce (page 359)

Cut chilies in half lengthwise and remove seeds and stems. In a nonstick skillet, sauté chilies in olive oil 3–4 minutes or until tender. In a blender or food processor, purée the chilies, garlic, pineapple juice, vinegar, salt and pepper. Stir in Hot Chili Sauce.

NOTE: Anaheim chilies, also called Texas, California, New Mexico, Colorado, guajillo, long red or long green chilies, are usually available in Spanish and Mexican markets and in most supermarkets. Although the flavor will be slightly different, any other fresh hot chilies may be substituted.

SERVING SUGGESTION: Try Hot Chili Marinade on grilled steaks, barbecued turkey and chicken, lamb and pork roast. Two excellent recipes are Red-Hot Chili Steak (page 419) and Hot-and-Spicy Southwest Turkey (page 409).

APPROXIMATE NUTRITIONAL CONTENT PER ¼ CUP

Total calories: 56
Fat: 2 g
Percentage of calories from fat: 25%

Carbohydrates: 10 g
Protein: 1 g
Cholesterol: Tr
Sodium: 495 mg
Dietary fiber: Tr

CHILI SALSA

Makes 3 quarts

 1   3-ounce package dried arbol chilies
 ⅔   cup distilled white vinegar
 6   cloves garlic
 ½   teaspoon ground cumin
 ½   teaspoon oregano
 1½ teaspoons salt
 3   28-ounce cans Italian plum tomatoes

In a saucepan, place chilies with water to cover and bring to a boil. Remove from heat and let chilies soak until soft. Remove stems and seeds.

In a blender or food processor, combine prepared chilies, vinegar, garlic, cumin, oregano, salt and tomatoes, and purée. (This entire mixture will not fit into a blender or food processor at one time. As each batch is puréed, remove to a large mixing bowl.) Stir with a wooden spoon until well blended. Pour into pint and quart jars. Refrigerate what you will use within two weeks; freeze remaining salsa.

NOTE: Arbol chilies, also called chimayo, Thai or bird chilies, are available in many supermarkets and Spanish or Mexican markets. Seeding the chilies is cumbersome but worth the effort.

SERVING SUGGESTION: This salsa is great. Especially good sauce with Red-Hot Chili Steak (page 419) and Hot-and-Spicy Southwest Turkey (page 409).

APPROXIMATE NUTRITIONAL CONTENT PER ½ CUP

Total calories: 30	Carbohydrates: 7 g
Fat: Tr	Protein: Tr
Percentage of calories from fat:	Cholesterol: 0
7%	Sodium: 330 mg
	Dietary fiber: Tr

TOMATO-AND-CHILI SALSA

Makes 1 pint

  1½ cups diced ripe tomatoes
  ¼ cup diced serrano or other mild fresh chilies
  8 green onions, diced (optional)
  3 cloves garlic, minced
  ½ cup diced white onion
  ⅓ cup Snappy Tom Bloody Mary mix
  1 tablespoon lemon juice
  ¼ teaspoon black pepper
  ¼ cup finely chopped cilantro

In a medium bowl, combine all ingredients. Use at once or chill. Store in refrigerator up to 3 days.

SERVING SUGGESTION: Excellent as a dip, sauce or salad dressing. Especially good with Vegetable Crudités (page 363).

APPROXIMATE NUTRITIONAL CONTENT PER ¼ CUP

Total calories: 20
Fat: Tr
Percentage of calories from fat:
  6%

Carbohydrates: 4 g
Protein: Tr
Cholesterol: 0
Sodium: 60 mg
Dietary fiber: Tr

VEGETABLE CRUDITÉS WITH TOMATO-AND-CHILI SALSA

Makes 4 servings

2 large carrots
2 stalks celery
1 turnip
½ English cucumber
1 bunch radishes
1 cup Tomato-and-Chili Salsa (page 362)

Cut carrots, celery, turnip and English cucumber into sticks. Cut radishes into flowers. Serve with Tomato-and-Chili Salsa.

APPROXIMATE NUTRITIONAL CONTENT PER SERVING WITHOUT SALSA

Total calories: 39
Fat: Tr
Percentage of calories from fat: 5%

Carbohydrates: 8 g
Protein: 1 g
Cholesterol: 0
Sodium: 55 mg
Dietary fiber: 2 g

Add 20 calories per tablespoon of salsa.

FISH & SHELLFISH

A NOTE ON FISH & SHELLFISH

Fish and shellfish are high in protein, and many are also low in fat. Unfortunately, varieties such as salmon and swordfish are rich in oil. Recipes that use oily fish can derive more than 30% of calories from fat. But a component of fish oil is Omega-3, which is beneficial to cardiac health, so eating a recipe that is over 30% fat from fish oil is not the same as eating one over 30% fat from red meat.

Though more healthful than saturated meat fat, fish oil is still rich in calories. Be sure to accompany oily fish with low-fat foods to control the fat content of the entire meal.

CRACKED DUNGENESS CRAB

Makes 4 servings

> 1 ripe tomato, finely chopped
> 3 tablespoons olive oil
> ½ cup fresh lemon juice
> ¾ teaspoon salt or to taste
> ½ teaspoon black pepper
> 1 bunch fresh parsley
> 2 pounds Dungeness crab, cooked, cracked and cleaned
> 1 lemon, cut into wedges

In a sauce dish or gravy boat, combine tomato, olive oil, lemon juice, salt and pepper. Line a platter with parsley and arrange crab on it. Garnish with lemon wedges. Pass the sauce.

SERVING SUGGESTION: Serve with Seafood Gazpacho (page 257), Napoleon Caesar Salad (page 342), Chocolate Angel Food Cake (page 483) with Chocolate, Orange or Vanilla Glaze (pages 484–486). For more elaborate fare, in addition to the above, include Mussels and Clams with Tomato and Basil (page 374), Cheese-and-Herb Flatbread (page 287), assorted seasonal fruit and Vanilla Angel Food Cake (page 482).

APPROXIMATE NUTRITIONAL CONTENT PER ¼-POUND SERVING OF CRABMEAT WITHOUT SAUCE

Total calories: 115
Fat: 2 g
Percentage of calories from fat: 14%

Carbohydrates: 3 g
Protein: 22 g
Cholesterol: 60 mg
Sodium: 1,217 mg
Dietary fiber: Tr

APPROXIMATE NUTRITIONAL CONTENT PER TABLESPOON OF SAUCE

Total calories: 26
Fat: 2 g
Percentage of calories from fat: 83%

Carbohydrates: 1 g
Protein: Tr
Cholesterol: 0
Sodium: 99 mg
Dietary fiber: Tr

Crab is high in sodium. Keep a balance for the day by selecting low-sodium foods for other meals.

TUNA WITH TOMATO-AND-BASIL SAUCE

Makes 4 servings

 2 tablespoons olive oil
 2 cloves garlic
 3 tomatoes, diced
 ¼ cup finely chopped fresh basil
 ½ teaspoon salt
 ¼ teaspoon black pepper
 1 pound fresh tuna (about ½ inch thick)
 1 bunch arugula or red leaf lettuce
    freshly ground pepper to taste

Prepare coals and cover the grill with foil.

In a blender or food processor, combine olive oil, garlic, tomatoes, basil, salt and ¼ teaspoon pepper, and purée until smooth.

Grill tuna over hot coals about 5 minutes or until done, turning only once. Line individual plates with arugula leaves. Arrange tuna on top. Grind black pepper over tuna. Pass with sauce.

SERVING SUGGESTION: Serve with Antipasto Vegetables (page 438), seasonal fruit and Lemon Ice (page 461).

APPROXIMATE NUTRITIONAL CONTENT PER SERVING WITHOUT SAUCE

Total calories: 198	Carbohydrates: 3 g
Fat: 7 g	Protein: 31 g
Percentage of calories from fat: 30%	Cholesterol: 49 mg
	Sodium: 59 mg
	Dietary fiber: 1 g

APPROXIMATE NUTRITIONAL CONTENT PER TABLESPOON OF SAUCE

Total calories: 5	Carbohydrates: Tr
Fat: Tr	Protein: Tr
Percentage of calories from fat:	Cholesterol: 0 mg
84%	Sodium: 17 mg
	Dietary fiber: Tr

TERIYAKI SALMON

Makes 4 servings

- 3 tablespoons reduced-sodium soy sauce
- ½ cup sake
- 1 teaspoon sugar
- 2 teaspoons olive oil
- 1 pound salmon fillets
- 2 bunches fresh spinach, washed
- 1 lemon, cut into wedges

In a bowl or covered jar, combine soy sauce, sake, sugar and olive oil. Pour over salmon and marinate at room temperature 30 minutes, basting frequently. Drain off marinade.

Prepare coals and cover the grill with foil.

Grill salmon, skin side up, over hot coals 5–6 minutes. Turn and cook 2–3 minutes or until salmon flakes easily when tested with a fork. Place on a bed of spinach. Garnish with lemon.

SERVING SUGGESTION: Serve with Mostaccioli with Tomatoes (page 451), Two-Mushroom Soup (page 251) and Lemon Ice (page 461).

APPROXIMATE NUTRITIONAL CONTENT PER SERVING

Total calories: 218	Carbohydrates: 5 g
Fat: 8 g	Protein: 28 g
Percentage of calories from fat:	Cholesterol: 46 mg
33%	Sodium: 363 mg
	Dietary fiber: 1 g

HICKORY-SMOKED SALMON

Makes 4 servings

    3 cups hickory chips
    1 pound salmon steaks
    1 teaspoon olive oil
    1 bunch fresh spinach
    ½ lemon, cut into wedges
    ½ lime, cut into wedges

Soak hickory chips in water about 1 hour. Drain thoroughly. Prepare coals and cover the grill with foil.

Rub salmon with olive oil. When coals are ready, sprinkle hickory chips over the coals. (The hickory will smoke for about 15 minutes, so put the seafood on at once.) Cook salmon on grill 10 minutes per inch of thickness of fish. If grill has a lid, keep it down during cooking.

Line serving platter with spinach leaves. Arrange cooked salmon on top. Garnish with lemon and lime wedges.

SERVING SUGGESTION: Serve with Barley with Pine Nuts (page 436), Grilled Herbed Tomatoes (page 440) and Lemon Ice (page 461).

APPROXIMATE NUTRITIONAL CONTENT PER SERVING

Total calories: 186	Carbohydrates: 2 g
Fat: 7 g	Protein: 27 g
Percentage of calories from fat:	Cholesterol: 46 mg
36%	Sodium: 115 mg
	Dietary fiber: Tr

MUSHROOM-STUFFED SALMON

Makes 10 servings

    2 tablespoons sake
    1 tablespoon sesame oil
    1 tablespoon olive oil or canola oil
    3 tablespoons reduced-sodium soy sauce
    1 jalapeño pepper, seeded and coarsely chopped
    2 ounces fresh ginger, peeled and chopped
    6 cloves garlic
    3 pounds whole salmon
    1 onion, sliced
    1 7-ounce package dried forest mushrooms
        (Shiitake), reconstituted in water until softened
    ⅓ pound button mushrooms, sliced

In a blender or food processor, combine sake, sesame oil, olive oil, soy sauce, jalapeño pepper, ginger and garlic to make a marinade.

Arrange salmon on aluminum foil. Stuff inside cavity to bulging with onions and mushrooms. Fold foil around salmon to form a bowl. Pour marinade over fish. Wrap fish in two thicknesses of foil.

Bake at 425°F. or grill over hot coals (preferably with lid down) 30–40 minutes or until fish is just cooked.

SERVING SUGGESTION: Serve with Shrimp-and-Spinach Salad (page 313), Wild and White Rice (page 429), Stir-Fried Snow Peas (page 443) and tangerines.

APPROXIMATE NUTRITIONAL CONTENT PER SERVING

Total calories: 228	Carbohydrates: 5 g
Fat: 8 g	Protein: 31 g
Percentage of calories from fat:	Cholesterol: 52 mg
34%	Sodium: 310 mg
	Dietary fiber: Tr

SWORDFISH STEAKS

Makes 4 servings

```
  2   teaspoons olive oil, plus oil for grill
  ¼   cup fresh lemon juice
  2   cloves garlic, minced
  1   tablespoon minced parsley
1 ½   tablespoons fresh rosemary sprigs
  1   pound swordfish steaks (about 1 inch thick)
      fresh rosemary and thyme (optional)
  1   lime, cut into wedges
  ¼   cup Calamata olives, pitted and chopped
  2   teaspoons capers
```

In a small bowl, combine 2 teaspoons olive oil, lemon juice, garlic, parsley and rosemary. Arrange swordfish in an 8 x 8-inch casserole. Pour marinade over swordfish and marinate at room temperature 35–40 minutes. Remove from marinade.

Prepare coals and oil grill rack.

Place swordfish on grill rack over hot coals. Grill, turning once, until just cooked, about 9–10 minutes.

Place swordfish on a bed of fresh herb sprigs, if desired. Garnish with lime. Sprinkle with olives and capers.

SERVING SUGGESTION: Serve with Roasted Red Potatoes with Lemon and Olive Oil (page 449) and Tomatoes with Spinach and Parmesan (page 447).

APPROXIMATE NUTRITIONAL CONTENT PER SERVING

Total calories: 198
Fat: 8 g
Percentage of calories from fat:
   35%

Carbohydrates: 4 g
Protein: 28 g
Cholesterol: 4 mg
Sodium: 378 mg
Dietary fiber: Tr

GRILLED RAINBOW TROUT

Makes 4 servings

> 1 pound fresh rainbow trout fillet
> juice of ½ lemon
> 2 teaspoons olive oil
> salt
> black pepper
> paprika
> 1 clove garlic, finely minced
> 1 teaspoon fresh thyme leaves
> 1 lemon, cut into wedges
> 1 lime, cut into wedges

Prepare coals, preferably mesquite.

Arrange trout fillet on a sheet of foil. Drizzle with lemon and olive oil. Sprinkle with salt, pepper, paprika, garlic and thyme.

Grill over hot coals about 8 minutes or until fish flakes easily when pricked with a fork. Serve with plenty of fresh lemon and lime wedges.

SERVING SUGGESTION: Serve with Georgetown Rice Salad (page 334), Grilled Corn in Husks (page 441), and Strawberry Sherbet with Strawberry Sauce (page 465).

APPROXIMATE NUTRITIONAL CONTENT PER SERVING

Total calories: 206	Carbohydrates: 6 g
Fat: 7 g	Protein: 30 g
Percentage of calories from fat: 31%	Cholesterol: 83 mg
	Sodium: 107 mg
	Dietary fiber: Tr

CALAMARI WITH LINGUINE

Makes approximately 16 cups

 1 28-ounce can Italian plum tomatoes, puréed in a blender or food processor
1½ tablespoons olive oil, plus ½ teaspoon
 ¼ cup dry white wine (Soave Bolla is good)
 2 6½-ounce cans chopped clams, drained
 1 tablespoon tomato paste
 ½ teaspoon oregano
 ½ teaspoon basil
 ½ teaspoon salt
 ½ teaspoon black pepper
 1 14-ounce can water-packed artichoke hearts, drained
 3 cloves garlic, minced
 1 pound squid tubes, cleaned and cut into ¼-inch rings
 1 pound fresh linguine cooked *al dente*
 3 tablespoons chopped fresh parsley
 ½ teaspoon crushed red pepper

In a large saucepan, combine puréed tomatoes, 1½ tablespoons olive oil, wine, clams, tomato paste, oregano, basil, salt and pepper. Heat just to boiling, reduce heat and simmer 20–30 minutes. Add artichokes.

In a nonstick skillet, heat the remaining ½ teaspoon olive oil. Add garlic and squid tubes, and sauté 3–4 minutes or until done. Drain. Add to tomato sauce. Divide pasta into bowls. Ladle sauce over top. Sprinkle with parsley and crushed red pepper.

SERVING SUGGESTION: Serve with Roasted Garlic Bread (page 291), Mediterranean Antipasto (page 329) and Berry-Filled Melon Rounds (page 489).

APPROXIMATE NUTRITIONAL CONTENT PER CUP

Total calories: 204
Fat: 3 g
Percentage of calories from fat:
   13%

Carbohydrates: 33 g
Protein: 12 g
Cholesterol: 86 mg
Sodium: 216 mg
Dietary fiber: 2 g

CALAMARI WITH STIR-FRIED VEGETABLES

Makes 4 servings

1 pound squid tubes, cleaned and cut into
   strips ¼ inch wide
1 tablespoon olive oil
1 tablespoon finely minced gingerroot
3 cloves garlic, slivered
1 medium white onion, thinly sliced
1 red pepper, seeded and thinly sliced
1 green pepper, seeded and thinly sliced
⅓ pound fresh mushrooms, thinly sliced
1 8-ounce can sliced water chestnuts, drained
3 stalks celery, thinly sliced
¼ cup bottled oyster sauce
1 tablespoon reduced-sodium soy sauce
½ teaspoon sesame oil

In a nonstick skillet, toss squid tubes with ½ teaspoon of the olive oil and sauté over medium heat 2–3 minutes or until squid turns white. Remove from heat.

In a wok, heat remaining 2½ teaspoons olive oil. Add gingerroot, garlic and onions, and stir-fry 3–4 minutes or until onions begin to soften. Add peppers, mushrooms, water chestnuts and celery, and stir-fry 2–3 minutes or just until peppers are crisp-tender. Add squid. Combine oyster sauce, soy sauce and sesame oil, and pour over vegetables and squid.

(continued on next page)

(continued from preceding page)

NOTE: Oyster sauce is available in most supermarkets and Oriental groceries.

SERVING SUGGESTION: Serve with Tomato Shrimp Soup (page 261), steamed rice and, for dessert, Fresh Pineapple with Papaya Purée (page 491).

APPROXIMATE NUTRITIONAL CONTENT PER SERVING

Total calories: 220
Fat: 6 g
Percentage of calories from fat:
   24%

Carbohydrates: 20 g
Protein: 21 g
Cholesterol: 264 mg
Sodium: 843 mg
Dietary fiber: 2 g

The sodium content of this menu is high. Keep a balance for the day by selecting low-sodium foods at other meals.

MUSSELS AND CLAMS WITH TOMATO AND BASIL

Makes 4 servings

  2 tablespoons fresh basil
  2 tablespoons olive oil
  ¼ cup minced parsley
  1 tablespoon minced garlic
  ½ cup white wine (Soave Bolla is good)
  ½ teaspoon salt
  ¼ teaspoon black pepper
  ½ teaspoon crushed red pepper
  4 large ripe tomatoes, diced
  3 pounds mussels, washed, soaked and bearded
  1 pound clams, soaked and cleaned

In a large steamer over boiling water, combine all the ingredients. Cover and steam 5–10 minutes, removing each clam and mussel as it opens.

SERVING SUGGESTION: Serve with pasta nests, Napoleon Caesar Salad (page 342), seasonal fruit and Lemon Ice (page 461).

APPROXIMATE NUTRITIONAL CONTENT PER SERVING

Total calories: 263
Fat: 8 g
Percentage of calories from fat:
   28%

Carbohydrates: 15 g
Protein: 29 g
Cholesterol: 67 mg
Sodium: 634 mg
Dietary fiber: 2 g

MUSSELS AND CLAMS IN WINE AND GARLIC

Makes 4 servings

¼ cup white wine (Soave Bolla is good)
2½ tablespoons olive oil
8 large cloves garlic
   juice of 1 lemon
½ teaspoon salt
¼ teaspoon black pepper
3 pounds clams, soaked and cleaned
1 pound fresh mussels, washed, soaked and bearded

In large steamer over boiling water, combine all ingredients. Cover and steam 5–10 minutes, removing each clam and mussel as it opens.

APPROXIMATE NUTRITIONAL CONTENT PER SERVING

Total calories: 207
Fat: 5 g
Percentage of calories from fat:
   23%

Carbohydrates: 9 g
Protein: 29 g
Cholesterol: 73 mg
Sodium: 470 mg
Dietary fiber: Tr

SEAFOOD GRILL

Makes 4 servings

3 cups hickory chips
1 salmon steak (about ½ pound)
1 black cod steak (about ½ pound)
2 teaspoons olive oil
1 bunch cilantro or parsley
2 lemons, cut into wedges

Soak hickory chips in water about 1 hour. Drain thoroughly. Prepare coals and cover the grill with foil.

Rub fish with olive oil. When coals are ready, sprinkle hickory chips over the coals. (The hickory will smoke for about 15 minutes, so put the seafood on at once.) Cook seafood on grill 10 minutes per inch of thickness of fish. If grill has a lid, keep it down during cooking.

Line serving platter with cilantro or parsley. Arrange cod and salmon on top. Split each steak in half lengthwise and garnish with lemons.

SERVING SUGGESTION: Serve with Vegetables with Chinese Noodles in Szechuan Sauce (page 444).

APPROXIMATE NUTRITIONAL CONTENT PER SERVING

Total calories: 153
Fat: 4 g
Percentage of calories from fat: 24%

Carbohydrates: 6 g
Protein: 25 g
Cholesterol: 50 mg
Sodium: 98 mg
Dietary fiber: Tr

SEA BASS WITH SHRIMP

Makes 5 servings

1 pound sea bass steaks
1 tablespoon olive oil
2 medium ripe tomatoes, diced
1 8-ounce can mushroom stems and pieces, drained
3 cloves garlic, thinly sliced
½ pound cooked shrimpmeat
¼ bunch fresh parsley
1 lemon, cut into wedges
2 medium tomatoes, cut into wedges

In a shallow baking pan, arrange sea bass in a single layer. Brush with 1 teaspoon of the olive oil. Combine remaining olive oil, diced tomatoes, mushrooms and garlic, and pour over sea bass.

Bake, uncovered, at 400°F. 10 minutes per inch of thickness of fish. Three to four minutes before fish is cooked, sprinkle shrimp over top. When sea bass turns white and flakes readily when touched with a fork, remove to a platter lined with parsley. Garnish with lemon and tomato wedges.

SERVING SUGGESTION: Serve with steamed rice or red potatoes, fresh asparagus and, for dessert, Vanilla Angel Food Cake (page 482) with Orange Glaze (page 486).

APPROXIMATE NUTRITIONAL CONTENT PER SERVING

Total calories: 207
Fat: 6 g
Percentage of calories from fat:
  24%

Carbohydrates: 10 g
Protein: 30 g
Cholesterol: 130 mg
Sodium: 183 mg
Dietary fiber: 3 g

SOLE WITH SHRIMP, CRAB AND MUSHROOMS

Makes 4 servings

> 1 cup Chicken Broth (page 272) or canned broth*
> ½ cup dry vermouth
> ¼ cup fresh lemon juice
> ¼ teaspoon salt
> ¼ teaspoon white pepper
> 1 pound sole fillets
> 1 teaspoon olive oil or canola oil
> 1 tablespoon finely chopped leek, white part only
> ¼ pound fresh mushrooms, sliced
> 1½ teaspoons arrowroot
> 3 tablespoons cold water
> ¼ pound cooked shrimpmeat
> ¼ pound cooked crabmeat
> ¼ cup freshly grated Parmesan cheese

In a skillet, combine chicken broth, vermouth and lemon juice, and bring to a boil. Add salt and white pepper. Place sole in the liquid; cover and poach 4–5 minutes or until fish is barely cooked. Remove sole from stock and drain on paper towels. Transfer stock to a saucepan and bring to a boil. Reduce heat and simmer, uncovered, 5 minutes to reduce to 1 cup.

In the same skillet, heat olive oil. Add leek and mushrooms, and sauté 3–4 minutes or until mushrooms are tender.

Bring fish stock back to boiling. Dissolve arrowroot in cold water and gradually add to fish stock. Cook and stir until stock begins to thicken. Add shrimpmeat, crabmeat, leek, mushrooms and half the cheese. Arrange sole in ovenproof baking dish. Pour sauce over sole. Sprinkle with remaining cheese. Broil 2–3 minutes or until cheese is melted.

*Canned broth is higher in sodium.

SERVING SUGGESTION: Serve with steamed tiny red potatoes, fresh asparagus and Frosty Lemon Supreme (page 468).

APPROXIMATE NUTRITIONAL CONTENT PER SERVING

Total calories: 261
Fat: 6 g
Percentage of calories from fat:
   20%

Carbohydrates: 4 g
Protein: 39 g
Cholesterol: 144 mg
Sodium: 568 mg
Dietary fiber: Tr

SCALLOPS AND PRAWNS WITH RISOTTO

Makes 6 servings

1	Risotto Milanese (page 434)
½	teaspoon olive oil
½	pound scallops, thawed if frozen, cut into halves if large
⅔	pound prawns, cooked, shelled and deveined

Prepare Risotto Milanese according to instructions. While risotto is cooking, in a nonstick skillet, sauté scallops in olive oil 4–6 minutes or until scallops are tender. Add scallops and prawns to risotto during the last 3–4 minutes of cooking.

SERVING SUGGESTION: Serve with fresh asparagus and seasonal fruit.

APPROXIMATE NUTRITIONAL CONTENT PER SERVING

Total calories: 447
Fat: 5 g
Percentage of calories from fat:
   10%

Carbohydrates: 72 g
Protein: 30 g
Cholesterol: 114 mg
Sodium: 497 mg
Dietary fiber: 2 g

SHRIMP-AND-VEGETABLE KABOBS

Makes 5 servings

½	teaspoon olive oil, plus oil for grill
1	8-ounce can tomato sauce
1	teaspoon ground cumin
¼	teaspoon chili powder
¼	teaspoon salt
¼	teaspoon black pepper
¾	pound medium prawns, cooked, shelled and deveined
1	large onion, cut into cubes
1	green pepper, cut into cubes
2	large tomatoes, cut into cubes
1 ½	cups fresh pineapple cubes

Prepare coals and brush the grill lightly with oil.

In a bowl, combine tomato sauce, cumin, chili powder, salt, pepper and olive oil. Set aside.

Alternate prawns, onion, green pepper, tomato and pineapple on each of five 15-inch metal skewers.

Barbecue kabobs 4–6 inches from heat, 8–10 minutes, turning frequently and basting several times with sauce.

VARIATION: Substitute chicken for prawns.

SERVING SUGGESTION: Serve with Wild and White Rice (page 429) and Fresh Lemon Ice Cream (page 462).

APPROXIMATE NUTRITIONAL CONTENT PER SERVING

Total calories: 134
Fat: 2 g
Percentage of calories from fat: 12%

Carbohydrates: 14 g
Protein: 16 g
Cholesterol: 133 mg
Sodium: 540 mg
Dietary fiber: 3 g

POULTRY

═══════════

A NOTE ON POULTRY
═══════════════════════

The versatility of chicken and turkey gives poultry the potential to be a part of an infinite number of low-fat meals—from main dishes to soups to salads.

The most healthful poultry is skinless white breast. Always remember to cook poultry without skin, since that's where the fat is contained. Three ounces of skinless chicken breast contains just 3 grams of fat; with skin, it contains twice that amount. It is the same for turkey. Three ounces of skinless breast has just 2.7 grams of fat; with skin, it has 8.7 grams of fat.

Not only is poultry appetizing by itself, but in many recipes it can be an excellent substitute for red meat. For example, ground turkey can replace hamburger in meat loaf. And a pounded chicken breast, grilled and served in a bun, is a great substitute for a hamburger of ground round.

CHICKEN TOSTADAS

Makes 6 servings

    2 chicken breasts, skinned and boned
    2 cups Chicken Stock (page 264) or canned broth*
 1 ½ teaspoons ground cumin
   ¾ teaspoon chili powder
    1 8-ounce can tomato sauce
   ¼ teaspoon salt
   ⅛ teaspoon black pepper
    1 small onion, diced
    1 large tomato, diced
    3 cups shredded lettuce
   ½ cup shredded low-fat Cheddar or part-skim
         mozzarella cheese
    6 8-inch flour tortillas,** warmed
    1 cup Black Bean Dip (page 348)

In a 2-quart saucepan, bring chicken and chicken stock to boiling. Reduce heat and simmer 20 minutes or until chicken is done. Remove chicken from stock. Dice and sprinkle with ½ teaspoon of the cumin and ½ teaspoon of the chili powder.

In a small saucepan, combine tomato sauce, the remaining teaspoon of cumin, the remaining ¼ teaspoon chili powder, salt and pepper, and warm over low heat.

Arrange chicken, onion, tomato, lettuce and cheese on a serving platter. Place warm tortillas in a napkin-lined basket, and put tomato sauce and Black Bean Dip into serving bowls.

To assemble, have each person spread a tortilla with bean dip, sprinkle with chicken, add sauce and then lettuce, tomato, onion and cheese.

*Canned broth is higher in sodium.

**Be sure to read the label when selecting a brand of flour tortillas. Do not buy tortillas that are prepared with lard or a saturated oil.

NOTE: To warm tortillas in a microwave, place tortillas between 2 slightly dampened paper towels. Microwave on high 1–2 minutes or until warm; keep wrapped until ready to serve. To warm tortillas on the stovetop, place them in a bamboo basket or vegetable steamer rack; steam in a covered pan over boiling water 3–5 minutes or until warm.

SERVING SUGGESTION: Serve with steamed rice, chilled watermelon and fresh berries.

APPROXIMATE NUTRITIONAL CONTENT PER SERVING

Total calories: 313
Fat: 7 g
Percentage of calories from fat:
  19%

Carbohydrates: 34 g
Protein: 29 g
Cholesterol: 54 mg
Sodium: 745 mg
Dietary fiber: 3 g

Chicken Tostadas are high in sodium. Serve with low-sodium accompaniments such as those suggested. To further reduce the sodium, rinse the beans in the Black Bean Dip and use salt-free tomato sauce.

CHICKEN FAJITAS

Makes 4 servings

¼ cup fresh lime juice
¼ cup reduced-sodium soy sauce
2 tablespoons olive oil
2 whole chicken breasts, skinned, boned and cut into thin strips
1 medium white onion, cut into thin wedges
1 medium green pepper, seeded and cut into thin strips
1 medium red pepper, seeded and cut into thin strips
1 large tomato, cut into thin strips
4 8-inch flour tortillas,* warmed
½ cup commercial or homemade tomato salsa

Prepare marinade by combining lime juice, soy sauce and olive oil. Pour ⅔ of the marinade over chicken and marinate in the refrigerator 1–2 hours, turning once or twice.

Prepare coals and cover the grill with foil.

Remove chicken from marinade with a slotted spoon; grill chicken over hot coals 4–5 minutes per side.

Meanwhile, in a wok or heavy skillet, heat remaining ⅓ marinade. Add onion and stir-fry 2–3 minutes. Add peppers and stir-fry 2–3 minutes. Toss with chicken and tomatoes, and serve immediately on a hot platter. Garnish with tomato salsa. Serve with warm tortillas.

*Be sure to read the label when selecting a brand of flour tortillas. Do not buy tortillas that are prepared with lard or a saturated oil.

NOTE: To warm tortillas in a microwave, place tortillas between 2 slightly dampened paper towels. Microwave on high 1–2 minutes or until warm; keep wrapped until ready to serve. To warm tortillas on the stovetop, place them in a bamboo basket or a vegetable steamer rack; steam in a covered pan over boiling water 3–5 minutes or until warm.

SERVING SUGGESTION: Serve with steamed rice, Refried Black Beans (page 425), and fresh berries, grapes and melons.

APPROXIMATE NUTRITIONAL CONTENT PER FAJITA

Total calories: 366
Fat: 14 g
Percentage of calories from fat:
   34%

Carbohydrates: 28 g
Protein: 32 g
Cholesterol: 78 mg
Sodium: 782 mg
Dietary fiber: 1 g

Chicken Fajitas are high in sodium. Serve low-sodium accompaniments such as those suggested.

GRILLED CHICKEN WITH SALSA

Makes 4 servings

   juice of 1 large lime (about ⅓ cup)
2 whole chicken breasts, skinned, boned and halved
1 cup commercial or homemade tomato salsa

In a medium bowl, pour lime juice over chicken and marinate at room temperature 1 hour, turning to coat. Drain off marinade.

Prepare coals and cover the grill with foil. Grill chicken over hot coals 10–12 minutes on each side or until done. Place chicken on serving plates and drizzle salsa over top.

SERVING SUGGESTION: Serve with Romaine Salad (page 343), Black Beans and Rice (page 426) and Spanish Flan (page 457).

APPROXIMATE NUTRITIONAL CONTENT PER SERVING

Total calories: 167
Fat: 5 g
Percentage of calories from fat:
   23%

Carbohydrates: 6 g
Protein: 27 g
Cholesterol: 73 mg
Sodium: 285 mg
Dietary fiber: 0

CHICKEN ENCHILADAS

Makes 8 servings

> 2 whole chicken breasts, skinned and boned
> 3 stalks celery, cut into chunks
> 1 medium onion, cut into chunks
> 2 cloves garlic
> 1½ cups Chicken Stock (page 264) or canned broth*

Filling
> ½ medium green pepper, diced
> ½ medium white onion, diced
> 1 large tomato, diced
> 1 3½-ounce can whole green chilies, diced
> ¼ cup Chicken Stock (page 264) or canned broth*
> ¼ teaspoon salt
> ¼ teaspoon black pepper
> 8 flour or corn tortillas**
> 2 ounces part-skim mozzarella cheese, thinly sliced
> ½ cup commercial or homemade enchilada sauce
>   (page 388)
> ½ cup commercial or homemade tomato salsa

In a medium stockpot, combine chicken, celery, onion chunks, garlic and chicken stock, and bring to a boil. Cover, reduce heat and simmer 30 minutes. Remove from heat. Let sit in stock 15 minutes. Remove celery, onion and garlic from stock and discard. (They will be grease-laden.) Reserve remaining stock for later use. Tear chicken into strips.

To Prepare Filling: In a medium stockpot, combine green pepper, diced onion, tomato, green chilies, ¼ cup chicken stock, salt and pepper. Cook over low heat 20 minutes or until vegetables are soft. Add chicken.

To Assemble: Place ¼ cup filling in each tortilla, along with a thin slice of mozzarella cheese and 1 teaspoon enchilada sauce. Roll and place seam side down in a lightly greased 9 x 13-inch ovenproof baking dish. Pour remaining enchilada sauce over top. Cover with foil. Bake at 350°F. 20–25 minutes or until hot. Accompany with tomato salsa.

*Canned broth is higher in sodium.

**Be sure to read the label when selecting a brand of flour tortillas. Do not buy tortillas that are prepared with lard or a saturated oil.

SERVING SUGGESTION: Serve with Refried Black Beans (page 425), steamed short-grain rice and fresh fruits.

APPROXIMATE NUTRITIONAL CONTENT PER ENCHILADA

Total calories: 220	Carbohydrates: 24 g
Fat: 5 g	Protein: 19 g
Percentage of calories from fat: 21%	Cholesterol: 41 mg
	Sodium: 428 mg
	Dietary fiber: 1 g

ENCHILADA CASSEROLE

Makes 8 servings

Enchilada Sauce
    1 8-ounce can tomato sauce
    1 teaspoon ground cumin
    ¼ teaspoon chili powder
    ¼ teaspoon salt
    ¼ teaspoon black pepper

Salsa
    1 14-ounce can Italian plum tomatoes, diced
    1 4-ounce can diced green chilies
    ⅛ teaspoon cayenne pepper
    ¼ teaspoon salt
    1 teaspoon ground cumin

    2 chicken breasts, skinned and boned
    2 cups Chicken Stock (page 264) or canned broth*
    ½ teaspoon olive oil or canola oil
    ¼ cup onion, chopped
    ½ teaspoon ground cumin
    ½ teaspoon chili powder
    ½ cup canned mushroom stems and pieces, drained
    2 tablespoons diced green chilies
    3 8-inch flour tortillas**
    ¾ cup freshly grated low-fat Cheddar cheese
    ¾ cup freshly grated part-skim mozzarella cheese

In a covered jar, combine all enchilada sauce ingredients. Set aside.

In a bowl, combine all salsa ingredients. Set aside.

In a 2-quart saucepan, bring chicken and chicken stock to a boil. Reduce heat and simmer 20 minutes or until chicken is done. Remove chicken from stock. Dice.

In a nonstick skillet, heat olive oil. Add onion and sauté until onion is tender.

Toss chicken with onion. Sprinkle with cumin and chili powder. Toss with mushrooms and green chilies. Combine Cheddar and mozzarella cheese.

Cover the bottom of a nonstick 9-inch round cake pan with some of the enchilada sauce. Place one of the tortillas over the sauce. Top with half the salsa, half the chicken mixture and a third of the cheese.

Top with a second tortilla, some enchilada sauce, remainder of salsa, chicken and a third more cheese. Top with final tortilla. Pour remaining enchilada sauce over top and sprinkle with remaining cheese. Bake at 350°F. 40–45 minutes.

*Canned broth is higher in sodium.

**Be sure to read the label when selecting a brand of flour tortillas. Do not buy those that are prepared with lard or a saturated oil.

SERVING SUGGESTION: Serve with Vegetable and Black Bean Antipasto (page 330), steamed rice and orange or lemon sherbet with mangos and papayas.

APPROXIMATE NUTRITIONAL CONTENT PER SERVING

Total calories: 204
Fat: 6 g
Percentage of calories from fat: 29%

Carbohydrates: 14 g
Protein: 22 g
Cholesterol: 49 mg
Sodium: 600 mg
Dietary fiber: 1 g

To further reduce the sodium, use fresh mushrooms in place of canned and omit the salt from the sauce and salsa.

MEXICAN CHICKEN

Makes 4 servings

- ¼ cup orange juice
- 1 tablespoon lime juice
- 2 teaspoons cider vinegar
- 1 tablespoon olive oil or canola oil
- ½ teaspoon oregano
- ½ teaspoon salt
- ¼ teaspoon black pepper
- 2 chicken breasts, skinned, boned and quartered

Prepare marinade by combining orange juice, lime juice, vinegar, olive oil and seasonings. Pour over chicken and marinate in the refrigerator at least 2 hours. Drain, reserving marinade.

Prepare coals and cover the grill with foil.

Grill chicken over hot coals 10–20 minutes on each side or until chicken is cooked. Baste frequently with reserved marinade during cooking.

SERVING SUGGESTION: Serve with black bean burritos (see page 392), Rice with Chilies (page 431) and fresh strawberries.

APPROXIMATE NUTRITIONAL CONTENT PER SERVING

Total calories: 171
Fat: 5 g
Percentage of calories from fat: 27%

Carbohydrates: 2 g
Protein: 27 g
Cholesterol: 73 mg
Sodium: 330 mg
Dietary fiber: Tr

CHICKEN CORTEZ

Makes 4 servings

1 6-ounce can pineapple juice
2 tablespoons lime juice
1 tablespoon distilled white vinegar
6 cloves garlic
½ teaspoon salt
½ teaspoon oregano
¼ teaspoon chili powder
¼ teaspoon black pepper
1 tablespoon olive oil or canola oil
2 chicken breasts, skinned, boned and halved

Prepare marinade by combining pineapple juice, lime juice, vinegar, garlic, salt, oregano, chili powder, pepper and olive oil. Pour over chicken and marinate in the refrigerator 2 hours or as long as overnight.

Prepare coals and cover the grill with foil.

Drain off marinade and reserve. Grill chicken over hot coals 6–8 minutes. Turn, baste with reserved marinade, and grill 6–8 minutes more. Turn and grill 5–10 minutes longer, turning frequently until chicken is cooked.

SERVING SUGGESTION: Serve with Beans Ranchero (page 424), warm tortillas (see page 383), Ensenada Salad (page 332) with Jalapeño Vinaigrette (page 357) and fresh strawberries.

APPROXIMATE NUTRITIONAL CONTENT PER SERVING

Total calories: 207
Fat: 7 g
Percentage of calories from fat:
  29%

Carbohydrates: 9 g
Protein: 27 g
Cholesterol: 73 mg
Sodium: 200 mg
Dietary fiber: Tr

CHICKEN BLACK BEAN BURRITOS

Makes 4 servings

  4   8-inch flour tortillas*
  2   chicken breasts, prepared as for Mexican
        Chicken (page 388)
  ½   head lettuce, shredded
  ½   cup Black Bean Dip* (page 348)
  ½   cup Chili Salsa (page 361) or commercial salsa

Heat tortillas according to instructions on page 383.

Slice chicken breasts into thin strips. Arrange lettuce, chicken and bean dip on serving platter. Accompany with salsa and warm tortillas.

To Prepare Burrito: Spoon bean dip along center of each tortilla. Divide chicken among tortillas and top with lettuce. Fold opposite sides of each tortilla over filling. Fold ends over folded sides.

*To reduce the sodium, rinse the beans in the bean dip and use corn tortillas instead of flour tortillas. Corn tortillas have no salt.

SERVING SUGGESTION: Serve with Rice with Chilies (page 431), Vegetable Antipasto of carrot, celery and sliced English cucumber sticks and, for dessert, Spanish Flan (page 457) or seasonal fruits.

APPROXIMATE NUTRITIONAL CONTENT PER BURRITO

Total calories: 338
Fat: 9 g
Percentage of calories from fat:
   24%

Carbohydrates: 31 g
Protein: 33 g
Cholesterol: 73 mg
Sodium: 599 mg
Dietary fiber: 3 g

The sodium content of this dish is high. Keep a balance for the day by selecting low-sodium foods at other meals.

MESQUITE-GRILLED CHICKEN

Makes 4 servings; sauce makes 2½ cups (enough for 3 pounds of chicken)

Sauce

- 1   15-ounce can tomato sauce
- 2   teaspoons olive oil or canola oil
- 1   tablespoon chili powder
- 1   teaspoon paprika
- 1   tablespoon Worcestershire sauce
- 1   teaspoon crushed red pepper
- ¼   teaspoon salt
- 2   tablespoons cider vinegar
- ½   teaspoon black pepper
- ½   teaspoon garlic powder
- ¾   teaspoon prepared mustard
- 3   tablespoons finely minced onion

- 1   pound chicken breasts, skinned and boned

In a jar with cover, combine all sauce ingredients. Refrigerate until ready to use. Sauce may be used at once, but the best flavors are achieved if made early in the day.

Prepare mesquite coals and cover the grill with foil.

Grill chicken over hot coals about 6 minutes. Turn and grill 6 minutes more. Turn again, baste with sauce and cook 4–5 minutes. Turn, baste, and grill 4–5 minutes or until chicken is done. Baste generously with sauce during last few minutes of cooking.

APPROXIMATE NUTRITIONAL CONTENT PER SERVING WITH ONE THIRD OF SAUCE

Total calories: 210	Carbohydrates: 4 g
Fat: 5 g	Protein: 36 g
Percentage of calories from fat: 22%	Cholesterol: 96 mg
	Sodium: 366 mg
	Dietary fiber: Tr

LOUISIANA CHICKEN STRIPS

Makes 4 servings

Sauce
- 1 egg
- ⅓ cup brown sugar
- ⅓ cup cider vinegar
- ⅓ cup dry mustard
- ¼ teaspoon salt

- 1 tablespoon oregano
- 2 teaspoons ground cumin
- 1 teaspoon chili powder
- 1 teaspoon powdered thyme
- ½ teaspoon cayenne
- 1 tablespoon potato starch
- 2 chicken breasts, skinned, boned and cut into strips
- 2 teaspoons olive oil
- 4 8-inch flour tortillas*
- ½ head iceberg lettuce, shredded

In the top of a double boiler, beat egg. Add sugar and beat; then add vinegar and dry mustard, and beat. Place top of double boiler over boiling water and cook 5–10 minutes, stirring often or until sauce thickens. Season with salt. Set aside.

In a pie plate, combine oregano, cumin, chili powder, thyme, cayenne and potato starch. Toss chicken strips in mixture until evenly coated.

In a nonstick skillet, heat olive oil. Add chicken strips and brown over high heat 4–5 minutes, stirring often. Reduce heat to low and continue cooking about 15 minutes or until chicken is cooked.

When chicken is nearly done, warm the tortillas (see page 00). Fold warmed tortillas into fourths and tuck into a napkin-lined basket.

Line an oval serving platter with shredded lettuce. Arrange chicken strips over lettuce. Place a dollop of sauce at each end of platter. Serve at once. To eat, fill each tortilla with lettuce and chicken, and dip into sauce.

*Be sure to read the label when selecting a brand of flour tortillas. Do not buy those that are prepared with lard or a saturated oil.

NOTE: Potato starch is available in most supermarkets or in Oriental groceries.

SERVING SUGGESTION: Good and quick to make as an hors d'oeuvre. For a light supper, serve with Pasta-and-Bean Salad (page 322) or rice and corn on the cob and seasonal fruit.

APPROXIMATE NUTRITIONAL CONTENT PER SERVING

Total calories: 430
Fat: 12 g
Percentage of calories from fat: 26%

Carbohydrates: 46 g
Protein: 35 g
Cholesterol: 126 mg
Sodium: 233 mg
Dietary fiber: 1 g

CHICKEN-AND-VEGETABLE CASSEROLE

Makes 6 servings

  2 chicken breasts, skinned, boned and quartered
  2 teaspoons powdered rosemary
  2 tablespoons dried parsley
  ½ teaspoon black pepper
  1 whole head garlic, separated into cloves and
     peeled
12 baby carrots
  1 large onion, cut into rings
  4 small red potatoes, halved
  1 pound fresh green beans, stemmed
  1 cup dry white wine (Soave Bolla is good)

In a covered casserole dish, arrange chicken on bottom. Combine rosemary, parsley and pepper. Sprinkle ⅓ of mixture over chicken. Top with garlic, carrots, onion and potatoes. Sprinkle ⅓ of seasoning mixture over potatoes. Top with green beans. Sprinkle remaining third of seasoning over top. Pour wine over all. Cover tightly with foil, then cover with lid. Bake at 350°F. 1 hour or until chicken is cooked and vegetables are tender.

    SERVING SUGGESTION: Serve with crusty French bread and Fresh Blackberry Pie (see page 478).

APPROXIMATE NUTRITIONAL CONTENT PER SERVING

Total calories: 242
Fat: 3 g
Percentage of calories from fat:
  9%

Carbohydrates: 28 g
Protein: 22 g
Cholesterol: 49 mg
Sodium: 93 mg
Dietary fiber: 5 g

CHICKEN WITH RICE

Makes 6 servings

> 2 teaspoons olive oil or canola oil
> 1 large onion, chopped
> 4 cloves garlic, minced
> ¼ cup all-purpose flour
> 1 teaspoon cayenne pepper
> 2 chicken breasts, skinned, boned, halved and cut into quarters
> 1 16-ounce can plum Italian tomatoes, chopped
> 2¾ cups Chicken Broth (page 272) or canned broth*
> ⅛ teaspoon powdered saffron
> ½ teaspoon salt or to taste
> 1⅓ cups uncooked long-grain rice
> 1½ cups cooked peas

In a skillet, heat olive oil. Add onion and garlic, and sauté 6–8 minutes or until onion is just tender.

Combine flour and cayenne. Dredge chicken in flour mixture. Add to skillet and brown 2–3 minutes on each side. Add tomatoes, chicken stock, saffron and salt, and bring to a boil. Stir in rice. Cover and simmer 30–45 minutes or until rice is tender and chicken is cooked. Stir in peas. Serve at once.

*Canned broth is higher in sodium.

SERVING SUGGESTION: Serve with Raspberry Pavlova (page 459).

APPROXIMATE NUTRITIONAL CONTENT PER SERVING

Total calories: 352
Fat: 5 g
Percentage of calories from fat: 13%

Carbohydrates: 49 g
Protein: 26 g
Cholesterol: 49 mg
Sodium: 626 mg
Dietary fiber: 3 g

THAI CHICKEN

Makes 8 servings

Marinade
½ cup olive oil
1 teaspoon sesame oil
3 tablespoons reduced-sodium soy sauce
⅓ cup rice vinegar
2 green onions, chopped
1 jalapeño pepper, chopped
4 large cloves garlic, minced
2 teaspoons freshly squeezed lime juice
2 teaspoons crushed red pepper
¼ teaspoon Tabasco sauce
¼ teaspoon white pepper
¼ teaspoon salt

2 chicken breasts skinned, boned and cut into strips
½ pound fresh spinach linguine, cooked *al dente*
½ pound fresh regular linguine, cooked *al dente*
¾ pound fresh asparagus, steamed 2–3 minutes or
    until crisp-tender and cut diagonally into thirds
½ cup fresh cilantro, chopped (optional)

In a small saucepan, combine marinade ingredients. Place the chicken breasts in a bowl with 3 tablespoons of the marinade and marinate 20–30 minutes at room temperature. In a nonstick pan, sauté the chicken 7 to 10 minutes or until cooked. Warm remaining marinade.

Meanwhile, arrange pasta in a large, low serving bowl; toss with 1 tablespoon warmed marinade. Spread chicken over top of pasta. Top with asparagus. Garnish with cilantro. Accompany with remaining warmed marinade.

VARIATION: Sprinkle with ¼ cup peanuts.

SERVING SUGGESTION: Serve with sliced, fresh peaches and apricots.

APPROXIMATE NUTRITIONAL CONTENT PER SERVING (INCLUDING THE 4 TABLESPOONS OF MARINADE CALLED FOR IN THE RECIPE INSTRUCTIONS)

Total calories: 415
Fat: 8 g
Percentage of calories from fat:
   17%

Carbohydrates: 58 g
Protein: 25 g
Cholesterol: 73 mg
Sodium: 112 mg
Dietary fiber: 6 g

APPROXIMATE NUTRITIONAL CONTENT PER ADDITIONAL TABLESPOON OF REMAINING MARINADE

Total calories: 67
Fat: 7 g
Percentage of calories from fat:
   94%

Carbohydrates: 1 g
Protein: Tr
Cholesterol: 0
Sodium: 149 mg
Dietary fiber: Tr

CHICKEN PRIMAVERA

Makes 4 servings

2 boneless chicken breasts, skinned and halved
¾ cup dry white wine (Soave Bolla is good)
1 cup Chicken Broth (page 272) or canned broth*
1 tablespoon tomato paste
1 tablespoon minced parsley
½ teaspoon powdered thyme
1 large white onion, sliced (about 2 cups)
3 large cloves garlic, minced
1 tablespoon olive oil or canola oil
2 green peppers, halved and sliced into half-rings
1 pint cherry tomatoes, halved

In a large nonstick skillet, brown chicken breasts 5–7 minutes on each side. In a saucepan, warm wine, chicken broth, tomato paste, parsley and thyme; pour over browned chicken breasts. Reduce heat and simmer, uncovered, 20–30 minutes, basting with sauce and turning often.

In a medium nonstick skillet, sauté onion and garlic in olive oil 7–10 minutes or until onions are softened. Remove from heat; add green peppers and tomatoes. Just before serving, add to chicken, raise heat to high, and cook 2–3 minutes or until sauce is bubbly and peppers and onions are warmed.

*Canned broth is higher in sodium.

SERVING SUGGESTION: Serve with Orzo with Saffron (page 433) and seasonal fruits.

APPROXIMATE NUTRITIONAL CONTENT PER SERVING

Total calories: 272	Carbohydrates: 14 g
Fat: 7 g	Protein: 30 g
Percentage of calories from fat: 25%	Cholesterol: 73 mg
	Sodium: 327 mg
	Dietary fiber: 3 g

TERIYAKI CHICKEN

Makes 4 servings

    2 chicken breasts skinned, boned and cut into
          1 ¼ - inch cubes
    ¼ cup reduced-sodium soy sauce
    ½ cup sake
    1 teaspoon granulated sugar
    2 teaspoons sesame oil
    1 red onion, cut into cubes
    1 green pepper, cut into cubes
    ¼ pound fresh mushroom buttons
    8 cherry tomatoes
    1 zucchini, peeled and cut into cubes
       olive oil for grill

Arrange chicken in a shallow dish. In a bowl, combine soy sauce, sake, sugar and sesame oil. Pour marinade over chicken and marinate 30 minutes at room temperature. Drain off marinade. On skewers, alternate chicken, onion, pepper, mushrooms, tomatoes and zucchini.

Prepare coals and brush the grill lightly with olive oil.

Grill kabobs 4–6 inches from heat, turning frequently and basting often, about 20 minutes or until chicken is done.

SERVING SUGGESTION: Serve with Oriental Rice (page 428) and Fresh Lemon Ice Cream (page 462).

APPROXIMATE NUTRITIONAL CONTENT PER SERVING

Total calories: 242	Carbohydrates: 11 g
Fat: 7 g	Protein: 30 g
Percentage of calories from fat:	Cholesterol: 73 mg
28%	Sodium: 371 mg
	Dietary fiber: 3 g

KUNG PAO CHICKEN

Makes 4 servings

- ½ cup Chicken Broth (page 272) or canned broth*
- ⅓ cup reduced-sodium soy sauce
- ½ cup sake
- 1 clove garlic, minced
- 1 teaspoon hot chili oil (LaYu)
- 2 chicken breasts, skinned, boned and cut into strips ¼ inch thick
- 2 tablespoons potato starch
- 1 tablespoon olive oil
- 2 dried negro or other hot red chilies, reconstituted in water
- 2 large cloves garlic
- ½ pound snow peas
- 1 8-ounce can whole water chestnuts, drained
- 6 green onions, cut diagonally into 1-inch pieces

In a 2-quart saucepan, combine chicken broth, soy sauce, sake, minced garlic and hot chili oil; let simmer while preparing the chicken.

Sprinkle chicken with 1 tablespoon of the potato starch. In a nonstick skillet, heat 2 teaspoons of the olive oil. Add chilies and garlic, and sauté 2–3 minutes. Add chicken and sauté about 10 minutes or until chicken is cooked. Remove chicken to a serving casserole.

Bring sauce to a boil. Dissolve remaining potato starch in 2 tablespoons cold water and gradually add to boiling broth. Cook and stir 2–3 minutes or until sauce thickens.

In the same nonstick skillet, heat remaining teaspoon of olive oil. Add snow peas and water chestnuts, and stir-fry until snow peas are crisp-tender, about 2 to 3 minutes. Add green onions. Combine with chicken. Pour sauce over and toss.

*Canned broth is higher in sodium.

NOTE: Potato starch is available in many supermarkets and in Oriental groceries.

SERVING SUGGESTION: Serve with short-grain rice and oranges, pineapple, papaya and fortune cookies.

APPROXIMATE NUTRITIONAL CONTENT PER SERVING

Total calories: 343	Carbohydrates: 24 g
Fat: 9 g	Protein: 29 g
Percentage of calories from fat:	Cholesterol: 73 mg
25%	Sodium: 990 mg
	Dietary fiber: 1 g

Due to the soy sauce, Kung Pao Chicken is high in sodium. Serve it with low-sodium accompaniments such as those suggested.

MUSHROOM-AND-ARTICHOKE CHICKEN

Makes 4 servings

- ¼ teaspoon black pepper
- ¼ teaspoon salt
- 1 teaspoon powdered rosemary
- 1 teaspoon paprika
- 2 chicken breasts, skinned and boned
- 2 teaspoons olive oil or canola oil
- 1 14-ounce can water-packed artichoke hearts, drained and cut into quarters
- ¼ pound fresh mushrooms, sliced
- 2 green onions, chopped
- ⅔ cup Chicken Stock (page 264) or canned broth*
- ¼ cup dry sherry
- 2 tablespoons all-purpose flour
- 2 tablespoons water

In a shallow pan, combine pepper, salt, rosemary and paprika, and dredge chicken in seasonings. In a nonstick skillet, heat olive oil. Add chicken and brown 3–5 minutes on each side.

Arrange chicken in a 2-quart baking dish. Tuck artichokes in between. To the skillet, add mushrooms and onions; sauté 2–3 minutes. Add chicken stock and sherry; bring to a boil. Combine flour with water. Add to stock mixture, stirring constantly 2–3 minutes. Pour sauce over chicken and artichokes. Cover with foil or lid. Bake at 375°F. 40 minutes.

*Canned broth is higher in sodium.

SERVING SUGGESTION: Serve with brown rice, fresh asparagus, Lettuce and Bermuda Onion Salad (page 341), Creamy Vinaigrette (page 354) and, for dessert, Berry Bavarian (page 460).

APPROXIMATE NUTRITIONAL CONTENT PER SERVING
Total calories: 231   Carbohydrates: 10 g
Fat: 6 g   Protein: 29 g
Percentage of calories from fat: Cholesterol: 73 mg
   23%   Sodium: 355 mg
                 Dietary fiber: 1 g

GARLIC CHICKEN

Makes 4 servings

6 large cloves garlic
3 tablespoons olive oil
1 teaspoon powdered rosemary
2 chicken breasts, skinned and boned
1 tablespoon grated orange zest

In a blender or food processor, purée garlic with olive oil. Add rosemary and whirl 20 seconds. Arrange chicken breasts in an 8 x 8-inch ovenproof baking dish. Sprinkle with orange zest. Pour marinade over all and marinate in the refrigerator 3–4 hours.

Drain off marinade. Bake chicken, uncovered, at 350°F. 30–35 minutes or until chicken is cooked.

SERVING SUGGESTION: Serve with Eggplant Parmigiana (page 448), Country Italian Bread (page 278) and Amaretto Oranges with Strawberries (page 492).

APPROXIMATE NUTRITIONAL CONTENT PER SERVING
Total calories: 194   Carbohydrates: 2 g
Fat: 8 g   Protein: 27 g
Percentage of calories from fat: Cholesterol: 73 mg
   39%   Sodium: 65 mg
                 Dietary fiber: 0

CHICKEN WITH TOMATOES AND PARMESAN

Makes 4 servings

1   teaspoon paprika
¾   teaspoon white pepper
½   teaspoon powdered rosemary
2   chicken breasts, skinned and boned
⅓   cup vermouth
2   tablespoons fresh lemon juice
1   cup Chicken Broth (page 272) or canned broth*
¼   teaspoon salt
1   tablespoon arrowroot
3   tablespoons cold water
1   14-ounce can water-packed artichoke hearts,
        drained
1   8-ounce can mushroom stems and pieces, drained
1   large ripe tomato, cut into 1-inch chunks
¼   cup freshly grated Parmesan cheese

Combine paprika, ½ teaspoon of the white pepper, and rosemary. Dredge chicken in seasonings to coat. Arrange chicken in a single layer in an 8 x 8-inch ovenproof baking dish. Bake at 375°F. 30 minutes or until chicken is cooked.

Meanwhile, in a 2-quart saucepan, combine vermouth, lemon juice, chicken broth, salt and remaining ¼ teaspoon white pepper, and bring to a boil. Reduce heat and simmer. When chicken is nearly cooked, bring mixture back to boiling. Combine arrowroot with cold water. Pour into broth; cook, stirring constantly, 2–3 minutes or until mixture thickens. Add artichokes and mushrooms.

Add tomatoes to chicken. Pour sauce over chicken and tomatoes. Sprinkle with cheese. Place under broiler 2–3 minutes or until cheese melts.

*Canned broth is higher in sodium.

SERVING SUGGESTION: Serve with tiny red potatoes, fresh green beans and, for dessert, Strawberry-Rhubarb Shortcake (page 470).

APPROXIMATE NUTRITIONAL CONTENT PER SERVING

Total calories: 285
Fat: 6 g
Percentage of calories from fat:
   18%

Carbohydrates: 20 g
Protein: 35 g
Cholesterol: 78 mg
Sodium: 532 mg
Dietary fiber: 2 g

STIR-FRIED CHICKEN

Makes 4 servings

  1 pound chicken breasts, skinned and boned
  1 tablespoon sake
  2 tablespoons potato starch
  2 teaspoons olive oil

Cut chicken breasts into cubes or strips. Toss with sake. Sprinkle with potato starch. In a nonstick skillet, heat olive oil over medium-high heat. Add chicken and stir-fry 8–10 minutes or until done.

NOTE: Potato starch is available in many supermarkets and in Oriental groceries.

SERVING SUGGESTION: Serve with Two-Mushroom Soup (page 251), Stir-Fried Vegetables (page 442), steamed rice and Fresh Pineapple with Papaya Purée (page 491).

APPROXIMATE NUTRITIONAL CONTENT PER SERVING

Total calories: 226
Fat: 7 g
Percentage of calories from fat:
   27%

Carbohydrates: 3 g
Protein: 35 g
Cholesterol: 96 mg
Sodium: 83 mg
Dietary fiber: Tr

TURKEY MEAT LOAF

Makes 8 servings

⅓ cup barley
2 8-ounce cans tomato sauce
¼ cup water
2 tablespoons dry mustard
3 tablespoons cider vinegar
¾ pound ground turkey breast
⅓ cup chopped green onions
1 egg
4 cloves garlic, finely minced
¼ teaspoon black pepper

In 1 cup of water, soak the barley overnight. Drain.

In a small bowl, combine tomato sauce, water, mustard and vinegar. Set aside. Combine barley, ground turkey, green onions, egg, garlic, pepper and ½ cup of the sauce. Mix thoroughly. Arrange in a loaf pan. Pour an additional ½ cup sauce over top. Bake at 325°F. 1 hour. Serve with remaining sauce.

NOTE: It is not essential to soak the barley overnight, but it will be more tender if you do.

SERVING SUGGESTION: Excellent for hot or cold sandwiches.

APPROXIMATE NUTRITIONAL CONTENT PER SERVING

Total calories: 128
Fat: 2 g
Percentage of calories from fat:
    13%

Carbohydrates: 13 g
Protein: 16 g
Cholesterol: 62 mg
Sodium: 401 mg
Dietary fiber: 2 g

Add 6 calories for each additional tablespoon of sauce.

HOT-AND-SPICY SOUTHWEST TURKEY

Makes 9 servings

> 1 2-pound fresh turkey breast
> 1 cup Hot Chili Sauce (page 359)
> ½ cup Chili Salsa (page 361)

Roast turkey on a rack in a 350°F. oven for 1½ hours; baste with ½ cup Hot Chili Sauce. Cook 45 minutes more or until turkey is cooked, basting frequently. In a small saucepan, combine remaining ½ cup Chili Sauce with Chili Salsa and heat. Pass the sauce with turkey.

NOTE: The leftovers make great sandwiches.

SERVING SUGGESTION: Serve with Rice with Chilies (page 431), Refried Black Beans (page 425), warm tortillas (see page 383) and fresh strawberries.

APPROXIMATE NUTRITIONAL CONTENT PER 3-OUNCE SERVING

Total calories: 140
Fat: 1 g
Percentage of calories from fat:
  5%

Carbohydrates: 4 g
Protein: 27 g
Cholesterol: 74 mg
Sodium: 264 mg
Dietary fiber: Tr

ROASTED CAJUN TURKEY

Makes 8 servings

    1 teaspoon garlic powder
    1 teaspoon ground thyme
    1 teaspoon dried basil
    1 teaspoon black pepper
    ½ teaspoon white pepper
    ½ teaspoon cayenne pepper
    2 pounds fresh turkey breast

Combine seasonings. Rub turkey with generous amounts of seasoning. Roast on a rack in a 350°F. oven for 1½ hours or until done.

SERVING SUGGESTION: Serve with Creole Rice (page 432) and Vanilla Angel Food Cake (page 482) with Vanilla Glaze (page 485).

APPROXIMATE NUTRITIONAL CONTENT PER SERVING

Total calories: 139
Fat: 1 g
Percentage of calories from fat:
  5%

Carbohydrates: Tr
Protein: 30 g
Cholesterol: 84 mg
Sodium: 53 mg
Dietary fiber: Tr

RED MEAT

A NOTE ON RED MEAT

Red meat is naturally high in fat. To keep it from becoming a dietary disaster, look for less-fat cuts such as "loin round" for beef and "loin/leg" for pork, lamb and veal on food labels. These terms indicate lean choices. Beef labeled USDA Select Grade is the leanest, followed by Choice and then Prime.

Because of the high-fat nature of red meat, it is very important to reduce fat in accompanying foods. By surrounding a leg of lamb, about 34% fat, with couscous, green beans and tomatoes, you can reduce the percentage of fat in the meal to about 22%.

Marinades are often used with leaner cuts of red meat to enhance flavor. In the nutritional calculations for our recipes, it is estimated that about one-half of any sodium or fat in the marinade will be left in the bowl. Be sure always to thoroughly drain the marinade before cooking.

LAMB WITH GARLIC

Makes 8 servings

- 1 3-pound leg of lamb, boned and butterflied
- 1 tablespoon minced parsley
- 1 tablespoon ground sage
- 1 tablespoon powdered rosemary
- 2 teaspoons olive oil
- 2 tablespoons fresh lemon juice
- ½ teaspoon salt
- ¼ teaspoon black pepper
- 8 cloves garlic, thinly sliced

Rub lamb on all sides with parsley, sage and rosemary.

In a bowl, combine olive oil, lemon juice, salt and pepper. Pour over seasoned lamb and rub into meat. Insert sliced garlic cloves in cracks and crevices.

Prepare coals and cover the grill with foil.

Place the lamb on a very hot grill. Turn every 10 minutes for a total cooking time of about 30 minutes for rare and 45 minutes for well done. Rare will register 160°F. on a meat thermometer; well done, 175°F. Just before serving, cut lamb into slices ½ inch thick and arrange on a platter.

SERVING SUGGESTION: Serve with Bulgur with Parmesan (page 435), Green Beans with Pimiento (page 445) and Grilled Herbed Tomatoes (page 440).

APPROXIMATE NUTRITIONAL CONTENT PER SERVING

Total calories: 249	Carbohydrates: 3 g
Fat: 11 g	Protein: 34 g
Percentage of calories from fat:	Cholesterol: 106 mg
39%	Sodium: 217 mg
	Dietary fiber: Tr

Serving the lamb with low-fat accompaniments such as couscous, green beans and tomatoes will reduce the total fat content of the meal to about 25%.

ROAST VEAL WITH ROSEMARY AND GARLIC

Makes 8 servings

2 pounds veal loin roast, boned
½ teaspoon coarsely ground black pepper
8 cloves garlic
8 sprigs fresh rosemary

Rub roast with black pepper. Insert garlic at intervals over roast. Tuck sprigs of rosemary in with the garlic. Roast on a rack in a 325°F. oven about 30 minutes per pound or to desired doneness.

SERVING SUGGESTION: Serve with Potatoes with Mushrooms and Tomatoes (page 439) and Green Beans with Pimiento (page 445).

APPROXIMATE NUTRITIONAL CONTENT PER SERVING

Total calories: 176	Carbohydrates: 1 g
Fat: 5 g	Protein: 29 g
Percentage of calories from fat:	Cholesterol: 108 mg
25%	Sodium: 55 mg
	Dietary fiber: Tr

GRILLED VEAL TENDERLOINS

Makes 4 servings

2 tablespoons olive oil
4 cloves garlic
¼ teaspoon salt
⅛ teaspoon black pepper
1 pound veal tenderloins

In a blender or food processor, combine olive oil, garlic and seasonings. Pour marinade over veal and marinate in the refrigerator 6–8 hours. Remove from marinade and thoroughly drain off excess.

Prepare coals and cover the grill with foil.

Grill tenderloins over hot coals 5–6 minutes or to desired doneness.

SERVING SUGGESTION: Serve with Roasted Potatoes with Garlic (page 450), Asparagus with Lemon Vinaigrette (page 437) and fresh seasonal fruits.

APPROPRIATE NUTRITIONAL CONTENT PER SERVING

Total calories: 189
Fat: 7 g
Percentage of calories from fat: 33%

Carbohydrates: 1 g
Protein: 30 g
Cholesterol: 76 mg
Sodium: 220 mg
Dietary fiber: Tr

MEDALLIONS OF PORK WITH LEMON

Makes 4 servings

1½	tablespoons olive oil
3	cloves garlic
¼	teaspoon powdered rosemary
1	pound lean boneless pork tenderloins, thinly sliced
2½	tablespoons fresh lemon juice
¼	teaspoon salt
¼	teaspoon black pepper

In a blender or food processor, combine olive oil and garlic. Add rosemary and whirl 1 minute more. Arrange pork tenderloins in an 8 x 8 x 2-inch casserole. Pour marinade over pork and marinate in refrigerator 1–2 hours. Drain off marinade thoroughly.

Heat a nonstick skillet. Add tenderloins and brown 2 minutes on each side. Reduce heat, add lemon juice and cook, turning often, 3–5 minutes more or until pork is cooked. Season with salt and pepper.

SERVING SUGGESTION: Serve with Barley with Pine Nuts (page 436), Spinach-Stuffed Tomatoes (page 446) and sliced apples or applesauce.

APPROXIMATE NUTRITIONAL CONTENT PER SERVING

Total calories: 138	Carbohydrates: 2 g
Fat: 6 g	Protein: 18 g
Percentage of calories from fat: 39%	Cholesterol: 57 mg
	Sodium: 176 mg
	Dietary fiber: Tr

Serving the pork with the low-fat accompaniments suggested above will reduce the total fat content of the meal to about 25%.

BEEF-AND-VEAL LOAF WITH RED PEPPER SAUCE

Makes 10 servings

   1 cup diced French bread with crust
  ½ cup non-fat milk
   1 pound extra-lean ground round steak
   1 pound extra-lean ground veal
   2 eggs
  ¼ teaspoon black pepper
  ¼ teaspoon ground thyme
  ¼ teaspoon ground rosemary
  ¾ cup freshly grated Parmesan cheese

Red Pepper Sauce
   1 red pepper, halved and seeded
   1 tablespoon olive oil
   1 teaspoon fresh lemon juice
  ¾ teaspoon balsamic vinegar
  ¾ teaspoon salt or to taste
  ¼ teaspoon cayenne pepper

Soften the bread in milk for 10–15 minutes. Meanwhile, combine ground round, veal, eggs, pepper, thyme, rosemary and Parmesan cheese. Squeeze bread dry (discard milk), add to meat mixture and mix. Shape into a loaf and put into an 8-inch loaf pan. Bake at 375°F. 1 hour.

A few minutes before meat loaf is cooked, in a microwave or a steamer basket over boiling water, steam red pepper 4 minutes or until softened. Put into a blender or food processor; add olive oil, lemon juice, vinegar, salt and cayenne pepper. Purée. Pass the sauce with the loaf.

SERVING SUGGESTION: Serve with Risotto Milanese (page 434). The leftovers make great sandwiches.

APPROXIMATE NUTRITIONAL CONTENT PER SERVING

Total calories: 247
Fat: 10 g
Percentage of calories from fat:
   35%

Carbohydrates: 12 g
Protein: 27 g
Cholesterol: 114 mg
Sodium: 477 mg
Dietary fiber: Tr

This dish is high in sodium. Keep a balance for the day by selecting low-sodium foods at other meals.

STEAK AND ONIONS

Makes 4 servings

  1 pound top round cubed steak
  2 teaspoons olive oil
  6 cloves garlic, chopped
  1 white onion, halved and sliced
  1 green pepper, cut into thin strips
  1 red pepper, cut into thin strips

Slice the steak into thin, stir-fry strips following the lines made in the meat by the butcher's tenderizing machine.

In a nonstick pan, heat olive oil. Add steak and garlic, and brown 1–2 minutes. Add onion and cook 3–4 minutes or until onions begin to soften. Add peppers and cook 2–3 minutes. Serve at once.

SERVING SUGGESTION: Good with steamed rice and, for dessert, fresh strawberries with Vanilla or Chocolate Angel Food Cake (pages 482–483).

APPROXIMATE NUTRITIONAL CONTENT PER SERVING

Total calories: 204
Fat: 8 g
Percentage of calories from fat:
   35%

Carbohydrates: 5 g
Protein: 27 g
Cholesterol: 71 mg
Sodium: 55 mg
Dietary fiber: Tr

STIR-FRIED BEEF AND ASPARAGUS

Makes 4 servings

> 1 pound fresh asparagus
> ¾ pound eye of round steak, thinly sliced into stir-fry strips
> 1 tablespoon sake
> 1 tablespoon reduced-sodium soy sauce
> 1 teaspoon olive oil

Sauce

> 1 tablespoon oyster sauce
> 2 tablespoons sake
> ¼ teaspoon granulated sugar
> 1 tablespoon reduced-sodium soy sauce
> ¼ cup water
> ½ teaspoon hot chili oil (LaYu)
> ½ teaspoon potato starch

In a covered steamer rack over boiling water, steam asparagus 1½ minutes. Set aside. Pour sake and soy sauce over beef and marinate at room temperature 20–30 minutes.

In a bowl, combine sauce ingredients and stir well. In a wok or nonstick skillet, heat olive oil. Add beef and stir-fry 4–5 minutes. Add asparagus and sauce. Cook, stirring constantly, 2–3 minutes or until very hot.

NOTE: Oyster sauce is available in the Oriental section of most supermarkets.

SERVING SUGGESTION: Serve with short-grain rice or Chinese noodles and fresh pineapple, papaya and fortune cookies.

APPROXIMATE NUTRITIONAL CONTENT PER SERVING

Total calories: 211
Fat: 7 g
Percentage of calories from fat:
   30%

Carbohydrates: 7 g
Protein: 27 g
Cholesterol: 62 mg
Sodium: 500 mg
Dietary fiber: 1 g

RED-HOT CHILI STEAK

Makes 6 servings

1½ pounds top round steak
¾ cup Hot Chili Marinade (page 360)
½ cup Hot Chili Sauce (page 359)

Marinate round steak in Hot Chili Marinade in the refrigerator at least 2 hours and as long as overnight. Drain off marinade and reserve.

Prepare the coals and cover the grill with foil.

Grill steak over hot coals 6 minutes on each side, basting 2–3 times with reserved marinade. Cut steak on the diagonal into long strips. Accompany with Hot Chili Sauce.

SERVING SUGGESTION: Serve with Black Bean Soup (page 245), Ensenada Salad (page 332) and Spanish Flan (page 457) or fresh fruit. Or substitute Black Beans and Rice for Black Bean Soup.

APPROXIMATE NUTRITIONAL CONTENT PER SERVING

Total calories: 200
Fat: 6 g
Percentage of calories from fat:
   28%

Carbohydrates: 8 g
Protein: 27 g
Cholesterol: 70 mg
Sodium: 434 mg
Dietary fiber: Tr

TACO PIZZA

Makes 8 servings

1	white onion, chopped
1	pound extra-lean ground round
1	tablespoon chili powder
¼	teaspoon garlic powder
½	teaspoon ground cumin
¼	teaspoon cayenne pepper
¼	teaspoon black pepper
½	teaspoon paprika
½	teaspoon salt
½	cup commercial or homemade tomato salsa
⅓	cup Red Bean Dip (see page 348)
1	Easy Pizza Crust (page 279)
2	medium tomatoes, diced
1 ½	cups lettuce, shredded
½	cup grated low-fat Cheddar cheese

In a nonstick skillet, sauté onion and ground round. Season with chili powder, garlic powder, cumin, cayenne pepper, black pepper, paprika and salt. Add salsa and toss.

Spread Red Bean Dip over cooked pizza crust. Top with ground round mixture. Arrange diced tomatoes over top. Cover with lettuce and sprinkle with cheese. Place under the broiler for 1–2 minutes or just until cheese begins to melt.

SHORTCUT SUGGESTION: In place of homemade dough, purchase a heart-healthy, uncooked crust from a local pizza parlor. Be sure it's made with olive oil or an unsaturated, nonhydrogenated oil such as safflower, soybean or corn oil. Do not use a crust made with hydrogenated shortening, lard, palm oil or coconut oil. (You may wish to purchase several crusts at one time to keep on hand in the freezer.)

SERVING SUGGESTION: Serve with seasonal fruits.

APPROXIMATE NUTRITIONAL CONTENT PER SERVING

Total calories: 249	Carbohydrates: 25 g
Fat: 10 g	Protein: 14 g
Percentage of calories from fat:	Cholesterol: 32 mg
36%	Sodium: 457 mg
	Dietary fiber: 3 g

MARINATED GRILLED STEAK

Makes 8 servings

- ½ cup reduced-sodium soy sauce
- ½ cup vermouth
- 2 tablespoons olive oil
- 2 tablespoons brown sugar
- 1 tablespoon Worcestershire sauce
- 2 cloves garlic, minced
- 1 fresh gingerroot, peeled and sliced
- 2 pounds top round or eye of round steak

In a bowl, combine soy sauce, vermouth, olive oil, brown sugar, Worcestershire sauce, garlic and gingerroot. Pour marinade over meat and marinate in the refrigerator 3–24 hours. Thoroughly drain off marinade.

Prepare coals and cover the grill with foil.

Grill over hot coals about 6 minutes on each side or to desired doneness.

SERVING SUGGESTION: Serve with Vegetable Antipasto Salad (page 328), corn on the cob and fresh berries with Vanilla Angel Food Cake (page 482).

APPROXIMATE NUTRITIONAL CONTENT PER SERVING

Total calories: 171	Carbohydrates: 2 g
Fat: 6 g	Protein: 24 g
Percentage of calories from fat:	Cholesterol: 64 mg
31%	Sodium: 206 mg
	Dietary fiber: 0

SPAGHETTI SAUCE BOLOGNESE

Makes 3 quarts

 2 teaspoons olive oil or canola oil
 1 onion, coarsely chopped
 2 cloves garlic, chopped
 ½ pound extra-lean ground round steak
 ¼ pound extra-lean ground pork
 ½ pound fresh mushrooms, sliced
 ½ cup dry white wine (Soave Bolla is good)
 2 28-ounce cans Italian plum tomatoes
 2 tablespoons tomato paste
 ½ cup warm water
 ½ teaspoon salt
 ¼ teaspoon black pepper
 1 teaspoon basil

In a nonstick skillet, heat olive oil. Add onions and garlic and sauté 4–5 minutes. Add beef and pork, and sauté 5–6 minutes. Add mushrooms and sauté 3–4 minutes. Add white wine and simmer, covered, 4–5 minutes.

Drain tomatoes and finely chop; reserve juice for later use. Dissolve tomato paste in ½ cup warm water. Add diced tomatoes and tomato paste to meat. Simmer over low heat 30–40 minutes. Season with salt, pepper and basil.

SERVING SUGGESTION: Serve over fresh pasta. Accompany with Mediterranean Antipasto Salad (page 329) and Roasted Garlic Bread (page 291).

APPROXIMATE NUTRITIONAL CONTENT PER 1-CUP SERVING

Total calories: 86	Carbohydrates: 8 g
Fat: 3 g	Protein: 7 g
Percentage of calories from fat: 28%	Cholesterol: 15 mg
	Sodium: 344 mg
	Dietary fiber: 1 g

Add 190 calories per cup of spaghetti.

BEANS, RICE & OTHER GRAINS

A NOTE ON BEANS AND RICE

Beans and rice are excellent as side dishes or as components of hearty, appetizing meals. They satisfy without overloading on calories, provide fiber and complex carbohydrates, and are low in fat.

In many recipes for beans, there is an option to use canned beans in order to cut preparation and cooking time. Many brands (Progresso, for one) offer a variety (black beans, red kidney beans, cannellini beans) that are virtually as good as homemade. Commercially prepared beans, however, are generally higher in sodium. Rinsing them before use will reduce the sodium by one-half.

Brown rice has three times the amount of fiber as white rice and can be substituted for white rice in most recipes.

Try short-grain (Oriental) rice as a flavorful side dish. It can be purchased at Japanese and Chinese markets, or in the Oriental section of most grocery stores.

BEANS RANCHERO

Makes 14 cups

         4   dried pasilla chilies
    1½   cups water
         1   medium tomato
         1   cup chopped white onion
         5   cloves garlic
         1   teaspoon oregano
         1   teaspoon salt
         6   cups Beef Stock (page 268) or canned broth*
         1   6-ounce can tomato paste
         2   fresh jalapeño peppers, seeded and chopped
    ¼   teaspoon thyme
    1¼   cups lentils
         6   cups cooked Seville Rice (page 430)

Soak dried chilies in 1½ cups water 30–60 minutes or until soft. Pour chilies with soaking liquid into a blender or food processor; add tomato, ½ cup of the chopped onion, garlic and oregano, and purée. Add salt. Set aside.

In a stockpot, combine beef stock, tomato paste, remaining ½ cup chopped onion, peppers and thyme, and bring just to boiling. Add lentils, reduce heat, cover and simmer 1½–2 hours or until lentils are tender. Stir in hot-chili mixture. Simmer 10 minutes. Serve over Seville Rice.

NOTE: Pasilla chilies, also called poblano, negro or chilaca, are available in Mexican markets or in the Mexican or Spanish section of many supermarkets. Ancho chilies may be substituted.

*Canned broth is higher in sodium.

SERVING SUGGESTION: Good with Chicken Cortez (page 389).

APPROXIMATE NUTRITIONAL CONTENT PER CUP

Total calories: 173
Fat: Tr
Percentage of calories from fat:
 5%

Carbohydrates: 34 g
Protein: 6 g
Cholesterol: Tr
Sodium: 643 mg
Dietary fiber: 2 g

REFRIED BLACK BEANS

Makes 1 cup

    1 15-ounce can black beans, drained*
    1 tablespoon chili powder
    ½ teaspoon cumin
    2 teaspoons olive oil

In a blender or food processor, purée beans. Add chili powder and cumin. Blend.

In a nonstick skillet, heat olive oil. Add bean mixture and cook, stirring constantly, until beans are warm.

*Rinsing will reduce the sodium in the black beans by one-half.

SERVING SUGGESTION: Good with Chicken Enchiladas (page 386) or Chicken Fajitas (page 384).

APPROXIMATE NUTRITIONAL CONTENT PER TABLESPOON

Total calories: 28
Fat: 1 g
Percentage of calories from fat:
 23%

Carbohydrates: 4 g
Protein: 1 g
Cholesterol: 0
Sodium: 90 mg
Dietary fiber: 1 g

BLACK BEANS AND RICE

Makes 7 cups

> 1   tablespoon olive oil or canola oil
> 1   small onion, chopped
> 3   serrano chilies, halved and seeded
> 2   15-ounce cans black beans*
> ¼   teaspoon ground cumin
> ⅛   teaspoon cayenne pepper
> 1   cup uncooked long-grain white rice
> 1¾   cups Chicken Broth (page 272) or canned broth**
> 3   cloves garlic, crushed

In a nonstick skillet over medium heat, heat olive oil. Add onion and chilies, and sauté 6–8 minutes or until tender. Drain beans, reserving ½ cup liquid. Add beans with ½ cup liquid to onions and chilies. Cook, uncovered, 20–30 minutes or until about half the liquid is absorbed. Season with cumin and cayenne pepper.

Meanwhile, rinse rice until water runs clear; drain. Add chicken broth and garlic, and bring to a boil. Stir. Reduce heat, cover and simmer 20–30 minutes or until broth is absorbed and rice is tender. Ladle black beans over rice.

*Rinsing will reduce the sodium in the black beans by one-half.

**Canned broth is higher in sodium.

SERVING SUGGESTION: Good with Chicken with Salsa (page 385).

APPROXIMATE NUTRITIONAL CONTENT PER ½-CUP SERVING

Total calories: 116	Carbohydrates: 21 g
Fat: 1 g	Protein: 5 g
Percentage of calories from fat: 11%	Cholesterol: Tr
	Sodium: 238 mg
	Dietary fiber: 2 g

RICE PILAF

Makes 7 servings (about ½ cup each)

> ½   teaspoon olive oil or canola oil
> 3   cloves garlic, minced
> 1   small onion, diced
> 1 ½ cups Chicken Broth (page 272) or canned broth*
> 1   cup uncooked short-grain white rice
> ¼   teaspoon dry mustard
> ½   teaspoon Tabasco sauce
> 1   tablespoon chopped fresh parsley

In a nonstick skillet, heat olive oil. Add garlic and onion, and sauté 6–8 minutes or until onion is tender. Spoon into a 3-quart saucepan. Add chicken broth, rice, dry mustard and Tabasco. Heat to boiling, stirring once or twice. Reduce heat, cover and steam for 20 minutes or until rice is tender and broth is absorbed. Add parsley. Toss.

   *Canned broth is higher in sodium.

APPROXIMATE NUTRITIONAL CONTENT PER ½ CUP

Total calories: 114
Fat: Tr
Percentage of calories from fat:
   7%

Carbohydrates: 22 g
Protein: 3 g
Cholesterol: Tr
Sodium: 147 mg
Dietary fiber: Tr

ORIENTAL RICE

Makes 3 cups

1 teaspoon olive oil or canola oil
1 small white onion, finely chopped
2 cloves garlic, minced
1 cup long-grain white rice
3 cups Beef Broth (page 274) or canned broth*
1 teaspoon paprika
1 teaspoon soy sauce
2 tablespoons chopped fresh parsley

In a nonstick skillet, heat olive oil. Add onion and garlic, and sauté 4–6 minutes or until onion is crisp-tender. Add rice and brown 2–3 minutes. Add beef broth, paprika and soy sauce, and bring to a boil. Reduce heat, cover and simmer 20–30 minutes or until broth is absorbed and rice is tender. Add parsley and toss.

*Canned broth is higher in sodium.

SERVING SUGGESTION: Good with Teriyaki Chicken (page 401) and grilled beef or salmon.

APPROXIMATE NUTRITIONAL CONTENT PER ½ CUP

Total calories: 131
Fat: 1 g
Percentage of calories from fat:
  9%

Carbohydrates: 26 g
Protein: 3 g
Cholesterol: Tr
Sodium: 334 mg
Dietary fiber: Tr

WILD AND WHITE RICE

Makes approximately 7 cups

1⅓ cups wild rice
  1 cup beef consommé
  1 cup short-grain white rice

Steam wild rice according to package directions, substituting 1 cup beef consommé for 1 of the cups of water. Allow 45–60 minutes cooking time.

In a separate pan, steam short-grain rice according to package directions. Allow 20–30 minutes cooking time.

Combine both cooked rices in a bowl and toss to make a colorful accompaniment.

APPROXIMATE NUTRITIONAL CONTENT PER ½ CUP

Total calories: 114
Fat: Tr
Percentage of calories from fat: 2%

Carbohydrates: 25 g
Protein: 2 g
Cholesterol: Tr
Sodium: 57 mg
Dietary fiber: Tr

SEVILLE RICE

Makes 3 cups

>   1   cup uncooked long-grain white rice
>   1 ¾   cups Chicken Broth (page 272) or canned broth*
>   3   cloves garlic, crushed

Rinse rice until water runs clear; drain. In a saucepan, combine rice, chicken broth and garlic, and bring to a boil. Stir. Reduce heat; cover and simmer 20–30 minutes or until broth is absorbed and rice is tender.

*Canned broth is higher in sodium.

APPROXIMATE NUTRITIONAL CONTENT PER ½ CUP

Total calories: 125
Fat: Tr
Percentage of calories from fat:
   3%

Carbohydrates: 25 g
Protein: 3 g
Cholesterol: Tr
Sodium: 152 mg
Dietary fiber: Tr

RICE WITH CHILIES

Makes 6 cups

> 1 tablespoon olive oil
> 1 cup long-grain white rice
> 1 small onion, chopped
> 3 cloves garlic, sliced
> 2 cups Chicken Broth (page 272) or canned broth*
> ½ teaspoon salt
> 1 4-ounce can diced green chilies
> 1 small tomato, diced
> ½ cup freshly grated low-fat Cheddar cheese

In a nonstick skillet, heat olive oil; add rice, onion and garlic, and stir-fry 6–8 minutes or until rice is lightly browned and onion is tender. Add chicken broth and salt; cover and simmer until most of liquid is absorbed. Add green chilies and tomatoes, and sprinkle with cheese. Cover and steam 2–3 minutes or until cheese is melted.

*Canned broth is higher in sodium.

SERVING SUGGESTION: Good with Chicken Black Bean Burritos (page 392).

APPROXIMATE NUTRITIONAL CONTENT PER ¾-CUP SERVING

Total calories: 135	Carbohydrates: 22 g
Fat: 3 g	Protein: 5 g
Percentage of calories from fat: 20%	Cholesterol: Tr
	Sodium: 365 mg
	Dietary fiber: 1 g

CREOLE RICE

Makes 3 cups

1 ¾	cups Chicken Broth (page 272) or canned broth*
½	teaspoon cayenne pepper
½	teaspoon ground cumin
½	teaspoon oregano
½	teaspoon black pepper
¼	teaspoon white pepper
1	cup long-grain white rice
2	teaspoons olive oil or canola oil
3	large cloves garlic
1	cup chopped white onion
¾	cup diced eggplant (optional)
¾	cup diced green pepper

In a saucepan, bring chicken broth to a boil; add cayenne, cumin, oregano, and black and white pepper. Stir in rice. Reduce heat, cover and simmer 20–30 minutes or until broth is absorbed and rice is tender.

Meanwhile, in a nonstick skillet, heat olive oil. Add garlic, onion and eggplant, if using, and sauté 4–5 minutes or until onion is just tender and eggplant is softened. Add green pepper and cook 2–3 minutes. Toss with the cooked rice.

*Canned broth is higher in sodium.

NOTE: This rice is very spicy. For a milder flavor, reduce each of the seasonings by one-half.

APPROXIMATE NUTRITIONAL CONTENT PER ½ CUP

Total calories: 156	Carbohydrates: 29 g
Fat: 2 g	Protein: 4 g
Percentage of calories from fat: 13%	Cholesterol: Tr
	Sodium: 165 mg
	Dietary fiber: 2 g

ORZO WITH SAFFRON

Makes 8 cups

  4 cups Chicken Stock (page 264) or canned broth*
10 cups water
  1 pound orzo
  3 cloves garlic
  ¼ teaspoon powdered saffron

In a saucepan, bring chicken stock and water to a boil. Add orzo and garlic. Boil 15–20 minutes or until orzo is cooked *al dente*. Drain. Rinse lightly so as not to lose the chicken stock flavor. Pour into serving bowl. Toss with saffron.

    *Canned broth is higher in sodium.

    SERVING SUGGESTION: Especially good with Chicken Primavera (page 400).

APPROXIMATE NUTRITIONAL CONTENT PER CUP

Total calories: 221
Fat: 2 g
Percentage of calories from fat:
  7%

Carbohydrates: 42 g
Protein: 10 g
Cholesterol: Tr
Sodium: 148 mg
Dietary fiber: 2 g

RISOTTO MILANESE

Makes 8 servings

 6 cups Chicken Stock (page 264) or canned broth*
 1 small onion, chopped
 1 teaspoon olive oil
 1 16-ounce box long-grain Italian risotto
    (Arborio rice)
⅓ teaspoon powdered saffron
¼ cup dry white wine (Soave Bolla is good)
⅓ pound fresh mushrooms, sliced
 1 7-ounce can water-packed artichoke hearts,
    drained
    salt (optional)

In a saucepan, bring chicken stock just to boiling; reduce heat and let simmer.

In a large nonstick skillet, sauté onion in olive oil 4–6 minutes. When onion is tender, stir in rice; sauté 3–4 minutes, stirring often. Add saffron, wine and ¼ cup of the simmering stock. When the liquid is absorbed, add ½ cup additional stock. Stir and cook until liquid is absorbed, then add another ½ cup stock. Repeat the process until all the stock is used. Add mushrooms and artichokes when last half-cup of stock is added. Remove from heat. Cover and let sit 5–10 minutes or until all the liquid is absorbed. Season with salt, if desired.

*Canned broth is higher in sodium.

NOTE: Risotto is similar to stir-fried rice. It is not boiled rice, so it is important to add the liquid very gradually and regulate the heat so that the liquid does not evaporate too quickly. Total cooking time should be about 30 minutes. Risotto is found in the gourmet sections of many supermarkets and in Italian markets.

APPROXIMATE NUTRITIONAL CONTENT PER SERVING

Total calories: 272
Fat: 3 g
Percentage of calories from fat:
  9%

Carbohydrates: 54 g
Protein: 9 g
Cholesterol: 1 mg
Sodium: 250 mg
Dietary fiber: 1 g

BULGUR WITH PARMESAN

Makes 4 servings

1 ½ cups Beef Broth (page 274) or canned broth*
¼ teaspoon Tabasco sauce
⅛ teaspoon salt
1 cup cracked wheat bulgur
¼ cup freshly grated Parmesan cheese

In a large saucepan, combine beef broth, Tabasco sauce and salt, and bring to a boil. Stir in bulgur. Remove from heat and cover. Let sit until broth is absorbed and bulgur is tender. Add Parmesan and toss.

*Canned broth is higher in sodium.

VARIATION: Substitute couscous for bulgur.

SERVING SUGGESTION: Good with chicken, lamb and seafood.

APPROXIMATE NUTRITIONAL CONTENT PER SERVING

Total calories: 191
Fat: 3 g
Percentage of calories from fat:
  13%

Carbohydrates: 35 g
Protein: 7 g
Cholesterol: 5 mg
Sodium: 363 mg
Dietary fiber: 8 g

BARLEY WITH PINE NUTS

Makes 4 cups

    1   cup pearl barley
    2   cups water
    1 ½ cups Beef Stock (page 268) or canned broth*
    1 ½ cups Chicken Stock (page 264) or canned broth*
    2   tablespoons leek, white part only
    ⅓   pound fresh mushrooms, sliced
    ⅓   cup pine nuts
    2   tablespoons chopped fresh parsley

Soak barley overnight in water. About 45–60 minutes before dinner, in a saucepan bring beef and chicken stocks to a boil. Add barley along with soaking liquid and boil 1–2 minutes. Add leek. Reduce heat, cover and simmer 30–45 minutes or until most of liquid is absorbed. Add mushrooms. Continue to simmer 5–10 minutes or until mushrooms are tender and liquid is absorbed. Stir in pine nuts and parsley.

*Canned broth is higher in sodium.

SERVING SUGGESTION: Good with pork.

APPROXIMATE NUTRITIONAL CONTENT PER ½ CUP

Total calories: 137

Fat: 3 g

Percentage of calories from fat: 23%

Carbohydrates: 22 g

Protein: 5 g

Cholesterol: Tr

Sodium: 225 mg

Dietary fiber: 4 g

VEGETABLES & PASTA

ASPARAGUS WITH LEMON VINAIGRETTE

Makes 4 servings

    1 pound fresh asparagus
    ¼ cup fresh lemon juice
    2 teaspoons olive oil
    ½ teaspoon salt
    ¼ teaspoon black pepper

Microwave or steam asparagus until crisp-tender. Combine lemon juice, olive oil, salt and pepper. Pour over asparagus while asparagus is still warm.

VARIATION: Substitute ½ pound fresh broccoli for asparagus.

APPROXIMATE NUTRITIONAL CONTENT PER SERVING

Total calories: 52
Fat: 2 g
Percentage of calories from fat:
    38%

Carbohydrates: 6 g
Protein: 3 g
Cholesterol: 0
Sodium: 271 mg
Dietary fiber: 1 g

ANTIPASTO VEGETABLES

Makes 6 servings

- 4 small carrots, peeled and thinly sliced on the diagonal
- 1 small zucchini, peeled and sliced on the diagonal into matchstick strips
- ¼ pound broccoli florets
- 6 baby red potatoes, quartered
- ⅓ pound fresh green beans
- 1 clove garlic, minced
- ¼ cup fresh lemon juice
- 1 tablespoon olive oil
- ½ teaspoon salt
- ¼ teaspoon black pepper

In a steamer rack over boiling water, steam vegetables one type at a time until crisp-tender: carrots, zucchini and broccoli about 2 minutes each; potatoes and green beans about 6–10 minutes. As each vegetable is cooked, remove to a large, low serving bowl.

While vegetables are steaming, in a small saucepan combine garlic, lemon juice, olive oil, salt and pepper, and simmer 5–10 minutes. Pour sauce over cooked vegetables.

SERVING SUGGESTION: Great with grilled entrées.

APPROXIMATE NUTRITIONAL CONTENT PER SERVING

Total calories: 126
Fat: 2 g
Percentage of calories from fat: 17%

Carbohydrates: 24 g
Protein: 3 g
Cholesterol: 0
Sodium: 199 mg
Dietary fiber: 4 g

POTATOES WITH MUSHROOMS AND TOMATOES

Makes 8 servings

⅓ cup beef consommé
2 tablespoons dry white wine (Frascati is good)
2 teaspoons chervil
1 tablespoon chopped parsley
1 tablespoon olive oil
½ teaspoon salt
¼ teaspoon black pepper
1 ½ pounds tiny red potatoes, cooked and halved
¼ pound fresh mushrooms, cooked and sliced, or 1 8-ounce can mushroom stems and pieces, drained
1 large tomato, diced

In a small bowl, combine consommé, white wine, chervil, parsley, olive oil, salt and pepper. Pour over potatoes while potatoes are still warm. Arrange in a low salad bowl. Toss with mushrooms and tomatoes. Thoroughly drain excess marinade. Serve hot or cold.

APPROXIMATE NUTRITIONAL CONTENT PER SERVING

Total calories: 100
Fat: 2 g
Percentage of calories from fat: 18%

Carbohydrates: 18 g
Protein: 2 g
Cholesterol: Tr
Sodium: 174 mg
Dietary fiber: 1 g

GRILLED HERBED TOMATOES

Makes 6 servings

3 large ripe tomatoes, halved
¼ teaspoon olive oil
½ teaspoon powdered rosemary
¼ teaspoon salt
¼ teaspoon black pepper
3 cloves garlic, slivered

Brush tomato halves with olive oil, then sprinkle with rosemary, salt and pepper. Divide slivered garlic among tomatoes, pushing each sliver all the way into the tomato. Grill herb side up 8–10 minutes.

APPROXIMATE NUTRITIONAL CONTENT PER HALVED TOMATO

Total calories: 16
Fat: Tr
Percentage of calories from fat: 16%

Carbohydrates: 3 g
Protein: Tr
Cholesterol: 0
Sodium: 94 mg
Dietary fiber: 1 g

GRILLED CORN IN HUSKS

Remove outside husks, leaving light green inner husks. Reserve some of the outer husks. Remove and discard silk. Lay inner husks back in place around corn. Tear several reserved outer husks into ¼-inch strips and tie around tops of corn to secure. Soak corn in a pan of cold water to cover for 30 minutes. Drain. Grill 15–20 minutes, turning occasionally.

NOTE: If you have a low fire and place corn away from the flame, you can omit the soaking step. This, of course, will increase the cooking time.

VARIATION: Instead of using butter on corn, try lime juice or lemon juice, or even barbecue or stir-fry sauce.

APPROXIMATE NUTRITIONAL CONTENT PER EACH 5 x 1¾-INCH EAR OF CORN

Total calories: 83	Carbohydrates: 19 g
Fat: Tr	Protein: 2 g
Percentage of calories from fat: 9%	Cholesterol: 0
	Sodium: 13 mg
	Dietary fiber: 6 g

STIR-FRIED VEGETABLES

Makes 4 servings (1⅓ cups sauce)

½ small head cauliflower
½ pound broccoli
½ cup freshly squeezed lemon juice,
      plus 1 tablespoon
4 tablespoons water
1 cup Chicken Broth (page 272) or canned broth*
¼ teaspoon soy sauce
1 tablespoon grated lemon rind
1 clove garlic, minced
2 tablespoons cornstarch

Break cauliflower and broccoli into florets. In a wok or heavy skillet, heat 1 tablespoon of the lemon juice and 2 tablespoons of the water. Add cauliflower and stir-fry 3–4 minutes. Add broccoli and stir-fry 2–3 minutes longer or just until cauliflower and broccoli are crisp-tender.

In a medium saucepan, combine chicken broth, remaining lemon juice, soy sauce, lemon rind and garlic, and heat just to boiling. In a covered jar, shake together cornstarch and remaining 2 tablespoons water. Gradually add to broth, stirring constantly until thickened. Pass sauce with vegetables.

*Canned broth is higher in sodium.

SERVING SUGGESTION: Especially good with Stir-Fried Chicken (page 407).

APPROXIMATE NUTRITIONAL CONTENT PER SERVING

Total calories: 61
Fat: Tr
Percentage of calories from fat:
   8%

Carbohydrates: 12 g
Protein: 4 g
Cholesterol: Tr
Sodium: 239 mg
Dietary fiber: 3 g

STIR-FRIED SNOW PEAS

Makes 4 servings

> 2 teaspoons olive oil
> 1 teaspoon finely minced garlic
> 1 teaspoon minced fresh ginger
> ¼ teaspoon crushed red pepper
> ½ pound snow peas

In a nonstick skillet, heat olive oil, garlic, ginger and red pepper; sauté 2–3 minutes. Add snow peas. Stir-fry 2–3 minutes or just until crisp-tender.

APPROXIMATE NUTRITIONAL CONTENT PER SERVING

Total calories: 45	Carbohydrates: 5 g
Fat: 2 g	Protein: 2 g
Percentage of calories from fat:	Cholesterol: 0
46%	Sodium: 3 mg
	Dietary fiber: 1 g

Don't be too concerned with the percentage of calories from fat. The calories in the snow peas are so low that even a small amount of fat elevates the percentage.

VEGETABLES WITH CHINESE NOODLES IN SZECHUAN SAUCE

Makes 8 servings

Sauce

¼ cup soy sauce
1 tablespoon Dijon mustard
¼ cup sesame oil
1 teaspoon olive oil
½ teaspoon hot chili oil (LaYu)
1 tablespoon mayonnaise

Noodles

2 cups Chicken Stock (page 264) or canned broth*
4 cups water
1 8-ounce package buckwheat (Soba) noodles
½ cup sliced bamboo shoots, drained
1 5-ounce can baby corn, drained and sliced
1 cup fresh snow peas, steamed until crisp-tender
½ red pepper, diced
1 carrot, peeled and diced
3 green onions, chopped

In a jar with cover, combine ingredients for sauce. Set aside.

In a saucepan, bring chicken stock and water to a boil. Add noodles and cook until *al dente*. Drain, rinse and arrange in a serving bowl. Drizzle with desired amount of sauce. Toss with remaining ingredients.

*Canned broth is higher in sodium.

SERVING SUGGESTION: Excellent with grilled seafood or chicken.

APPROXIMATE NUTRITIONAL CONTENT PER SERVING WITHOUT SAUCE

Total calories: 142
Fat: 1 g
Percentage of calories from fat:
  8%

Carbohydrates: 27 g
Protein: 6 g
Cholesterol: Tr
Sodium: 145 mg
Dietary fiber: 2 g

APPROXIMATE NUTRITIONAL CONTENT PER TABLESPOON OF SAUCE

Total calories: 65
Fat: 7 g
Percentage of calories from fat:
  96%

Carbohydrates: Tr
Protein: Tr
Cholesterol: 1 mg
Sodium: 272 g
Dietary fiber: 0

Most of the fat and sodium are in the dressing. Remember to use a moderate amount.

GREEN BEANS WITH PIMIENTO

Makes 4 servings

½ pound fresh green beans
1 2-ounce jar pimiento strips, drained

Microwave or steam green beans until crisp-tender. Drain. Arrange in symmetrical bundles of three on a serving tray. Place a pimiento strip around the center of each bundle.

APPROXIMATE NUTRITIONAL CONTENT PER SERVING

Total calories: 77
Fat: Tr
Percentage of calories from fat:
  6%

Carbohydrates: 14 g
Protein: 4 g
Cholesterol: 0
Sodium: 3 mg
Dietary fiber: 0

SPINACH-STUFFED TOMATOES

Makes 4 servings

> 4 large ripe tomatoes
> 6 cups fresh spinach leaves
> 1 teaspoon Tabasco sauce

Scoop pulp and seeds from tomatoes (reserve for soup). Drain tomatoes upside down for a few minutes.

In a nonstick skillet or in a microwave, steam spinach leaves, covered, 1–2 minutes or just until leaves begin to soften. (It is not necessary to use additional moisture or oil since there is already enough moisture in the spinach.) Set aside.

Arrange tomatoes in an 8 x 8 x 2-inch ovenproof casserole dish. Place under broiler 5–10 minutes or until tomatoes are hot. Drizzle cavity of each tomato with ¼ teaspoon Tabasco. Fill each tomato with spinach. Serve at once.

VARIATION: Just before serving, sprinkle with freshly grated Parmesan cheese.

APPROXIMATE NUTRITIONAL CONTENT PER SERVING

Total calories: 42
Fat: Tr
Percentage of calories from fat: 10%

Carbohydrates: 8 g
Protein: 3 g
Cholesterol: 0
Sodium: 81 mg
Dietary fiber: 8 g

TOMATOES WITH SPINACH AND PARMESAN

Makes 4 servings

2 bunches fresh spinach leaves
2 cloves garlic, minced
1 egg, beaten
2 tablespoons bread crumbs
1 teaspoon olive oil
⅛ teaspoon powdered thyme
½ teaspoon black pepper
⅛ teaspoon cayenne pepper
2 tablespoons fresh Parmesan cheese
1 large tomato, cut into 4 thick slices

Microwave or steam spinach with garlic 2–3 minutes or until spinach is just wilted. Cool. Wring out excess moisture. Chop. Add egg, bread crumbs, olive oil, thyme, black pepper, cayenne pepper and Parmesan cheese, and toss. Arrange tomato slices in an 8 x 8-inch ovenproof casserole dish. Top with spinach mixture. Bake at 350°F, 20 minutes or until spinach is hot.

APPROXIMATE NUTRITIONAL CONTENT PER SERVING

Total calories: 87
Fat: 4 g
Percentage of calories from fat:
   37%

Carbohydrates: 8 g
Protein: 6 g
Cholesterol: 55 mg
Sodium: 183 mg
Dietary fiber: 3 g

Don't be too concerned with the percentage of calories from fat. The calories in the spinach and tomatoes are so low that even a small amount of fat elevates the percentage.

EGGPLANT PARMIGIANA

Makes 6 servings

        2 teaspoons olive oil
        2 cloves garlic, sliced
        1 onion, chopped
        2 cups tomato, chopped
        ½ cup Chicken Broth (page 272) or canned broth*
        1 teaspoon basil
        1 teaspoon parsley
        1 teaspoon oregano
        ¼ teaspoon salt
        ¼ teaspoon black pepper
        2 eggs, slightly beaten
        ⅓ cup Parmesan cheese
        1 eggplant, cut into ⅛-inch slices
        ½ cup shredded part-skim mozzarella cheese

In a medium nonstick skillet, heat 1 teaspoon of the olive oil. Add garlic and onion, and sauté 6–8 minutes or until onion is tender; add tomato, chicken broth, basil, parsley, oregano, salt and pepper. Simmer, uncovered, over low heat 20 minutes, stirring often. Set aside.

Combine beaten eggs with 2 tablespoons of the Parmesan cheese. Dip eggplant into egg mixture. In a large nonstick skillet, heat remaining teaspoon of olive oil. Cook eggplant 1 minute on each side or until eggplant is lightly browned. Remove to platter as eggplant is cooked.

Pour ¼ of the tomato mixture on the bottom of a 8 x 8 x 2-inch ovenproof casserole dish. Layer eggplant over top. Sprinkle eggplant with ¼ more sauce, then with ⅓ mozzarella, then with ⅓ Parmesan. Repeat layers. Pour remaining sauce over top and sprinkle with remaining mozzarella and Parmesan. Cover with foil and bake in a 350°F. oven 30 minutes.

*Canned broth is higher in sodium.

SERVING SUGGESTION: Good with chicken and seafood.

APPROXIMATE NUTRITIONAL CONTENT PER SERVING

Total calories: 169
Fat: 8 g
Percentage of calories from fat:
   44%

Carbohydrates: 13 g
Protein: 11 g
Cholesterol: 86 mg
Sodium: 376 mg
Dietary fiber: 4 g

Because of the cheese, Eggplant Parmigiana is high in fat. Serve with low-fat accompaniments or select low-fat foods at other meals to keep a low-fat balance for the day.

ROASTED RED POTATOES WITH LEMON AND OLIVE OIL

Makes 4 servings

  1 pound tiny red potatoes, halved
¼ cup fresh lemon juice
  1 tablespoon olive oil
½ teaspoon salt
¼ teaspoon black pepper

In a 13 x 9 x 2-inch ovenproof casserole dish, arrange potatoes. Combine lemon juice, olive oil, salt and pepper; pour over potatoes. Roast in a 350°F. oven 30–40 minutes or until potatoes are tender, turning 3–4 times to baste.

APPROXIMATE NUTRITIONAL CONTENT PER SERVING

Total calories: 157
Fat: 3 g
Percentage of calories from fat:
   19%

Carbohydrates: 30 g
Protein: 2 g
Cholesterol: 0
Sodium: 275 mg
Dietary fiber: 3 g

ROASTED POTATOES WITH GARLIC

Makes 8 servings

    1 pound tiny red potatoes, halved
    1 head garlic, cloves separated but not peeled
    2 tablespoons olive oil
    ½ teaspoon salt
    ¼ teaspoon black pepper

In a 9 x 13 x 2-inch ovenproof casserole dish, arrange potatoes in a single layer. Tuck garlic cloves among potatoes. Drizzle with olive oil, salt and pepper.

Bake at 350°F. 30–40 minutes or until potatoes are tender and garlic is soft.

Squeeze garlic from peels onto potatoes. Toss potatoes with pan drippings.

APPROXIMATE NUTRITIONAL CONTENT PER SERVING

Total calories: 92
Fat: 3 g
Percentage of calories from fat:
  25%

Carbohydrates: 16 g
Protein: 1 g
Cholesterol: 0
Sodium: 139 mg
Dietary fiber: 1 g

MOSTACCIOLI WITH TOMATOES

Makes approximately 4 quarts

¼	cup olive oil
2	tablespoons balsamic vinegar
3	cloves garlic
2	ounces fresh basil
1	teaspoon salt
¼	teaspoon black pepper
1	pound mostaccioli or other tube-shaped pasta, cooked *al dente*
1 ½	pounds ripe tomatoes, cut into 1-inch cubes
1	cup Calamata olives, pitted and halved

In a blender or food processor, combine olive oil, vinegar and garlic. Add ½ of the basil and whirl 1 minute. Add salt and pepper. Pour over mostaccioli while pasta is still warm. Add tomatoes and olives; toss. Garnish with remaining whole basil leaves.

SERVING SUGGESTION: Especially good with salmon.

APPROXIMATE NUTRITIONAL CONTENT PER CUP

Total calories: 167	Carbohydrates: 27 g
Fat: 5 g	Protein: 5 g
Percentage of calories from fat:	Cholesterol: 0
27%	Sodium: 306 mg
	Dietary fiber: 2 g

Calamata olives are high in fat as well as sodium. If you choose to omit them, the calories change to 159, the sodium to 138 mg and the percentage of calories from fat to 23%. And the recipe will still taste good.

PASTA WITH FRESH TOMATO, BASIL AND MOZZARELLA

8 servings

> 1   pound fresh, ripe tomatoes
> 6   cups fresh basil
> 1   tablespoon olive oil
> ½   teaspoon salt
> ¼   teaspoon black pepper
> 1   pound ziti or tube-shaped pasta, cooked *al dente*
> 1½ cups grated part-skim mozzarella cheese

Plunge tomatoes into boiling water for 1–2 minutes to soften skins, then into ice water; peel and coarsely chop. Coarsely chop 4 cups of the basil leaves; reserve remaining whole leaves for garnish.

   In a nonstick skillet, heat olive oil and add tomatoes. Bring to a boil. Reduce heat to simmer and add chopped basil, salt and pepper. While pasta is still warm, toss with sauce and mozzarella. Turn pasta over and over to mix ingredients and melt cheese. Garnish with remaining 2 cups basil.

   SERVING SUGGESTION: An excellent main meal pasta. Serve with Italian Pizza Bread with Rosemary and Garlic (page 280) and fresh fruit.

APPROXIMATE NUTRITIONAL CONTENT PER SERVING

Total calories: 365
Fat: 10 g
Percentage of calories from fat:
   24%

Carbohydrates: 51 g
Protein: 19 g
Cholesterol: 24 mg
Sodium: 336 mg
Dietary fiber: 3 g

PENNE PUTTANESCA

Makes 8 servings

> 1 tablespoon olive oil
> 1 cup chopped white onion
> 5 cloves garlic, minced
> 1 28-ounce can Italian plum tomatoes, coarsely chopped
> ½ teaspoon crushed red pepper
> ½ teaspoon salt
> 1 cup Calamata olives, pitted and chopped
> 1 2-ounce can anchovy fillets, drained and finely chopped
> 3 tablespoons drained capers
> 1 pound penne or other tube-shaped pasta, cooked *al dente*
> ⅓ cup Parmesan cheese

In a nonstick skillet, heat olive oil. Add onions and garlic, and sauté 6–8 minutes. Pour into a small stockpot. Add tomatoes, crushed red pepper and salt. Heat just to boiling; reduce heat and simmer 10 minutes. Add olives, anchovies and capers. Serve over pasta. Sprinkle with Parmesan.

SERVING SUGGESTION: Serve with tossed green salad, crusty French bread and seasonal fruits.

APPROXIMATE NUTRITIONAL CONTENT PER SERVING

Total calories: 309	Carbohydrates: 49 g
Fat: 8 g	Protein: 13 g
Percentage of calories from fat: 23%	Cholesterol: 3 mg
	Sodium: 840 mg
	Dietary fiber: 4 g

Penne Puttanesca is high in sodium. Be sure to serve it with low-sodium accompaniments.

PASTA STUFFED WITH BASIL AND TOMATO

Makes 8 servings

Sauce

  1 28-ounce can plum tomatoes
  1 carrot, chopped
  1 small white onion, chopped
  4 large cloves garlic
  ½ teaspoon salt
  ¼ teaspoon black pepper
  1 cup fresh basil leaves

Filling

  1 15-ounce container part-skim ricotta cheese
  2 cups freshly grated Parmesan cheese
  1 cup fresh basil leaves
  2 eggs
  ½ teaspoon salt
  ¼ teaspoon black pepper

  1 12-ounce package jumbo pasta shells, cooked
     very *al dente*
  ¼ cup grated part-skim mozzarella cheese

To Make the Sauce: In a saucepan, combine tomatoes, carrot, onion, garlic, salt and pepper; simmer sauce 30 minutes. Add basil leaves and simmer 10 minutes longer.

To Make Filling: In a blender or food processor, combine ricotta, Parmesan, basil, eggs, salt and pepper. Stuff mixture into cooked jumbo pasta shells.

Arrange shells in a single layer in a 9 x 13 x 2-inch ovenproof dish. Cover with sauce. (Be sure each shell is completely covered with sauce, or pasta will dry out.) Sprinkle with mozzarella. Bake, uncovered, at 425°F. 20–25 minutes or until sauce is bubbly.

SERVING SUGGESTION: Serve with Pepper, Onion and Tomato Salad (page 340) with Light Italian Vinaigrette (page 356) and Chilled Anisette Melons (page 493).

APPROXIMATE NUTRITIONAL CONTENT PER SHELL

Total calories: 109
Fat: 4 g
Percentage of calories from fat: 33%

Carbohydrates: 11 g
Protein: 7 g
Cholesterol: 25 mg
Sodium: 270 mg
Dietary fiber: 1 g

DESSERTS

A NOTE ON DESSERTS

While most of the emphasis in a low-fat eating pattern is on main meals, soups and salads, desserts can also play an important role. Low-fat desserts can avert feelings of deprivation and provide satisfaction. They can give needed psychological support, particularly to those with a strong "fat tooth."

Many of the desserts in this section are made with non-fat milk. Not only do they satisfy the need for "dessert," but they also provide calcium without unwanted dairy fat. Donvier ice-cream makers and milk-shake blenders are recommended for making homemade non-fat frozen yogurt, ice milk, and milk shakes in minutes.

A few standard recipes from *Don't Eat Your Heart Out Cookbook,* including Applesauce and Baked Apples, are so popular that I've repeated them here.

SPANISH FLAN

Makes six ½-cup servings

⅓ cup granulated sugar, plus 6 tablespoons
4 whole eggs
4 egg whites
1 teaspoon vanilla extract*
2 cups non-fat milk
sprigs of fresh mint (optional)

In a small, nonstick skillet, spread ⅓ cup of the sugar. Cook over medium heat, stirring constantly, just until sugar is completely melted and forms a caramel syrup that is clear amber in color. Pour syrup immediately into 6 individual 1-cup custard cups. Tilt so syrup coats bottom of each cup. Set cups on a baking rack.

In a large bowl, using a whisk, beat eggs, additional egg whites, the remaining 6 tablespoons sugar and vanilla until well blended but not frothy. Add milk and stir. Pour egg mixture into custard cups.

Arrange custard cups in a 9 x 13 x 2-inch pan. Pour boiling water into the pan, filling bottom to a depth of about 1 inch. Bake at 350°F. 40 minutes or until knife inserted near edge of cup comes out clean. Cool on wire rack 30 minutes. Serve at once or chill.

To serve, run a knife around edge of flan; invert cup onto dessert plate. Caramel syrup will flow over flan. Garnish with mint sprig or small fresh flower.

*Use Mexican vanilla, if available.

SERVING SUGGESTION: Good with Mexican and Cajun dishes.

APPROXIMATE NUTRITIONAL CONTENT PER SERVING

Total calories: 177
Fat: 3 g
Percentage of calories from fat: 18%

Carbohydrates: 27 g
Protein: 9 g
Cholesterol: 143 mg
Sodium: 121 mg
Dietary fiber: 0

LEMON CUSTARD

Makes 6 servings

  3 egg whites
  2 egg yolks
 ⅔ cup non-fat milk
 ¼ cup freshly squeezed lemon juice
  1 teaspoon grated lemon zest
 ¼ teaspoon salt
 ¾ cup granulated sugar
 ¼ cup all-purpose flour

In a bowl, beat egg whites until stiff peaks form; set aside. In another bowl, lightly beat egg yolks; beat in milk, lemon juice and lemon zest. Add salt, sugar and flour, and beat until smooth. Fold yolk mixture into egg whites. Pour into six individual 1-cup custard cups. Place the cups in a 9 x 13 x 2-inch baking pan. Pour boiling water into baking pan to a depth of about 1 inch. Bake at 350°F. 20–30 minutes or until golden and top springs back. Serve warm.

APPROXIMATE NUTRITIONAL CONTENT PER SERVING

Total calories: 149
Fat: 2 g
Percentage of calories from fat:
   10%

Carbohydrates: 30 g
Protein: 4 g
Cholesterol: 71 mg
Sodium: 133 mg
Dietary fiber: Tr

RASPBERRY PAVLOVA

Makes 6 servings

> 5 egg whites
> ½ teaspoon cream of tartar
> 2 teaspoons vanilla extract
> ⅔ cup granulated sugar
> ½ cup low-fat vanilla yogurt
> 1 10-ounce package fresh frozen raspberries in
> heavy syrup, thawed

In a bowl, beat egg whites until foamy; add cream of tartar and vanilla. Beat 1 minute. Gradually add sugar, 1 tablespoon at a time, and beat until egg whites form stiff peaks. Line a 10-inch round pizza pan with a paper lunch bag trimmed to pan size. Spread mixture evenly over covered baking sheet to form a circle. Use a spoon to smooth center and edges. (A cookie sheet may be used in place of a pizza pan but spread mixture to form a circle.) Bake in a 275°F. oven for 1 hour. Cool on wire rack for 1 hour. Remove to serving plate. Spread vanilla yogurt over meringue. Top with berries. Serve at once.

APPROXIMATE NUTRITIONAL CONTENT PER SERVING

Total calories: 145
Fat: Tr
Percentage of calories from fat:
   4%

Carbohydrates: 29 g
Protein: 4 g
Cholesterol: 1 mg
Sodium: 59 mg
Dietary fiber: 2 g

BERRY BAVARIAN

Makes 10 servings

1 cup skim evaporated milk
2 3-ounce packages cherry gelatin dessert mix
1⅓ cup boiling water
2 cups thinly sliced fresh strawberries

Into a mixing bowl, pour evaporated milk. Chill in freezer until ice crystals form around edges, about 1½ hours. (Chill beater blades also.)

Dissolve gelatin mix in boiling water. Chill until syrupy, about 1 hour.

Beat chilled milk on high speed 5–8 minutes or until it is the consistency of whipped cream. Gently fold gelatin and sliced berries into whipped milk. Pour into stemmed glasses. Garnish with additional berries, if desired.

APPROXIMATE NUTRITIONAL CONTENT PER SERVING

Total calories: 85
Fat: Tr
Percentage of calories from fat:
  2%

Carbohydrates: 18 g
Protein: 3 g
Cholesterol: 1 mg
Sodium: 29 mg
Dietary fiber: Tr

LEMON ICE

Makes 1½ quarts

> 2 cups granulated sugar
> 4 cups water
> 2 cups fresh lemon juice

In a 3-quart saucepan, combine sugar with 2 cups of the water. Bring to a boil over high heat and continue to boil, uncovered, for 5 minutes. Let cool. Combine lemon juice with remaining 2 cups water. Mix well. Stir into syrup mixture. Chill. Pour into ice-cream freezer and process according to manufacturer's directions.

For best flavor and texture, serve within 6 weeks. To serve, let hard frozen ice stand at room temperature until slightly softened before serving.

SERVING SUGGESTION: Good with fresh berries and Ladyfingers (page 469).

APPROXIMATE NUTRITIONAL CONTENT PER ½-CUP SERVING

Total calories: 130	Carbohydrates: 53 g
Fat: 0	Protein: Tr
Percentage of calories from fat: 0	Cholesterol: 0
	Sodium: 3 mg
	Dietary fiber: Tr

FRESH LEMON ICE CREAM

Makes 1½ quarts

⅓ cup fresh lemon juice
1½ teaspoons lemon zest
1⅓ cups evaporated skim milk
1 egg
1½ cups granulated sugar
¾ cup non-fat milk
1 cup fresh blueberries or raspberries (optional)

Combine lemon juice and lemon zest. Chill in refrigerator. Pour evaporated milk into a mixing bowl. Chill in freezer until ice crystals form around edges, about 1½ hours or shorter if milk is already cold. (Chill beater blades also.) Beat chilled milk with egg on high speed until it is the consistency of heavy cream, about 5 minutes. Gradually add sugar and beat until mixture thickens. Add lemon juice and lemon zest; beat 2 minutes. Add milk and beat 1 minute more.

Pour into ice-cream freezer and process according to manufacturer's directions.

Scoop into stemmed glasses. Top with blueberries or raspberries, if desired.

APPROXIMATE NUTRITIONAL CONTENT PER ½-CUP SERVING

Total calories: 127
Fat: Tr
Percentage of calories from fat: 3%

Carbohydrates: 29 g
Protein: 3 g
Cholesterol: 19 mg
Sodium: 39 mg
Dietary fiber: Tr

LEMONADE

Makes 3 quarts

> 2 cups granulated sugar
> 4 cups water
> 2 cups freshly squeezed lemon juice
> 1 quart carbonated mineral water
> 1 lemon, sliced

In a 3-quart saucepan, combine sugar with 2 cups of the water. Bring to a boil over high heat and continue to boil, uncovered, for 5 minutes. Let cool. Combine lemon juice with remaining 2 cups water. Mix well. Stir into syrup mixture; chill.

To serve, pour lemonade into a drinking glass or pitcher with ice. Stir in equal parts of mineral water. Garnish with a slice of lemon.

APPROXIMATE NUTRITIONAL CONTENT PER ¾-CUP SERVING

Total calories: 88	Carbohydrates: 24 g
Fat: 0	Protein: Tr
Percentage of calories from fat: 0	Cholesterol: 0
	Sodium: 3 mg
	Dietary fiber: Tr

CHERRY LEMON ICE

Makes 4 servings

> 2 cups Fresh Lemon Ice Cream (page 462)
> 1 10-ounce bottle low-calorie natural cherry seltzer
>   or mineral water (Winterbrook is good)
> 4 strawberries
>   sprigs of fresh mint

Scoop ½ cup lemon ice cream into each of 4 stemmed glasses. Pour cherry seltzer over the top. Garnish with a strawberry and a sprig of mint.

SERVING SUGGESTION: Very refreshing—especially during hot summer weather.

APPROXIMATE NUTRITIONAL CONTENT PER SERVING

Total calories: 131
Fat: Tr
Percentage of calories from fat:
  4%

Carbohydrates: 31 g
Protein: 3 g
Cholesterol: 19 mg
Sodium: 39 mg
Dietary fiber: Tr

Strawberry Sherbet with Strawberry Sauce

Makes 1½ quarts

3 egg yolks, beaten
1 cup granulated sugar
3 cups non-fat milk
¼ teaspoon salt
4 cups fresh strawberries
1 teaspoon vanilla extract

In a 2-quart saucepan, combine egg yolks, ½ cup of the sugar, 1 cup of the non-fat milk, and salt. Cook over medium heat, stirring often, until bubbles form around edges, about 15 minutes. Chill at least 4 hours.

In a blender or food processor, purée berries. Remove half the puréed berries to a small serving bowl and chill in refrigerator. To remaining puréed berries, add remaining ½ cup sugar and whirl 1 minute to blend.

Pour chilled egg mixture, sugared berries, vanilla and remaining 2 cups milk into ice-cream freezer. Process according to manufacturer's directions.

Serve in bowls. Top with remaining puréed berries.

APPROXIMATE NUTRITIONAL CONTENT PER ½-CUP SERVING

Total calories: 112	Carbohydrates: 22 g
Fat: 1 g	Protein: 3 g
Percentage of calories from fat: 12%	Cholesterol: 54 mg
	Sodium: 78 mg
	Dietary fiber: 1 g

ANY FLAVOR FROZEN YOGURT

Makes 3 cups

> 24-ounce apricot, blueberry, cherry or
> raspberry non-fat yogurt (Yoplait fat-
> free is good)

Pour chilled yogurt into ice-cream freezer. Process according to manufacturer's directions. Enjoy as is or top with Strawberry Sauce (page 467) or Peach Sauce (page 468).

NOTE: This is so simple and yet so good, as well as heart-healthy. I have tried several recipes for frozen non-fat yogurt, and none is as good or as easy as this.

APPROXIMATE NUTRITIONAL CONTENT PER ½-CUP SERVING

Total calories: 100
Fat: 0
Percentage of calories from fat:
   0

Carbohydrates: 20 g
Protein: 4 g
Cholesterol: 3 mg
Sodium: 63 mg
Dietary fiber: 0

FROZEN YOGURT PARFAIT WITH FRUIT SAUCES

Makes 4 servings

- ¼ cup Strawberry Sauce (page 467)
- ½ cup Cherry Frozen Yogurt (see page 466)
- ¼ cup Peach Sauce (page 468)
- ½ cup Blueberry Frozen Yogurt (see page 466)
- ½ cup Apricot Frozen Yogurt (see page 466)
    sprigs of mint

Spoon a dab of strawberry sauce in a narrow parfait or champagne glass. Top with a small scoop (use a melon baller or very small ice-cream scoop) of cherry frozen yogurt; then, in order, peach sauce, blueberry frozen yogurt, strawberry sauce, apricot frozen yogurt and strawberry sauce. Garnish with mint.

VARIATION: Arrange small scoops of each kind of frozen yogurt on chilled dessert plates. Top each with a fruit sauce for a simple but very refreshing dessert, especially in hot weather.

APPROXIMATE NUTRITIONAL CONTENT PER SERVING

Total calories: 102
Fat: Tr
Percentage of calories from fat:
  1%

Carbohydrates: 22 g
Protein: 4 g
Cholesterol: 2 mg
Sodium: 47 mg
Dietary fiber: 1 g

FROSTY LEMON SUPREME

Makes 8 servings

½ cup crushed graham cracker crumbs
2 egg whites
⅓ cup very cold water
⅓ cup non-fat dry milk
1 egg yolk
1 teaspoon grated lemon zest
¼ cup fresh lemon juice
¼ cup granulated sugar

Line a 9-inch pie plate with ¼ cup of the graham cracker crumbs. Beat egg whites, water and milk to stiff peaks. Add egg yolk, lemon zest and lemon juice; beat 1 minute, gradually adding sugar. Spoon into pie plate. Sprinkle remaining crumbs over top. Freeze at least 2 hours.

NOTE: When selecting a brand of graham crackers, be sure to read the label. Heart-healthy brands use unsaturated oils such as safflower, soybean, cottonseed, rapeseed or canola. Do not buy a brand that uses saturated fat such as lard, palm oil or coconut oil.

APPROXIMATE NUTRITIONAL CONTENT PER SERVING

Total calories: 61
Fat: 1 g
Percentage of calories from fat:
    15%

Carbohydrates: 11 g
Protein: 2 g
Cholesterol: 27 mg
Sodium: 47 mg
Dietary fiber: Tr

LADYFINGERS

Makes 3 dozen

3 whole eggs, separated
2 egg whites
⅔ cup granulated sugar
1 teaspoon vanilla extract
¾ cup all-purpose flour, plus 1 tablespoon
¼ teaspoon tub-style safflower margarine
1 teaspoon cornmeal
   confectioners' sugar (optional)

In a large bowl of an electric mixer, beat egg whites to soft peaks; gradually beat in ⅓ cup of the sugar and beat until stiff peaks form.

In a small bowl, whisk egg yolks until thick and lemon-colored. Whisk in vanilla. Fold into egg whites.

In a flour sifter, combine remaining ⅓ cup sugar with flour. Sift into egg mixture and carefully fold. Grease lady-finger pans or small muffin tins with margarine. Sprinkle with cornmeal. Spoon batter into pans until each section or cup is about two-thirds full.

Bake in a 375°F. oven about 12 minutes or until nicely browned on outside. Cool on racks. If desired, sprinkle with confectioners' sugar.

APPROXIMATE NUTRITIONAL CONTENT PER COOKIE

Total calories: 31
Fat: Tr
Percentage of calories from fat:
   13%

Carbohydrates: 6 g
Protein: 1 g
Cholesterol: 18 mg
Sodium: 9 mg
Dietary fiber: Tr

STRAWBERRY-RHUBARB SHORTCAKE

Makes 12 miniature servings

1	24-ounce container low-fat vanilla yogurt
2	cups sliced rhubarb
3	cups strawberries, hulled and halved
2	tablespoons water
2	tablespoons cornstarch
½	cup granulated sugar
1	cup all-purpose flour
1½	teaspoons baking powder
½	teaspoon salt
3	tablespoons olive oil or canola oil
⅓	cup non-fat milk

Pour yogurt into an ice-cream freezer. Process according to manufacturer's directions.

In a 2-quart saucepan, combine rhubarb, strawberries, water, cornstarch and sugar. Bring to a boil. Reduce heat, cover and simmer, stirring often, about 10 minutes or until rhubarb is tender.

Meanwhile, in a mixing bowl, combine flour, baking powder and salt. In a small jar, combine olive oil and milk; add all at once to flour mixture. Stir with a fork until dough forms. Pour into miniature nonstick muffin tins and bake at 475°F. 10–12 minutes.

To serve, cut biscuits in half. Ladle warm sauce over biscuit. Top with a scoop of frozen yogurt, then top biscuit with other half. Ladle additional rhubarb sauce over top.

VARIATION: Use angel food cake in place of biscuits.

SHORTCUT: Substitute Vanilla Angel Food Cake (page 482), or a heart-healthy brand of angel food cake mix for homemade, and a heart-healthy commercially prepared frozen yogurt or low-fat ice cream for the vanilla yogurt.

APPROXIMATE NUTRITIONAL CONTENT PER SERVING

Total calories: 186
Fat: 5 g
Percentage of calories from fat:
  21%

Carbohydrates: 32 g
Protein: 4 g
Cholesterol: 3 mg
Sodium: 174 mg
Dietary fiber: 2 g

ALMOND MACAROONS

Makes 1½ dozen

> ½   pound almond paste (Bordon's Red-E is good;
>   so is Solo Brand)
> ⅔   cup granulated sugar
> ¼   cup egg white (about 2–3 eggs)

In a mixing bowl, cut almond paste into small pieces. Blend with sugar. Add egg whites and beat 4–5 minutes or until mixture is smooth. Drop by tablespoons or use a pastry bag with star tube (tablespoon size) and pipe cookies onto baking sheets lined with brown paper or parchment paper. Leave about 1-inch space between each cookie.

Bake at 350°F. 18–20 minutes or until golden. Allow to cool 5 minutes. Remove from pans and cool on wire racks. If cookies stick, dampen the back of the paper with a moist cloth; after a few minutes, remove the cookies from the paper.

APPROXIMATE NUTRITIONAL CONTENT PER COOKIE

Total calories: 86
Fat: 3 g
Percentage of calories from fat:
  32%

Carbohydrates: 14 g
Protein: 2 g
Cholesterol: 0
Sodium: 8 mg
Dietary fiber: Tr

EASY PASTRY CRUST

Makes two 9-inch crusts

> 2   cups all-purpose flour
> ¼   teaspoon salt
> ⅓   cup olive oil or canola oil
> ½   cup very cold non-fat milk, plus 1 tablespoon

In a mixing bowl, combine flour and salt. Pour olive oil and milk into a small bowl (do not stir); add all at once to flour mixture. Stir lightly with a fork or pastry blender. Using hands, form dough into two balls.

Place each ball between two sheets of waxed paper; press into a thick, flat disk about 5 inches in diameter. Place into zip-lock bags and chill 15 minutes.

Roll each disk of dough into a circle on a well-floured pastry cloth. Place in a 9-inch pie plate. Adjust crust. Flute edges.

If a baked shell is needed, prick bottom and sides generously with tines of a fork (prick where bottom and sides meet all around pie shell). If filling and crust are to be baked together, do not prick crust. Bake at 450°F. 8–10 minutes or until golden. Cool on wire rack.

For single-crust recipes: place one of the flattened 5-inch disks in the freezer. It will keep several weeks.

NOTE: Oil-based pastry crusts do not have the same rich flavor nor the same light, flaky texture as shortening-based crusts. Crusts made with oil, however, are a great improvement from a heart-health standpoint. For example, this homemade oil-based recipe has 794 calories, 37 grams of fat, and 304 mg of sodium. A shortening-based crust has 900 calories, 60 grams of fat and 1,100 mg of sodium.

APPROXIMATE NUTRITIONAL CONTENT PER CRUST

Total calories: 794
Fat: 37 g
Percentage of calories from fat:
42%

Carbohydrates: 98 g
Protein: 15 g
Cholesterol: 1 mg
Sodium: 304 mg
Dietary fiber: 3 g

OLD-FASHIONED APPLE PIE

Makes 8 servings

    6   cups apples, pared and sliced
1 ¼ tablespoons lemon juice
  ¼ cup granulated sugar
  ⅛ teaspoon salt
  ½ teaspoon cinnamon
   2 tablespoons all-purpose flour
   2 Easy Pastry Crusts, unbaked (page 472)

In a bowl, toss apples with lemon juice. Combine sugar, salt, cinnamon and flour, and mix with apples. Spoon into pastry-lined pie plate. Adjust top crust, flute edges, and prick. Bake at 450°F. 10 minutes. Reduce heat to 375°F. and continue baking 40–50 minutes.

APPROXIMATE NUTRITIONAL CONTENT PER SERVING

Total calories: 293
Fat: 10 g
Percentage of calories from fat:
29%

Carbohydrates: 50 g
Protein: 4 g
Cholesterol: Tr
Sodium: 110 mg
Dietary fiber: 3 g

APPLE-CRANBERRY PIE

Makes 8 servings

3 large red Delicious apples, peeled, cored and cut
   into eighths
1 cup fresh cranberries, picked over and rinsed
½ cup fresh raisins
½ cup granulated sugar, plus 1 tablespoon
1½ tablespoons cornstarch
1 teaspoon cinnamon
2 Easy Pastry Crusts, unbaked (page 472)
1 egg, slightly beaten
1 tablespoon water

In a bowl, combine apples, cranberries and raisins; toss with ½ cup of the sugar, cornstarch and cinnamon. Pour into a 9-inch pastry-lined pie plate. Arrange crust over top and flute edges. Using a sharp knife, make slits in top of crust to create steam vents. Combine egg with water and brush over pie crust. Sprinkle with remaining 1 tablespoon sugar. Bake at 400°F. for 20 minutes. Reduce heat to 350°F. and bake 30 minutes more. Remove to rack to cool. Serve warm or cold.

APPROXIMATE NUTRITIONAL CONTENT PER SERVING

Total calories: 229
Fat: 5 g
Percentage of calories from fat:
   21%

Carbohydrates: 44 g
Protein: 3 g
Cholesterol: 27 mg
Sodium: 47 mg
Dietary fiber: 2 g

LEMON CHIFFON PIE

Makes 10 servings

> ⅓ cup fresh lemon juice
> ⅔ cup water
> 1 envelope unflavored gelatin
> ¼ cup granulated sugar, plus 2 tablespoons
> 3 egg yolks, slightly beaten
> 1 tablespoon lemon zest
> 5 egg whites
> ½ teaspoon cream of tartar
> 1 Easy Pastry Crust, baked (page 472)
> 10 strawberries, thinly sliced (optional)

In a saucepan, combine lemon juice, water, gelatin, ¼ cup of the sugar, and egg yolks. Heat just to boiling, stirring constantly. Remove from heat. Stir in lemon zest. Place saucepan in a larger saucepan filled with ice and water. Refrigerate 20 minutes or until mixture mounds when dropped from a spoon.

Beat egg whites and cream of tartar to soft peaks; gradually add remaining 2 tablespoons sugar and beat to stiff peaks. Fold in lemon mixture. Mound into pie shell and chill at least 3 hours.

Just before serving, layer top of each piece with sliced strawberries, if desired.

APPROXIMATE NUTRITIONAL CONTENT PER SERVING

Total calories: 133	Carbohydrates: 17 g
Fat: 5 g	Protein: 5 g
Percentage of calories from fat: 35%	Cholesterol: 64 mg
	Sodium: 61 mg
	Dietary fiber: Tr

LEMON MERINGUE PIE

Makes 10 servings

- ¼ cup all-purpose flour
- 5 tablespoons cornstarch
- 1 teaspoon salt
- 1¼ cups granulated sugar
- 2¼ cups boiling water
- 3 egg yolks, lightly beaten
- ½ cup freshly squeezed lemon juice, plus 1 tablespoon
- 1 teaspoon lemon zest
- 1 Easy Pastry Crust, baked (page 472)

Meringue
- 7 egg whites
- ½ teaspoon cream of tartar
- ½ teaspoon vanilla extract
- ⅓ cup granulated sugar

In the top of a double boiler, combine flour, cornstarch, salt, sugar and boiling water. Cook over simmering water 10–15 minutes or until thickened and clear, stirring constantly. Add egg yolks and cook 2 minutes more. Remove from heat. Add lemon juice and lemon zest. Cool. (Do not stir filling while it is cooling.) Turn into cooled baked pie shell.

To make meringue, beat egg whites until fluffy. Add cream of tartar and vanilla. Continue beating, gradually adding sugar. Beat until stiff peaks are formed. Spoon meringue over filling. Mound in peaks, covering filling completely. Bake at 400°F. 8–12 minutes or until peaks are golden.

APPROXIMATE NUTRITIONAL CONTENT PER SERVING

Total calories: 253
Fat: 5 g
Percentage of calories from fat:
   18%

Carbohydrates: 48 g
Protein: 5 g
Cholesterol: 64 mg
Sodium: 288 mg
Dietary fiber: Tr

STRAWBERRY-RHUBARB PIE

Makes 8 servings

½ cup granulated sugar
¼ cup all-purpose flour
¼ teaspoon salt
¼ teaspoon nutmeg
3 cups rhubarb, cut into ½-inch pieces
1 cup sliced strawberries
2 Easy Pastry Crusts, unbaked (page 472)

In a bowl, combine sugar, flour, salt and nutmeg. Add fruit and toss to coat. Let stand 20 minutes. Spoon into pastry-lined pie plate. Adjust top crust, flute edges, and prick. Bake at 400°F. 40–45 minutes.

APPROXIMATE NUTRITIONAL CONTENT PER SERVING

Total calories: 274
Fat: 10 g
Percentage of calories from fat:
   31%

Carbohydrates: 43 g
Protein: 5 g
Cholesterol: Tr
Sodium: 145 mg
Dietary fiber: 2 g

FRESH BERRY PIE

Makes 8 servings

 2 Easy Pastry Crust, unbaked (page 472)
 2 tablespoons all-purpose flour
 ½ cup granulated sugar
 ⅛ teaspoon salt
 4 cups fresh raspberries, strawberries or
    blackberries
 1 teaspoon lemon juice

Line a 9-inch pie plate with pastry. Mix together flour, sugar and salt; sprinkle ¼ of the mixture on uncooked bottom crust. Coat berries with lemon juice and toss with remaining sugar mixture. Spoon into pie plate. Adjust top crust, flute edges, and prick. Bake at 450°F. 15 minutes. Reduce heat to 350°F. and continue baking 25–30 minutes.

APPROXIMATE NUTRITIONAL CONTENT PER SERVING

Total calories: 281
Fat: 9 g
Percentage of calories from fat:
   30%

Carbohydrates: 45 g
Protein: 5 g
Cholesterol: Tr
Sodium: 110 mg
Dietary fiber: 4 g

BERRY COBBLER

Makes 8 servings

¾ cup water
2 tablespoons cornstarch
½ cup granulated sugar
3 cups strawberries, raspberries, blueberries or
     blackberries

Topping
1 cup all-purpose flour, sifted
½ teaspoon salt
1½ teaspoons baking powder
⅓ cup non-fat milk
3 tablespoons safflower oil

In a medium saucepan, combine water, cornstarch and sugar, and bring to a boil. Cook 1 minute, stirring constantly. Add berries and remove from heat. Pour into a 9- or 10-inch pie plate.

Combine flour, salt and baking powder. Mix milk with oil and add to flour. Using a fork or pastry blender, work dough into a ball. Drop by spoonfuls onto fruit cobbler.

Bake at 425°F. 25–30 minutes or until topping is lightly browned.

APPROXIMATE NUTRITIONAL CONTENT PER SERVING

Total calories: 172
Fat: 5 g
Percentage of calories from fat:
   28%

Carbohydrates: 29 g
Protein: 2 g
Cholesterol: Tr
Sodium: 203 mg
Dietary fiber: 2 g

PUDDING CAKE

Makes 12 servings

      1 Vanilla Angel Food Cake (page 482)
      ¾ cup freshly squeezed orange juice
      1 tablespoon gelatin
      ¼ cup all-purpose flour
      ⅔ cup granulated sugar, plus 3 tablespoons
      ¼ teaspoon salt
      2 cups skim milk
      3 eggs, separated
      1 tablespoon grated orange zest

Prepare the cake according to instructions.

Combine orange juice and gelatin; set aside. In a double boiler over boiling water, combine flour, ⅔ cup of the sugar, salt and milk. Cook and stir until thickened, about 10 minutes. Stir in gelatin, egg yolks and orange zest. Remove from heat at once and cool. Cut cooled cake into bite-size pieces.

Beat egg whites to soft peaks. Add the remaining 3 tablespoons sugar and beat 2–3 minutes. Fold into custard. Alternate layers of cake and custard in a nonstick bundt pan. Refrigerate at least 6 hours. Unmold.

VARIATION: Garnish with raspberries. This is also beautiful served in a glass dish. And it can be turned into an English trifle by layering with fruit and sherry or other spirits.

APPROXIMATE NUTRITIONAL CONTENT PER SERVING

Total calories: 245
Fat: 1 g
Percentage of calories from fat: 5%

Carbohydrates: 51 g
Protein: 8 g
Cholesterol: 54 mg
Sodium: 224 mg
Dietary fiber: Tr

VANILLA ANGEL FOOD CAKE AND FRESH STRAWBERRIES WITH STRAWBERRY SAUCE

Makes 12 servings

1 Vanilla Angel Food Cake (page 482)
4 cups strawberries, sliced
1 Strawberry Sauce, chilled (page 467)

Arrange cake on a platter lined with a paper doily. Surround with bowls of sliced strawberries and Strawberry Sauce. Top cake slices with sliced berries, then sauce.

VARIATION: Substitute sliced peaches for strawberries and Peach Sauce (page 468) for Strawberry Sauce.

APPROXIMATE NUTRITIONAL CONTENT PER SERVING

Total calories: 174
Fat: Tr
Percentage of calories from fat: 2%

Carbohydrates: 39 g
Protein: 4 g
Cholesterol: 0
Sodium: 143 mg
Dietary fiber: 2 g

VANILLA ANGEL FOOD CAKE

Makes 12 servings

1¾	cups egg whites (about 12 eggs)
1½	teaspoons cream of tartar
¼	teaspoon salt
1½	cups granulated sugar
1¼	cups sifted cake flour
2	teaspoons vanilla extract
¾	teaspoon almond extract
¾	teaspoon fresh lemon juice

In a large mixing bowl, combine egg whites, cream of tartar and salt. Beat egg whites just to very soft peaks. Turn mixer to lowest speed (use a balloon whisk attachment if available) and gradually add sugar, 1 tablespoon at a time.

Keeping mixer on lowest speed, add flour, 1 tablespoon at a time. Do not overmix. Fold in vanilla, almond extract and lemon juice.

Using a spatula, transfer the batter to a nonstick angel food cake pan. Run the spatula down deep through the batter to break any air pockets. Bake on bottom rack of a 350°F. oven 45–50 minutes or until cake is golden and cracks on top feel dry.

Invert pan and let cool. Remove from pan onto serving platter.

NOTE: Angel food cake is the cake of choice at our house because it is so low in fat. If you've never had a homemade angel food cake, be sure to try this one.

SERVING SUGGESTION: Serve with fresh raspberries, strawberries or peaches, or glaze cake with Chocolate, Orange or Vanilla Glaze (pages 484–486).

APPROXIMATE NUTRITIONAL CONTENT PER SERVING

Total calories: 148

Fat: Tr

Percentage of calories from fat:
    1%

Carbohydrates: 33 g

Protein: 4 g

Cholesterol: 0

Sodium: 99 mg

Dietary fiber: Tr

CHOCOLATE ANGEL FOOD CAKE

Makes 12 servings

1 package angel food cake mix (choose a one-step mix; Betty Crocker is good)

⅓ cup unsweetened cocoa powder (Ghiradelli and Dröste are good)

Prepare cake mix according to package directions. After ingredients are moistened, begin to beat and add cocoa powder gradually, 1 tablespoon at a time. Do not overbeat the mixture; stay within the time limit designated on the package. Scrape sides and bottom of bowl with a spatula to mix in any extra cocoa powder. Pour into a nonstick bundt or angel food cake pan. Bake according to package directions.

SERVING SUGGESTION: Good with Orange, Chocolate or Vanilla Glaze (pages 484–486).

APPROXIMATE NUTRITIONAL CONTENT PER SERVING

Total calories: 158

Fat: 1 g

Percentage of calories from fat:
    7%

Carbohydrates: 35 g

Protein: 5 g

Cholesterol: 0

Sodium: 142 mg

Dietary fiber: Tr

CHOCOLATE GLAZE

Makes ½ cup

1 cup confectioner's sugar, sifted
2 tablespoons cold non-fat milk
1 teaspoon unsweetened cocoa powder (Ghiradelli and Dröste are good)

In a small bowl, combine confectioner's sugar and milk. Stir until smooth. Add cocoa powder and stir until smooth.

NOTE: The best way to glaze a cake is to spread the frosting over the top and allow it to drizzle down the sides.

SERVING SUGGESTION: Good on Vanilla or Chocolate Angel Food Cake (pages 482–483).

APPROXIMATE NUTRITIONAL CONTENT PER TABLESPOON

Total calories: 51
Fat: Tr
Percentage of calories from fat: 2%

Carbohydrates: 13 g
Protein: Tr
Cholesterol: Tr
Sodium: 2 mg
Dietary fiber: Tr

VANILLA GLAZE

Makes 1 cup

- 1½ cups confectioners' sugar, sifted
- 1 egg white
- 1 teaspoon vanilla extract
- 1 teaspoon fresh lemon juice
- dash salt
- 2–2½ tablespoons non-fat milk

In a small bowl, whisk together powdered sugar, egg white, vanilla, lemon juice and salt. Gradually add milk to reach desired thickness.

APPROXIMATE NUTRITIONAL CONTENT PER TABLESPOON

Total calories: 38	Carbohydrates: 9 g
Fat: Tr	Protein: Tr
Percentage of calories from fat: 0	Cholesterol: Tr
	Sodium: 12 mg
	Dietary fiber: 0

ORANGE GLAZE

Makes ½ cup

1 cup confectioner's sugar, sifted
2 tablespoons fresh orange juice, chilled
1 tablespoon orange zest

In a small bowl, combine sugar, orange juice and orange zest. Stir until smooth.

Drizzle over cake or rolls, or pour into small serving dish and serve on the side.

NOTE: For best flavor, squeeze the orange juice in advance and chill thoroughly. Combine it with the sugar and orange zest just before serving.

SERVING SUGGESTION: Good on Vanilla or Chocolate Angel Food Cake (pages 482–483) and on Hot Cross Buns (page 288).

APPROXIMATE NUTRITIONAL CONTENT PER TABLESPOON

Total calories: 49
Fat: Tr
Percentage of calories from fat: 0

Carbohydrates: 13 g
Protein: Tr
Cholesterol: 0
Sodium: Tr
Dietary fiber: Tr

STRAWBERRY SAUCE

Makes 1 cup

2½ cups strawberries
2 tablespoons granulated sugar
1 teaspoon fresh lemon juice

In a blender or food processor, combine strawberries, sugar and lemon juice. Purée until very smooth.

VARIATION: Substitute raspberries for strawberries.

SERVING SUGGESTION: Good as a sauce with peaches, apricots, melons and berries, and also on Vanilla Angel Food Cake (page 482), Strawberry Sherbet (see page 465) or any flavor frozen yogurt.

APPROXIMATE NUTRITIONAL CONTENT PER TABLESPOON

Total calories: 13
Fat: Tr
Percentage of calories from fat: 6%

Carbohydrates: 3 g
Protein: Tr
Cholesterol: Tr
Sodium: Tr
Dietary fiber: Tr

PEACH SAUCE

Makes 1½ cups

>   4   ripe peaches, peeled and pitted
> 1 ½   teaspoons fresh lemon juice
>   ¼   cup granulated sugar
>   1   teaspoon almond extract

In a blender or food processor, combine peaches, lemon juice and sugar. Purée until very smooth. Add almond extract.

SERVING SUGGESTION: Good as a sauce with fresh peaches, apricots, melons or berries. Excellent with sliced peaches over Vanilla Angel Food Cake (page 482).

APPROXIMATE NUTRITIONAL CONTENT
PER TABLESPOON

Total calories: 14
Fat: Tr
Percentage of calories from fat: 1%

Carbohydrates: 3 g
Protein: Tr
Cholesterol: 0
Sodium: Tr
Dietary fiber: Tr

BERRY-FILLED MELON ROUNDS

Makes 4 servings

> ½ cantaloupe, peeled, seeded and cut crosswise
          into rounds 1 inch thick
> 1 ½ cups fresh raspberries
> ½ lime, cut into wedges

Arrange melon rounds on chilled dessert plates. Fill with berries. Garnish with lime wedges.

VARIATION: Freeze raspberries. Just before serving, purée raspberries in a blender or food processor. The berries will taste almost like sorbet when blended.

APPROXIMATE NUTRITIONAL CONTENT PER SERVING

Total calories: 28
Fat: Tr
Percentage of calories from fat: 8%

Carbohydrates: 7 g
Protein: Tr
Cholesterol: 0
Sodium: 1 mg
Dietary fiber: 2 g

PEACHES SUPREME

Makes 4 servings

- ½ cup Peach Sauce (page 468)
- 4 fresh ripe peaches
- ½ cup fresh raspberries
- ½ cup fresh blueberries

Divide peach sauce among 4 chilled dessert plates. Slice peaches into quarters only deep enough to remove the pits and still leave sections attached. Center 1 peach on each plate. Sprinkle with raspberries and blueberries.

APPROXIMATE NUTRITIONAL CONTENT PER SERVING

Total calories: 83
Fat: Tr
Percentage of calories from fat: 3%

Carbohydrates: 21 g
Protein: 1 g
Cholesterol: 0
Sodium: 1 mg
Dietary fiber: 3 g

FRESH PINEAPPLE WITH PAPAYA PURÉE

Makes 4 servings

1 large ripe papaya, peeled, halved and seeded
  juice of ½ lime (approximately 2 tablespoons)
  grated zest of ½ lime (about ¼ teaspoon)
1 small fresh pineapple, peeled and cut into cubes
1 banana, sliced
1 mandarin orange, sectioned

In a blender or food processor, purée papaya, lime juice and lime zest. Chill. Divide papaya purée equally among dessert plates; arrange pineapple cubes, banana slices and orange sections over top.

VARIATION: Accompany with a scoop of Frozen Yogurt (see page 466). Or freeze the papaya. Just before serving, purée the frozen papaya with lime juice and lime zest. The purée will taste almost like sorbet when blended.

APPROXIMATE NUTRITIONAL CONTENT PER SERVING

Total calories: 79
Fat: Tr
Percentage of calories from fat:
  5%

Carbohydrates: 20 g
Protein: Tr
Cholesterol: 0
Sodium: Tr
Dietary fiber: 2 g

AMARETTO ORANGES WITH STRAWBERRIES

Makes 4 servings

3 large navel oranges, peeled, sliced into thin rings and then torn or cut into sections
2 tablespoons amaretto liqueur
6 strawberries, thinly sliced
4 whole strawberries

Arrange oranges in a shallow bowl; pour amaretto over oranges and toss. Chill 2 hours or overnight. Just before serving, line the edges of 4 small dessert plates with sliced strawberries. Arrange orange sections in center. Top with whole strawberries.

VARIATION: Substitute 4 maraschino cherries for the whole strawberries. The sweetness of the cherries is an excellent flavor with the oranges, although the recipe will still taste good if the cherries are omitted.

APPROXIMATE NUTRITIONAL CONTENT PER SERVING

Total calories: 81
Fat: Tr
Percentage of calories from fat: 2%

Carbohydrates: 16 g
Protein: 1 g
Cholesterol: 0
Sodium: Tr
Dietary fiber: 2 g

CHILLED ANISETTE MELONS

Makes 6 servings

½ cantaloupe
7 tablespoons anisette liqueur
3½ tablespoons water
¼ watermelon
sprigs of fresh mint

Using a melon baller, form balls from cantaloupe. Combine 3 tablespoons of the anisette with 1½ tablespoons of the water; pour over cantaloupe balls. Cover and chill 1–2 hours.

Remove rind from watermelon. Cut melon into wedges. Combine remaining 4 tablespoons anisette with remaining 2 tablespoons water; pour over melon. Chill 1–2 hours.

To serve, arrange watermelon triangles symmetrically on chilled individual dessert plates. Top each triangle with a melon ball. Garnish with remaining melon balls and mint.

APPROXIMATE NUTRITIONAL CONTENT PER SERVING

Total calories: 117
Fat: Tr
Percentage of calories from fat:
    5%

Carbohydrates: 19 g
Protein: 1 g
Cholesterol: 0
Sodium: 6 mg
Dietary fiber: 1 g

APPLESAUCE

Makes 8 servings

8–10 large cooking apples, peeled, cored and cut into
      chunks
  ½ cup water
  ½ cup or less granulated sugar
  1 teaspoon cinnamon

In a saucepan, combine apples and water. Cover and simmer, stirring frequently, until apples are barely tender, about 6–10 minutes. Add sugar and continue cooking about 30 minutes or until sugar dissolves. Stir in cinnamon.

NOTE: For a smooth rather than chunk-type sauce, purée apples in a blender or food processor before adding sugar. Proceed as for chunk-style.

If using a crockpot, combine all ingredients. Cover and cook on low heat 8 hours or overnight.

APPROXIMATE NUTRITIONAL CONTENT PER SERVING

Total calories: 136
Fat: Tr
Percentage of calories from fat:
  3%

Carbohydrates: 36 g
Protein: Tr
Cholesterol: 0
Sodium: 1 mg
Dietary fiber: 3 g

BAKED APPLES

Makes 8 servings

- ¼ cup or less brown sugar
- 1 teaspoon cinnamon
- 1 tablespoon safflower oil
- ⅓ cup raisins
- 6–8 medium baking apples, cored

In a bowl, mix sugar, cinnamon, oil and raisins. Fill center of apples and place upright in a baking dish. Pour 1 cup water around apples. Bake at 375°F. 45–60 minutes, basting frequently.

NOTE: If using a crockpot, reduce water to ½ cup. Cook on low heat 8 hours or overnight.

APPROXIMATE NUTRITIONAL CONTENT PER SERVING

Total calories: 141
Fat: 2 g
Percentage of calories from fat: 13%

Carbohydrates: 33 g
Protein: Tr
Cholesterol: 0
Sodium: 4 mg
Dietary fiber: 3 g

BIBLIOGRAPHY

Acheson, K. J., et al. "Glycogen Storage Capacity and De Novo Lipogenesis During Massive Carbohydrate Overfeeding in Man." *American Journal of Clinical Nutrition* 48, 1988.

Alabaster, Oliver. *What You Should Know to Prevent Cancer*. New York: Simon & Schuster, 1985.

Alpert, Joseph. *The Heart Attack Handbook*. Boston: Little, Brown, 1984.

Ames, B. "Dietary Carcinogens and Anticarcinogens." *Science* 221, 1983.

Anderson, J. W., et al. "Effects of Oat Bran or Bean Intake for Hypercholesterolemic Men." *American Journal of Clinical Nutrition* 40, 1984.

Aronson, Virginia. "Effective Weight Control." *Runner's World*, March 1984.

Assembly of Life Sciences, National Research Council. "Diet, Nutrition, and Cancer Committee Report on Diet, Nutrition, and Cancer." Washington, D.C.: GPO, 1984.

Barnett, Robert. "Why Fat Makes You Fatter." *American Health*, May 1986.

Beauchamp, G. K., and B. J. Cowart. "Development of Sweet Taste." In: *Sweetness* (J. Dubbing, ed.). Berlin: Springer-Verlag, 1987.

Block, G., et al. "Nutrient Sources in the American Diet: Quantitative Data from the NHANES II Survey. II: Macronutrients and Fats." *American Journal of Epidemiology* 122, 1985.

Bennett, William, and Joel Gurin. *The Dieter's Dilemma: Eating Less and Weighing More*. New York: Basic Books, 1982.

Benson, Herbert. *The Relaxation Response*. New York: William Morrow, 1975.

Blondhein, S. H., et al. "Comparison of Weight Loss on Low-Calorie (800–1,200) and Very-Low-Calorie (300–600) Diets." *International Journal of Obesity* 5, 1981.

Booth, D. A., M. T. Connor, and S. Marie. "Sweetness and Food Selection: Measurement of Sweeteners' Effect on Acceptance." In: *Sweetness* (J. Dubbing, ed.). Berlin: Springer-Verlag, 1987.

Bray, G. A. "Obesity—A Disease of Nutrient or Energy Balance?" *Nutrition Reviews* 45, 1987.

———. "Obesity in America." National Institutes of Health, 1979.

Brody, Jane. *Jane Brody's Nutrition Book*. New York: Bantam Books, 1982.

Brown, M. S., and J. L. Goldstein. "How LDL Receptors Influence Cholesterol and Atherosclerosis." *Scientific American* 251, 1984.

———. "Lowering Plasma Cholesterol by Raising LDL Receptors." *New England Journal of Medicine* 305, 1981.

Brownell, K. D., et al. "Changes in Plasma Lipid and Lipoprotein Levels in Men and Women After a Program of Moderate Exercise." *Circulation* 65, 1982.

——— and J. P. Foreyt (eds.). *Handbook of Eating Disorders: Physiology, Psychology, and Treatment of Obesity, Anorexia, and Bulemia*. New York: Basic Books, 1986.

Burkitt, D. *Don't Forget Fiber in Your Diet*. New York: Arco Publishing, 1984.

Caggiula, A. W., et al. "The Multiple Risk Intervention Trial (MRFIT). IV. Intervention on Blood Lipids." *Preventive Medicine* 10, 1981.

Castelli, William P., et al. "Incidence of Coronary Heart Disease and Lipoprotein Cholesterol Levels—The Framingham Study." *Journal of the American Medical Association*, Vol. 256, 1986.

Cooper, Kenneth H. *The New Aerobics*. New York: M. Evans, 1970.

———. *The Aerobics Way*. New York: M. Evans, 1977.

———. *Controlling Cholesterol*. New York: Bantam Books, 1988.

Dazzi, A., and J. Dwyer. "Nutritional Analyses of Popular Weight Reduction Diets in Books and Magazines." *International Journal of Eating Disorders* 3, 1984.

Doll, R., and R. Petro. *The Causes of Cancer*. Oxford, U.K.: Oxford University Press, 1981.

Dreher, Henry. *Your Defense Against Cancer*. New York: Harper & Row, 1988.

Drewnowski, Adam. "Cognitive Structure in Obesity and Dieting." In: *Contemporary Issues in Clinical Nutrition* (M.R.C. Greenwood, ed.). New York: Churchill Livingston, 1983.

———. "Fats and Food Texture: Sensory and Hedonic Evaluations." In: *Food Texture* (H. R. Moskowitz, ed.). New York: Marcel Dekker, 1987.

——— and M. Greenwood. "Cream and Sugar: Human Preferences for High-Fat Foods." *Physiological Behavior* 30, 1983.

——— and H. R. Moskowitz. "Sensatory Characteristics of Foods: New Evaluation Techniques." *American Journal of Clinical Nutrition* 42, 1985.

——— et al. "Sweet Tooth Reconsidered: Taste Responsiveness in Human Obesity." *Psychology & Behavior*, Vol. 35, 1985.

——— et al. "Taste and Eating Disorders." *American Journal of Clinical Nutrition*, 1987.

Dwyer, J. "Sixteen Popular Diets: Brief Nutritional Analyses." In: *Obesity* (A. J. Stunkard, ed.). Philadelphia: W. B. Saunders, 1980.

Dychtwald, Ken. *The Age Wave*. Los Angeles: Jeremy P. Tarcher, 1989.

"Facts about Blood Cholesterol." U.S. Dept. of Health and Human Services, National Institutes of Health.

Farb, Peter, and G. Armelagos. *Consuming Passions: The Anthropology of Eating.* Boston: Houghton Mifflin, 1980.

Ferguson, J. M. *Habits, Not Diets: The Real Way to Weight Control.* Palo Alto, Calif.: Bull Publishing, 1976.

"Fish, Fatty Acids, and Human Health." Editorials, *New England Journal of Medicine* 7, 1985.

"Fish Oils and Colon Cancer." *Nutrition Research Newsletter*, July 1986.

Fisher, Marc, et al. "The Effect of Vegetarian Diets on Plasma Lipid and Platelet Level." *Archives of Internal Medicine* 146, 1986.

Flatt, J. P. "Dietary Fat, Carbohydrate Balance, and Weight Maintenance: Effects of Exercise." *American Journal of Clinical Nutrition* 45, 1987.

———. "Effect of Carbohydrate and Fat Intake on Postprandial Substrate Oxidation and Storage." Topics in *Clinical Nutrition* 45, 1987.

Food and Nutrition Board, National Research Council, National Academy of Sciences. *Recommended Dietary Allowances.* Washington, D.C., 1980.

Gale, J. C., R. L. Huenemann, and R. J. Brand. "Food Choices of Obese and Non-Obese Persons." *Journal of the American Dietetic Association* 67, 1975.

Geiselman, Paula J. "Appetite, Hunger and Obesity as a Function of Dietary Sugar Intake: Can These Effects Be Mediated by Insulin-Induced Hypoglycemia? A Reply to Commentaries." *Appetite*, 1985.

———. "Carbohydrates Do Not Always Produce Satiety: An Explanation of the Appetite- and Hunger-Stimulating Effects of Hexoses." *Progress in Psychological Psychology*, Vol. 12, 1987.

———. "Dietary Implications for the Control of Food Intake and Body Weight." *Nutrition and Behavior*, 1984.

——— and D. Novin. "The Role of Carbohydrates in Appetite, Hunger and Obesity." *Appetite*, 1982.

—— and D. Novin. "Sugar Infusion Can Enhance Feeding." *Science*, 1982.

Gershoff, Stanley (ed.). *The Tufts University Guide to Total Nutrition.* New York: Harper & Row, 1990.

Giovanni, M. E. "Category Scaling and Magnitude Estimation of Fat in Milk and Sucrose in Lemonade as a Function of Food Intake." Davis, Calif.: University of California, 1981.

Goldstein, Joseph L., and Michael S. Brown. "The Low-Density Lipoprotein Pathway and Its Relation to Atherosclerosis." *Annual Review of Biochemistry*, Vol. 46, 1977.

Gordon, T., et al. "High Density Lipoprotein as a Protective Factor Against Coronary Heart Disease: The Framingham Study." *American Journal of Medicine* 62, 1977.

Gray, D. S., et al. "Effects of Repeated Weight Loss and Regain on Body Composition in Obese Rats." *American Journal of Clinical Nutrition* 47, 1988.

Grinker, J. A. "Obesity and Sweet Taste." *American Journal of Clinical Nutrition* 31, 1978.

—— et al. "Studies of Taste in Childhood Obesity." In: *Hunger: Basic Mechanisms and Clinical Implications* (D. Novin et al., eds.). New York: Raven Press, 1976.

Grundy, Scott M. "Comparison of Monounsaturated Fatty Acids and Carbohydrates for Lowering Plasma Cholesterol." *New England Journal of Medicine* 314, 1986.

Hammer, R. L., et al. "Calorie Restricted Low-Fat Diet and Exercise in Obese Women." *American Journal of Clinical Nutrition* 49, 1989.

Hamilton, C. L. "Rats' Preference for High Fat Diets." *Journal of Physiological Psychology* 58, 1964.

Hausman, Patricia. *Jack Spratt's Legacy: The Science and Politics of Fat and Cholesterol.* New York: Richard Marek, 1981.

Holleb, Arthur I. *The American Cancer Society Cancer Book.* Garden City, N.Y.: Doubleday, 1986.

Kannel, W. B., et al. "Serum Cholesterol, Lipoproteins, and the Risk of Coronary Heart Disease: The Framingham Study." *Annals of Internal Medicine* 74, 1971.

Katch, F., and W. D. McArdle. *Nutrition, Weight Control, and Exercise.* Philadelphia: Lea & Febiger, 1988.

Kato, H., et al. "Epidemiologic Studies of Coronary Heart Disease and Stroke in Japanese Men Living in Japan, Hawaii, and California. Serum Lipids and Diet." *American Journal of Epidemiology* 97, 1973.

Keys, A. (ed.). "Coronary Heart Disease in Seven Countries." *Circulation* 41, 1970.

Kromhout, Daan, et al. "The Inverse Relation between Fish Consumption and 20-Year Mortality from Coronary Heart Disease." *New England Journal of Medicine* 312, 1985.

Laszlo, J. *Understanding Cancer.* New York: Harper & Row, 1987.

Levenson, F. B. *The Causes and Prevention of Cancer.* New York: Stein & Day, 1985.

Lewis, Barry. "Relationship of High-Density Lipoproteins to Coronary Artery Disease." *American Journal of Cardiology* 52, 1983.

Lipid Research Clinics Program. "The Lipid Research Clinics Coronary Primary Prevention Trial Results. I: Reduction in Incidence of Coronary Heart Disease. II: The Relationship of Reduction in Incidence of Coronary Heart Disease to Cholesterol Lowering." *Journal of the American Medical Association* 25, 1984.

Malcom, R., et al. "Taste Hedonics and Thresholds in Obesity." *International Journal of Obesity* 4, 1980.

Manson, J. E., et al. "Body Weight and Longevity." *Journal of the American Medical Association* 257, 1987.

Mirkin, G. *Getting Thin.* Boston: Little, Brown, 1983.

Morgan, K. J., and M. E. Zabik. "Amount and Food Sources of Total Sugar Intake by Children Aged 5 to 12." *American Journal of Clinical Nutrition* 34, 1981.

Nutrition and Cancer: Cause and Prevention. New York: American Cancer Society, 1984.

Ornish, Dean. *Dr. Dean Ornish's Program for Reversing Heart Disease.* New York: Random House, 1990.

Pangborn, R. M., K. E. Bos, and J. Stern. "Dietary Fat Intake and Taste Responses to Fat in Milk by Under-, Normal-, and Overweight Women." *Appetite* 6, 1985.

Pollock, M., J. Wilmore, and S. Fox. *Health and Fitness Through Physical Activity.* New York: Wiley Publishing, 1978.

"Provisional Dietary Fiber Table." *Journal of the American Dietetic Association* 86, 1986.

Rippe, J. M., et al. "Walking for Health and Fitness." *Journal of the American Medical Association* 259, 1988.

Rodin, J., H. R. Moskowitz, and G. A. Bray. "Relationship Between Obesity, Weight Loss, and Taste Responsiveness." *Physiological Behavior* 17, 1976.

Schutz, Y., J. P. Flatt, and E. Jequier. "Failure of Dietary Fat Intake to Promote Fat Oxidation: A Factor Favoring the Development of Obesity." *American Journal of Clinical Nutrition,* 1989.

Shepherd, R., and L. Stockley. "Fat Consumption and Attitudes Toward Food with a High Fat Content." *Human Nutrition: Applied Nutrition* 39, 1985.

Shrager, E. E., et al. "Hedonistic Responses to Mixtures of Sucrose and Fat in a Solid Food Unit (SFU)." Paper presented at the Eastern Psychological Association Meeting, Baltimore, Md., 1984.

Simko, V., and R. E. Kelley. "Physical Exercise Modifies the Effect of High Cholesterol-Sucrose Feeding in the Rat." *Eur. Journal of Applied Physiology* 40, 1979.

Simone, C. B. *Cancer and Nutrition.* New York: McGraw-Hill, 1983.

Smith, Everett L. *Exercise and Aging: The Scientific Basis.* Hillside, N.J.: Enslow Publishers, 1981.

Stamler, J. "Diet and Coronary Heart Disease." *Biometrics* 38, 1982.

Steen, S. N., R. A. Oppliger, and K. D. Brownell. "Metabolic Effects of Repeated Weight Loss and Regain in Adolescent Wrestlers." *Journal of the American Medical Association* 260, 1988.

Stunkard, A. J., et al. "An Adoption Study of Human Obesity." *New England Journal of Medicine* 314, 1986.

————, T. T. Foch, and Z. Hrubec. "A Twin Study of Human Obesity." *Journal of the American Medical Association* 256, 1986.

Sweetgall, Robert. *Rockport's Fitness Walking.* New York: Perigree Books, 1985.

U.S. Department of Agriculture. *Composition of Foods.* Agriculture Handbook No. 8. Washington D.C.: GPO, 1989.

————. *Nutritive Value of American Foods in Common Units.* Agriculture Handbook No. 456. Washington, D.C.: GPO, 1975.

U.S. Department of Health and Human Services. *Lowering Blood Cholesterol to Prevent Heart Disease.* National Institutes of Health Consensus Development Conference Statement 5, No. 7. Bethesda, Md.: National Institutes of Health, 1984.

————. *The Surgeon General's Report on Nutrition and Health.* DHHS (PHS) Publication No. 88–50210. Washington, D.C.: GPO, 1988.

Weil, Andrew, and W. Rosen. *Chocolate to Morphine. Understanding Mind-Active Drugs.* Boston: Houghton Mifflin, 1982.

Wooley, O. W., et al. "Calories and Sweet Taste: Effects on Sucrose Preference in the Obese and Non-Obese." *Physiological Behavior* 9, 1972.

Yudkin, J. "The Low Carbohydrate Diet." In *Obesity* (W. Butland et al., eds.). Edinburgh: Churchill Livingstone, 1973.

GENERAL INDEX

INDEX TO RECIPES

ABOUT THE AUTHORS

Joseph C. Piscatella is the author of two widely acclaimed books, *Don't Eat Your Heart Out Cookbook* and *Choices for a Healthy Heart*, which have been enthusiastically endorsed by health professionals. His recovery from open-heart surgery at age 32 and successful approach to healthy lifestyle changes are welcome news to those interested in improving health.

President of the Institute for Fitness and Health, Inc., in Tacoma, Washington, Mr. Piscatella lectures on lifestyle management skills and the control of health care costs to a variety of clients, including Fortune 500 companies, professional associations, educational institutions and health professionals. His seminar has been cited in *Time* for its effectiveness.

As a spokesman for a healthy lifestyle, he is a frequent guest on radio and television, contributes to national publications, and has hosted a television series on making healthy lifestyle changes. He is a member of the American Association for Cardiopulmonary Rehabilitation, the Association for Fitness in Business, and the National Wellness Association.

Bernie Piscatella is the vice president of the Institute for Fitness and Health and is responsible for all of the recipes in their books. They live in Tacoma with their two children.